PEDIATRIC

MEDICAL STUDENT
USMLE BOARD PARTS II AND III

PEARLS OF WISDOM

Robert M. Levin

Peter Emblad

Scott H. Plantz

Jonathan Adler

NOTE

The intent of Pediatric Medical Student Pearls of Wisdom is to serve as a study aid to improve performance on a standardized exam. It is not intended to be a source text of the knowledge base of pediatric medicine, nor to serve as a reference in any way for the practice of clinical pediatrics. Neither Boston Medical Publishing Corporation nor the editors warrant that the information in this text is complete. Readers are encouraged to verify each answer in several references. All drug use indications and dosages must be verified by the reader before administration of any compound.

The editors would like to extend thanks to Terri Lair for her excellent editorial and management support.

ISBN: 1-890369-24-1

DEDICATIONS

To my father, Sam S. Levin, who taught me to value knowledge.
To my mother, Beverly Imerman Levin, who encouraged me to pursue education.
To my uncle, David Goldfinger, M.D., who inspired me to become a physician.
To my wife, Lisa A. Solinar, M.D., who expects me to ask clear questions.
And to my children, Max, George, and Ana, who have taught me the value of a good answer.

Robert M. Levin

To Britte-Marie Evers, my mother and a woman of exceptional elegance, beauty, and character.

Peter Emblad

To Laura, Terri, Annessa, Judy, Sarah, Dasha, Brad, Vicki, and Robin.
Thank you for making this text a reality.

Scott H. Plantz

For Bug, Zach, and all the kids.

Jonathan Adler

EDITOR-IN-CHIEF

Robert M. Levin, M.D.
Professor and Chairman
Mt. Sinai Medical Center
Department of Pediatrics
Chicago, IL

ASSOCIATE EDITORS

Peter Emblad, M.D.
Boston Medical Center
Boston, MA

Scott H. Plantz, M.D.
Assistant Professor
Chicago Medical School
Mt. Sinai Medical Center
Chicago, IL

Jonathan Adler, M.D.
Instructor
Harvard Medical School
Boston, MA

CONTRIBUTING AUTHORS

Bobby Abrams, M.D.
Attending Physician
Macomb Hospital
Macomb, MI

Kristen Bechtel, M.D., MCP
Assistant Professor of Emergency Medicine
Allegheny University of the Health Sciences
Attending Physician
Department of Pediatric Emergency
St. Christopher's Hospital for Children
Philadelphia, PA

Michelle L. Bez, D.O.
Newcomb Medical Center
Vineland, NJ

David F. M. Brown, M.D.
Instructor in Medicine
Harvard Medical School
Massachusetts General Hospital
Boston, MA

Eduardo Castro, M.D.
Instructor in Medicine
Harvard Medical School
Massachusetts General Hospital
Boston, MA

Leslie S. Carroll, M.D.
Assistant Professor
Chicago Medical School
Toxicology Director
Mt. Sinai medical Center
Chicago, IL

Marjorie Chaparro, M.D.
Department of Pediatrics
Mount Sinai Hospital
Chicago, IL

Deandra Clark, M.D.
University of South Florida
Department of Pediatrics
Tampa, FL

David C. Cone, M.D.
Assistant Professor of Emergency Medicine
Chief, Division of EMS
Department of Emergency Medicine
Allegheny University of the Health Sciences
Philadelphia PA

C. James Corrall, M.D., MPH
Clinical Associate Professor of Pediatrics
Clinical Associate Professor of Emergency
Medicine
Indiana University School of Medicine
Indianapolis, IN

Judith A. Dattaro, M.D.
Attending Emergency Department
The New York Hospital
Instructor, Department of Surgery
Cornell V.A. Medical Center
New York, NY

Carl W. Decker, M.D.
Madigan Army Medical Center
Fort Lewis, WA

Phillip Fairweather, M.D.
Clinical Assistant Professor
Mount Sinai School of Medicine
New York, NY
Department of Emergency Medicine
Elmhurst Hospital Center
Elmhurst, NY

Craig Feied, M.D.
Clinical Associate Professor
George Washington University
Washington Hospital Center

Anne Freter, R.N., BSN
Intensive Care Unit
Hope Children's Hospital
Oak Lawn, IL

Lynn Garfunkel, M.D.
Assistant Professor of Pediatrics
Associate Director, Pediatric Residency Training
Program
Director, Combined Internal Medicine and
Pediatric Residency Training Program
University of Rochester School of Medicine and
Dentistry
Rochester, NY

Jay Gold, M.D.
MediStar
Madison, WI

Bill Gossman, M.D.
Chicago Medical School
Mt. Sinai Medical Center
Chicago, IL

John Graneto, D.O.
Director
Pediatric Emergency Medicine
Lutheran General Children's Hospital
Park Ridge, IL

Ned Hayes, M.D.
Chief, Epidemiology Section
Bacterial Zoonoses Branch
Division of Vector-Borne Infectious Diseases
Centers for Disease Control and Prevention
Fort Collins, CO

James F. Holmes, M.D.
University of California, Davis
School of Medicine
Sacramento, CA

Eddie Hooker, M.D.
Assistant Professor
University of Louisville
Louisville, KY

Ira Horowitz, M.D.
Director, Intermediate Intensive Care Unit
Department of Pediatrics
Division of Critical Care Medicine
Hope Children's Hospital
Christ Hospital and Medical Center
Oak Lawn, IL

Matt Kopp, M.D.
Department of Emergency Medicine
Rhode Island Hospital
Brown University School of Medicine
Providence, RI

Lance W. Kreplick, M.D.
Assistant Professor
University of Illinois
EHS Christ Hospital
Oak Lawn, IL

Deborah Lee, M.D.
Department of Neurology
Tulane University Medical Center
New Orleans, LA

Gillian Emblad, P.A., CMA
Physician Assistant
New England Medical Center
Boston, MA

Bernard Lopez, M.D.
Assistant Professor
Thomas Jefferson Medical College
Thomas Jefferson University Hospital
Philadelphia, PA

Mary Nan S. Mallory, M.D.
Instructor
University of Louisville
Louisville, KY

Bridget Ann Martell, M.D.
Yale New Haven hospital
New haven, CT

David Morgan, M.D.
University of Texas
Southwestern Medical Center
Parkland Memorial Hospital
Dallas, TX

Peter Noronha, M.D.
Associate Professor of Clinical of Pediatrics
Associate Program Director of Pediatrics
University of Illinois College of Medicine
Chicago, IL

Scott E. Olitsky, M.D.
Assistant Professor of Ophthalmology
State University of New York at Buffalo
The Children's Hospital of Buffalo
Buffalo, NY

Edward A. Panacek, M.D.
Associate Professor
University of California, Davis
School of Medicine
Sacramento, CA

Geraldo Reyes, M.D.
Director
Critical Care Training
Hope Children's Hospital
Oak Lawn, IL

Karen Rhodes, M.D.
University of Chicago Medical Center
Chicago, IL

Luis R. Rodriquez, M.D., FAAP
Assistant Professor of Pediatrics
Mount Sinai School of Medicine
New York, NY
Elmhurst Hospital Center
Elmhurst, NY

Carlo Rosen, M.D.
Instructor
Harvard Medical School
Massachusetts General Hospital
Boston, MA

Bruce K. Rubin, M.D.
Professor of Pediatrics, Physiology and
Pharmacology
Brenner Children's Hospital
Winston-Salem, NC

Girish D. Sharma, M.D., FCCP
Assistant Professor of Pediatrics
Section of Pediatric Pulmonology
The University of Chicago Children's Hospital
Chicago, IL

Rejesh Shenoy, M.D.
Department of Pediatrics
University of Illinois College of Medicine
Chicago, IL

Clifford S. Spanierman, M.D., FAAP
Pediatric Emergency Medicine Physician
Department of Emergency Medicine
Lutheran General Children's Hospital
Park Ridge, IL

Dana Stearns, M.D.
Instructor
Harvard Medical School
Massachusetts General Hospital

Jack Stump, M.D.
Attending Physician
Rogue Valley Medical Center
Medford, OR

Joan Surdukowski, M.D.
Assistant Professor
Chicago Medical School
Mount Sinai Hospital
Chicago, IL

Loice Swischer, M.D.
Medical College of Pennsylvania
Philadelphia, PA

Nicholas Tapas, M.D.
General Pediatrician
Lutheran General Hospital
Park Ridge, IL

Hector Trujillo, M.D.
General Pediatrician
Miami Children's Hospital Miami, FL

Michael Zevitz, M.D.
Assistant Professor
Chicago Medical School Chicago, IL

Stan Zuba, M.D.
Assistant Professor of Pediatrics
RUSH/ The Chicago Medical School
Chicago, IL

WE APPRECIATE YOUR COMMENTS!

We appreciate your opinion and encourage you to send us any suggestions or recommendations. Please let us know if you discover any errors, or if there is any way we can make our *Pearls of Wisdom* Text more helpful to you. We are also interested in recruiting new authors and editors. Please call, write, fax, or e-mail. We look forward to hearing from you.

R.M.L., S.H.P., J.N.A., & P.W.E.

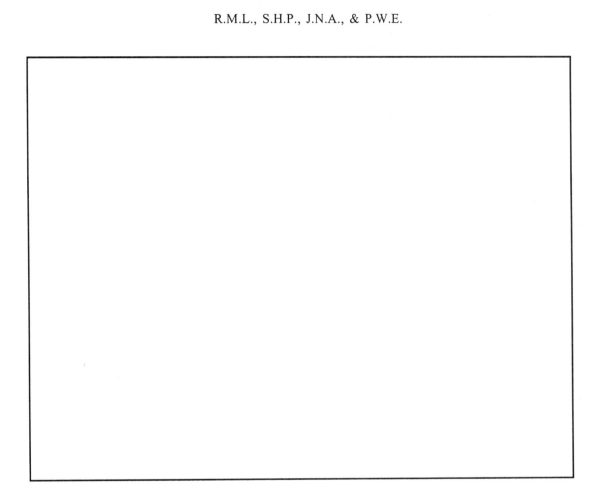

Return to:

Boston Medical Publishing Corporation
237 S. 70th Street, Suite 206, Lincoln, NE 68510

888-MBOARDS
402-484-6118
FAX: 402-484-6552
E-MAIL: bmp@emedicine.com

www.emedicine.com

INTRODUCTION

Welcome! Pediatric *Pearls of Wisdom*, has been written to help you learn and/or brush up on your pediatric medicine skills. Pearls of Wisdom has been designed as a study aid to improve your performance on the Pediatric Written Boards, recertification examination, or Pediatric In-service exam. *Pearls* is packed with practical, useful information intended for Pediatric specialists. However, in recent years, we have discovered that our unique format is of great use to house officers and medical students rotating in pediatric medicine as well. Before we begin, a few words are appropriate to discuss format, intent, limitations and use.

Since *Pearls* is primarily intended as a study aid, the text is written in rapid-fire question/answer format. This way, readers receive immediate gratification. Moreover, misleading or confusing "foils" are not provided. This eliminates the risk of erroneously assimilating an incorrect piece of information that made a big impression. Questions themselves often contain a pearl intended to reinforce the answer. Additional "hooks" are often attached to the answer in various forms, including mnemonics, evoked visual imagery, repetition, and humor. Additional information not requested in the question may be included in the answer. Emphasis has been placed on distilling trivia and key facts that are easily overlooked, that are quickly forgotten, and that somehow seem to be needed on board exams.

Many questions have answers without explanations. This enhances ease of reading and rate of learning. Explanations often occur in a later question/answer. Upon reading an answer, the reader may think "Hmm, why is that?" or "Are you sure?" If this happens to you, go check! Truly assimilating these disparate facts into a framework of knowledge absolutely requires further reading of the surrounding concepts. Information learned in response to seeking an answer to a particular question is retained much better than information that is passively observed. Take advantage of this! Use *Pearls* with your preferred source texts handy and open.

The first half of the text is presented in topic areas found on the Pediatric board exam. Information presented is mostly limited to straightforward, basic facts. The last section of the book, "Random Pearls," consists of questions grouped into small clusters by topic, presented in no particular order. This section repeats some of the factual information previously covered and builds on this foundation with emphasis on linking information and filling in gaps from the topical chapters.

Pearls has limitations. We have found many conflicts between sources of information. We have tried to verify in several references the most accurate information. Some texts have internal discrepancies further confounding clarification.

Pearls risks accuracy by aggressively pruning complex concepts down to the simplest kernel—the dynamic knowledge base and clinical practice of pediatric medicine is not like that! Furthermore, new research and practice occasionally deviates from that which likely represents the right answer for test purposes. This text is designed to maximize your score on a test. Refer to your most current sources of information and mentors for direction for practice.

Pearls is designed to be used, not just read. It is an interactive text. Use a 3x5 card and cover the answers; attempt all questions. A study method we recommend is oral, group study, preferably over an extended meal or pitchers. The mechanics of this method are simple and no one ever appears stupid. One person holds Pearls, with answers covered, and reads the question. Each person, including the reader, says "Check!" when he or she has an answer in mind. After everyone has "checked" in, someone states his/her answer. If this answer is correct, on to the next one, if not, another person says their answer or the answer can be read. Usually the person who "checks" in first gets the first shot at stating the answer. If this person is being a smarty-pants answer-hog, then others can take turns. Try it, it's almost fun!

Pearls is also designed to be re-used several times to allow, dare we use the word, memorization. Two check boxes are provided for any scheme of keeping track of questions answered correctly or incorrectly.

We welcome your comments, suggestions and criticism. Great effort has been made to verify these questions and answers. Some answers may not be the answer you would prefer. Most often this is attributable to variance between original sources. Please make us aware of any errors you find. We hope to make continuous improvements and would greatly appreciate any input with regard to format, organization, content, presentation, or about specific questions. We also are interested in recruiting new contributing authors and publishing new textbooks. Contact our managing editor at Boston Medical Publishing, 1-888-MBOARDS. We look forward to hearing from you!

Study hard and good luck!

R.M.L., S.H.P., J.N.A., & P.E

TABLE OF CONTENTS

SEDATION AND ANALGESIA

"All who drink of this remedy will recover... except those in whom it does not help, who will die. Therefore, it is obvious that it fails only in incurable cases."
- Galen

☐☐ **Explain the differences between the terms Opium, Opiate, and Opioid.**

Opium: From the Greek word for juice, applies to the juice extracted from the seeds of the poppy plant, the source for over 20 alkaloids.

Opiate: Any substance that is derived from the opium plant and can induce sleep, the naturally occurring medications from the opium plant are morphine and codeine.

Opioid: Any synthetic substance not derived from opium but that can induce narcosis. Synthetic opioids are meperidine (Demerol), and fentanyl (Sublimaze).

☐☐ **What is the most common adverse reaction caused by local anesthetics?**

Contact dermatitis is the most common local adverse reaction and is characterized by erythema and pruritus that could progress to vesiculation and oozing.

☐☐ **What is the half-life of acetaminophen (Tylenol)?**

Its half-life is 2-3 hours and is unaffected by renal disease as acetaminophen is metabolized in the liver.

☐☐ **On what specific sites in the CNS do the benzodiazepines act and where are they located?**

Benzodiazepine receptors are present in many regions of the brain including the thalamus, limbic structures and the cerebral cortex. They form part of a GABA receptor-chloride ion channel complex, and binding of benzodiazepines to this receptor facilitates the inhibitory actions of GABA, which are exerted through increased chloride ion conductance.

☐☐ **What are five non-pharmacologic methods used to reduce pain in pediatric patients?**

Biofeedback, desensitization, distraction, exercise and play are non-pharmacological interventions with demonstrated efficacy.

☐☐ **What is the principle behind biofeedback, and when is it useful?**

Biofeedback teaches the child with pain to distinguish between relaxed and tense body states. It is useful when pain is temporarily associated with stress or tension.

☐☐ **What is the fentanyl lollipop and what is its main side effect?**

The lollipop is a pediatric pre-anesthetic medication to be used by children as a self-administered drug. Some series report up to 50% incidence of vomiting making it impractical in children with "full stomachs" such as in an emergency department.

☐☐ **Describe the pharmacokinetics of codeine.**

Codeine has adequate oral absorption and is metabolized in the liver to morphine. It has a half-life of 2.5-3.5 hours and is excreted in the urine.

☐☐ **How potent is fentanyl, when compared to morphine?**

Fentanyl is 50-100 times more potent.

❏❏   **What is the mechanism of action of acetaminophen?**

Acetaminophen inhibits the synthesis of prostaglandins in the central nervous system and peripherally blocks pain impulse generation. It also produces antipyresis by inhibiting the hypothalamic heat regulating center.

❏❏   **Why should codeine _not_ be given intravenously?**

When given intravenously, codeine causes a large histamine release which leads to palpitations, hypotension, bradycardia, and peripheral vasodilatation.

❏❏   **Compare the cardiovascular adverse effects of fentanyl when compared to morphine.**

Fentanyl has less hypotensive effects than morphine due to minimal or no histamine release.

❏❏   **How much sugar, and what kind, is found in each 5 ml suspension of ibuprofen?**

2.5 gm of sucrose. This is important if you plan to use this suspension in a diabetic patient.

❏❏   **What are some of the misconceptions about pain in children?**

One of the misconceptions about pain in children is that pain perception in children is decreased because of biologic immaturity and that children have a higher tolerance to pain. Other misconceptions are that children have little or no memory of pain and that not only are they more sensitive to the side effects of analgesics, but that they are at special risk for addiction to narcotics. These beliefs are false.

❏❏   **Name four ways the pain of subcutaneously injected lidocaine can be reduced.**

1) Use a solution buffered with sodium bicarbonate.
2) Administer slowly.
3) Administer with a small needle, e.g., <30 gauge.
4) Use a warmed solution.

❏❏   **In many prepubertal children, what appears in the urine after the patient receives succinylcholine?**

Myoglobin. About 40% of prepubertal children exhibit this effect; however, it is not related to the apparent severity of the fasciculations.

❏❏   **How long does anesthesia last from a perineural injection of lidocaine?**

When used alone it lasts 60-75 minutes and when used in combination with epinephrine, anesthesia lasts up to two hours.

❏❏   **How long does it take for a local injection of lidocaine to exert its effect?**

Its effect is immediate.

❏❏   **What are endorphins?**

Endogenous morphine.

❏❏   **What are Mu receptors?**

A specific subtype of opioid receptors that are responsible for supraspinal analgesia, euphoria, and respiratory and physical dependence effects.

❏❏   **Describe the anesthetic agent propofol (Diprivan).**

Propofol is chemically unrelated to any other anesthetic drugs, it most closely resembles the alcohol family and has sedative properties which are similar to the alcohols. It is anecdotally called _milk of amnesia_. It may cause apnea.

PULMONARY

"We can only instill principles, put the student in the right path, give him methods, teach him how to study, and early to discern between essentials and non-essential."
– Sir William Osler

□□   **What should you suspect if a patient has symptoms similar to those associated with emphysema but he/she is very young and is not a smoker?**

L-1-antitrypsin deficiency. Without L-1-antitrypsin, excess elastase accumulates resulting in lung damage. Treatment for this condition is the same as emphysema. An L-1 proteinase inhibitor may also be useful.

□□   **List two drugs that can cause ARDS.**

Heroin and aspirin.

□□   **How long after an initial insult does ARDS usually occur?**

12–72 hours.

□□   **A 14-year-old high school freshman attended three days of classes at his new high school last week before it was shut down because of the potential of asbestos exposure. The boy currently exhibits a non-productive cough and says his chest hurts. Does this boy have asbestosis?**

Although a non-productive cough and pleurisy are symptoms of asbestosis, other signs, such as exertional dyspnea, malaise, clubbed fingers, crackles, cyanosis, pleural effusion and pulmonary hypertension, should be displayed before making a diagnosis of asbestosis. In addition, asbestosis does not develop until 10-15 years after regular exposure to asbestos.

□□   **What procedures should be performed to confine aspiration in a patient who is continuously vomiting and at risk for aspiration pneumonia?**

Lie the patient on his right side in Trendelenburg. This will help confine the aspirate to the right upper lobe.

□□   **Where does aspiration generally occur as revealed by chest x-ray?**

The lower lobe of the right lung. This is the most direct path for foreign bodies in the lung.

□□   **A 16-year-old tri-athlete develops wheezing when exercising. Describe a relevant treatment program for this individual.**

A sodium cromoglycate (cromolyn sodium) inhaler is the prophylactic medication of choice. Sodium cromoglycate stabilizes mast cells that are involved in the early and late phase bronchoconstrictive reactions of asthma. Sodium cromoglycate is a prophylactic treatment and is not effective once the attack has begun.

□□   **What pulmonary function test is the most diagnostic for asthma?**

FEV1/FVC. The amount of air exhaled in 1 second, in comparison to the total amount of air in the lung that can be expressed, is determined by performing this test. A ratio of under 80% is diagnostic of asthma. Peak flow monitors are helpful in monitoring asthma at home.

□□   **Is wheezing an integral part of asthma?**

No. Thirty-three percent of children with asthma will have only cough variant asthma with no wheezing.

❑❑   Which is more effective for relieving an acute exacerbation of bronchial asthma in a conscious patient, nebulized albuterol or albuterol MDI administered via an aerosol chamber?

They are equally efficacious.

❑❑   What are the McConnochie criteria for the diagnosis of bronchiolitis?

1) Acute expiratory wheezing
2) Age 6 months or less
3) Signs of viral illness, such as fever or coryza
4) With or without pneumonia or atopy
5) The first such episode

❑❑   What is the most common pathogen isolated in children with bronchiolitis?

Respiratory syncitial virus.

❑❑   Foreign body aspiration occurs most commonly in which age group?

1-3 years of age, with slight male predominance.

❑❑   Name the most common offender in foreign body aspiration.

Organic substances such as nuts and corn.

❑❑   What will be the predominant symptom of a child who has aspirated a foreign body which is lodged in his/her trachea?

Stridor.

❑❑   The predominant ausculatatory finding in a child with a foreign body lodged in the right mainstem bronchus:

Expiratory wheezing.

❑❑   A child is born to two parents who are both asthmatic. What is risk factor of the child having asthma as well?

Up to 50%.

❑❑   Is extrinsic asthma more common in children or in adults?

Children.

❑❑   What are the most common extrinsic allergens that affect asthmatic children?

Dust and dust mites.

❑❑   What kind of medical family history are asthmatic patients most likely to have?

Asthma, allergies, and/or atopic dermatitis.

❑❑   Which type of exercise usually triggers an asthmatic episode in patients with exercise-induced asthma?

High intensity exercise for more than 5-6 minutes.

❑❑   What is the role of salmeterol in the asthmatic patient?

It is used for the long term management of these patients and not in the acute setting. Because of its long half-life, it may be ideal for chronic use in nocturnal break-through exacerbations.

❑❑   Sympathomimetic agents are used to treat asthma. What enzyme is activated by these agents?

Adenyl cyclase.

❑❑ **What effects do increased levels of cAMP have on bronchial smooth muscle and on the release of chemical mediators, such as histamine, proteases, platelet activation factor and chemotactic factors, from airway mast cells?**

Relaxes smooth muscle and decreases the release of mediators. Recall that the effects of cAMP are opposed by cGMP. Thus, another treatment approach can be provided by *decreasing* the levels of cyclic GMP via the use of anticholinergic (antimuscarinic) agents, such as ipratropium bromide.

❑❑ **As discussed above, stimulation of ß-adrenergic receptors increases cAMP availability and results in smooth muscle relaxation. Which flavor of ß-adrenergic receptors primarily control bronchiolar and arterial smooth muscle tone?**

ß2-adrenergic receptors.

❑❑ **Right upper lobe cavitation with parenchymal involvement is a classic indicator of what disease?**

TB. Lower lung infiltrates, hilar adenopathy, atelectasis, and pleural effusion are also common.

❑❑ **What is the most common postoperative respiratory complication?**

Atelectasis. Respiratory failure and aspiration pneumonia are other postoperative complications.

❑❑ **What percentage of patients who have had abdominal surgery also develop atelectasis?**

> 25%.

❑❑ **Atelectasis accounts for what percentage of postoperative fevers?**

90%.

❑❑ **Why do we care about postoperative atelectasis?**

If it persists for more than 72 hours, pneumonia may develop. Perioperative mortality rates are then 20%. Incentive spirometry is an important therapy for the prevention of atelectasis.

❑❑ **A chest x-ray shows "honeycombing," atelectasis, and increased bronchial markings. What is the diagnosis?**

Bronchiectasis. Bronchography will show dilations of the bronchial tree, but this method of diagnosis is not recommended for routine use.

❑❑ **Bronchiectasis occurs most frequently in patients with what conditions?**

Patients with cystic fibrosis, immunodeficiencies, lung infections, or foreign body aspirations.

❑❑ **Which is the most common type of pathogen in bronchiolitis?**

RSV. It generally affects infants younger than 2 years old. Bronchiolitis is rarely seen in adults.

❑❑ **What is the treatment for severe bronchiolitis?**

Ribavirin.

❑❑ **Where in the United States is coccidioidomycosis most prevalent?**

Southwestern United States. If severe, treat the afflicted patient with amphotericin B.

❑❑ **Which populations are predisposed to progressive infection with coccidioidomycosis?**

African-Americans and diabetics.

❑❑   **A 2-year-old patient presents with a sudden harsh cough that is worse at night, wheezing, and rhonchi/inspiratory stridor. What is the diagnosis?**

Croup (also known as laryngotracheitis). This condition is usually preceded by an URI and most frequently caused by the parainfluenza virus. A barking seal like cough is a characteristic of croup.

❑❑   **In treating a patient with a common cold, you prescribe an oral decongestant. Is it necessary to also suggest an antitussant?**

Most coughs arising from a common cold are caused by the irritation of the tracheobronchial receptors in the posterior pharynx by postnasal drip. Postnasal drip can be cleared up with decongestant therapy, thereby eliminating the need for cough suppressant therapy.

❑❑   **What are the most common etiologies of a chronic cough?**

Postnasal drip (40%), asthma (25%), and gastroesophageal reflux (20%). Other etiologies include bronchitis, bronchiectasis, bronchogenic carcinoma, esophageal diverticula, sarcoidosis, viruses, and drugs.

❑❑   **Your vitamin-crazed mother insists that her vitamin C a day has helped her avoid colds. Is there any validity to this statement?**

No. Studies have failed to show a prophylactic effect of vitamin C. However, it has been shown that consuming 1 g of vitamin C a day decreases the severity and duration of symptoms associated with the common cold by 23%.

❑❑   **Which condition must be ruled out when childhood nasal polyps are found?**

Cystic fibrosis.

❑❑   **What age group is afflicted with the most colds per year?**

Kindergardners win the top billing with an average of 12 colds per year. Second place goes to preschoolers with 6-10 per year. School children get an average of 7 per year, and adolescents and adults average only 2- 4 per year.

❑❑   **What is the duration of a common cold?**

3-10 day self-limited course.

❑❑   **Which age group usually contracts croup?**

6 months to 3 years. Croup is characterized by cold symptoms, a sudden barking cough, inspiratory and expiratory stridor, and a slight fever.

❑❑   **A newborn presents with poor weight gain, steatorrhea, and a GI obstruction arising from thick meconium ileus. What test should be performed?**

The "sweat test," which detects electrolyte concentrations in the sweat. The infant may have cystic fibrosis. Cystic fibrosis is an autosomal recessive defect affecting the exocrine glands. As a result, electrolyte concentrations increase in the sweat glands.

❑❑   **What is the classic triad of cystic fibrosis?**

1) COPD.
2) Pancreatic enzyme deficiency.
3) Abnormally high concentration of sweat electrolytes.

❑❑   **What is the most common presentation of newborns with cystic fibrosis?**

GI obstruction due to meconium ileus.

❑❑   **Empyema is most often caused by which organism?**

Staphylococcus aureus. Gram-negative organisms and anaerobic bacteria also cause empyema.

☐☐ **Which age group typically gets epiglottitis?**

The 3-7 year age group, although any group can get epiglottitis.

☐☐ **What is the difference between the "cough of croup" and the "cough of epiglottitis"?**

Croup has a seal like "barking" cough, while epiglottitis is accompanied by a minimal cough. Children with croup have a hoarse voice while those with epiglottitis have a muffled voice.

☐☐ **What is the "thumb print sign"?**

A soft tissue inflammation of the epiglottis on a lateral x-ray of the neck.

☐☐ **Should a 7-year-old girl who has never received her Hib vaccine be vaccinated now?**

No, most children are immune by the age of 5.

☐☐ **How is fetal lung maturity assessed?**

By measuring the ratio of lecithin to sphingomyelin (L/S). An L/S ratio greater than 2 and the presence of phosphatidyl glycerol verifies that the fetal lungs are mature.

☐☐ **Are aspirated foreign bodies more likely to be found in the right or left bronchus?**

Right.

☐☐ **Hantavirus occurs most commonly in what geographic location?**

In the Southwestern U.S., especially in areas with deer mice.

☐☐ **What is the definition for massive hemoptysis?**

Coughing, not vomiting, of more than 600 mL of blood in 24 hours.

☐☐ **When should life-threatening hemoptysis be suspected?**

1) When there us a large volume of blood.
2) When there is the appearance of a fungus ball in a pulmonary cavity via chest x-ray.
3) When there is hypoxemia.

☐☐ **What percentage of the people living in the Ohio and the Mississippi valley are infected with histoplasmosis?**

100% in endemic areas. However, only 1% of these individuals develop the active disease. The spores of *H. capsulatum* can remain active for 10 years. For unknown reasons, bird or bat feces promotes the growth of the actual fungus. The spores are then released and subsequently inhaled, which is how the disease is transmitted.

☐☐ **What is Horner's syndrome?**

Miosis, ptosis, and anhydrosis (lack of sweat).

☐☐ **Which type of bacteria is most commonly found in lung abscesses?**

Anaerobic bacteria.

☐☐ **Which single antibiotic is the most effective for treating uncomplicated lung abscess?**

Clindamycin.

☐☐ **T/F: Flora of lung abscesses are usually polymicrobial.**

True.

❑❑   **Which age group is usually afflicted by pertussis?**

Infants younger than 2.

❑❑   **Where does pain from pleurisy radiate?**

The shoulder, as a result of diaphragmatic irritation.

❑❑   **Which is the <u>most</u> <u>common</u> community-acquired pneumonia?**

Pneumococcal pneumonia. Streptococcus pneumonia are actually normal flora. Treatment includes penicillin G or erythromycin.

❑❑   **Pneumatoceles, thin-walled air-filled cysts, on an infant's x-ray are a sign of which type of pneumonia?**

Staphylococcal pneumonia.

❑❑   **What are the <u>most</u> <u>common</u> causes of Staphylococcal pneumonias?**

Drug use and endocarditis. This pneumonia produces high fever, chills, and a purulent productive cough.

❑❑   **What are the extrapulmonary manifestations of mycoplasma?**

Erythema multiforme, pericarditis, and CNS disease.

❑❑   **What is the most frequent etiology of nosocomial pneumonia?**

Pseudomonas aurignosa. There is a high mortality associated with pneumonia caused by *Pseudomonas*. It most frequently occurs in immunocompromised patients or patients on mechanical ventilation.

❑❑   **A 14-year-old comes to your office bragging, between coughs, about a 3-day Young Republicans convention she attended last week in Las Vegas. She is nauseous and coughing; she has chills and a fever of 103.5°F. She also has a minor gait problem and splints her chest when she breaths. Should you be concerned about your own health as she has just given a mighty cough in your direction?**

This patient most likely has Legionnaires' disease. Unless you attended the same convention in Las Vegas, you are unlikely to catch this pneumonia from her. *Legionella pneumophila* contaminates the water in air conditioning towers and moist soil. It is not spread from person to person.

❑❑   **Describe the classic chest x-ray findings in a patient with mycoplasma pneumonia.**

Patchy diffuse densities involving the entire lung are most common. Pneumatoceles, cavities, abscesses, and pleural effusions can occur, but are uncommon.

❑❑   **Describe the classic chest x-ray findings in Legionella pneumonia.**

Dense consolidation and bulging fissures. Expect elevated liver enzymes and hypophosphatemia.

❑❑   **Match the pneumonia with the treatment.**

1) *Klebsiella pneumoniae.*   a) Erythromycin, tetracycline, or doxycycline.
2) *Streptococcal pneumoniae.*   b) Penicillin G.
3) *Legionella pneumophila.*   c) Cefuroxime and clarithromycin.
4) *Haemophilus influenza pneumonia.* d) Erythromycin and rifampin.
5) *Mycoplasma pneumonia.*
Answers: (1) c, (2) b, (3) d, (4) c, and (5) a.

❑❑   **A 16-year-old male presents to your office complaining of pleurisy, sudden onset of fever and chills, and rust colored sputum. What is the diagnosis?**

Pneumococcal pneumonia caused by Streptococcus pneumonia, the most common community acquired pneumonia. It is a consolidating lobar pneumonia and can be treated with penicillin G or erythromycin.

❑❑   **A 17-year-old college student is home for winter break and comes to your office complaining of a 1.5-week history of a non-productive dry hacking cough, malaise, a mild fever, and no chills. What is the diagnosis?**

Mycoplasma pneumoniae, also known as walking pneumonia. Although this is the most common pneumonia that develops in teenagers and young adults, it is an atypical pneumonia and is most frequently found in close contact populations (e.g., schools and military barracks).

❑❑   **Describe the different presentations of bacterial and viral pneumonia.**

Bacterial pneumonia is typified by a sudden onset of symptoms, including pleurisy, fever, chills, productive cough, tachypnea, and tachycardia. The most common bacterial pneumonia is Pneumococcal pneumonia.

Viral pneumonia is characterized by gradual onset of symptoms, no pleurisy, chills or high fever, general malaise, and a non-productive cough.

❑❑   **What is the most common cause of pneumonia in children?**

Viral pneumonia. Infecting viruses include influenza, parainfluenza, RSV, and adenoviruses.

❑❑   **What is the most common pneumonia acquired in the hospital?**

Pneumonia caused by aerobic Gram-negative bacteria.

❑❑   **What is the most common lethal, inheritable disease in the Caucasian population?**

Cystic fibrosis, an autosomal recessive disease occurring in 1/2,000 births.

❑❑   **What is the most common community acquired Gram-negative rod pneumonia?**

Pneumonia induced by *Klebsiella pneumonia*.

❑❑   **What bacterial agent that frequently causes community acquired pneumonia is not covered by erythromycin?**

Haemophilus influenzae.

❑❑   **Which two antimicrobial agents are broadly effective against organisms that cause both typical and atypical pneumonias?**

Azithromycin and clarithromycin.

❑❑   **What percentage of upper respiratory infectious agents are non-bacterial?**

Non-bacterial agents account for over 90% of pharyngitis, laryngitis, tracheal bronchitis, and bronchitis.

❑❑   **Name two anti-viral medications that are useful for viral pneumonia.**

Amantadine, for influenza A, and aerosolized Ribavirin, for RSV.

❑❑   **If a patient has a patchy infiltrate on a chest x-ray and bullous myringitis, what antibiotic should be prescribed?**

Erythromycin for mycoplasma.

❑❑   **What secondary bacterial pneumonia often occurs following a viral pneumonia?**

Staphylococcus aureus pneumonia.

❑❑   **Should steroids be used in aspiration pneumonia?**

No.

☐☐   **What therapy may increase the body's absorption of a pneumothorax or pneumomediastinum?**

A high inspired FiO_2.

☐☐   **What is the profile of a classic patient with a spontaneous pneumothorax?**

Male, athletic, tall, slim, 15-35 years of age. Pneumothorax does not occur most frequently during exercise.

☐☐   **What accessory x-rays may be obtained for the diagnosis of pneumothorax?**

AP film and lateral decubitus film on the affected side. Classic teaching has us believe that an expiratory film is more sensitive, though the latest studies in radiology texts refute this. Just get a regular inspiratory xray, will ya.

☐☐   **Which types of pneumonia are commonly associated with pneumothorax?**

Staphylococcus, TB, Klebsiella, and PCP.

☐☐   **Primary pulmonary hypertension is most common in what population?**

Young females. It is rapidly fatal within a few years.

☐☐   **What heart sounds are heard with pulmonary hypertension?**

A shortened second heart sound split and a louder P2.

☐☐   **What is the major etiology of pulmonary hypertension?**

Chronic hypoxia

☐☐   **A newborn is breathing rapidly and grunting. Intercostal retractions, nasal flaring, and cyanosis are noted. Auscultation shows decreased breath sounds and crackles. What is the diagnosis?**

Newborn respiratory distress syndrome, also known as hyaline membrane disease. X-rays show diffuse atelectasis. Treatment involves artificial surfactant and O_2 administration through CPAP.

☐☐   **Other than avoiding prematurity, what can be done to prevent newborn respiratory distress syndrome?**

If the fetus is > 32 weeks, administer betamethasone 48–72 hours before delivery to augment surfactant production.

☐☐   **Which type of rhinitis is associated with anxious patients?**

Vasomotor rhinitis. This is a non-allergic rhinitis of unknown etiology that involves nasal vascular congestion.

☐☐   **Which sinuses are fully formed in children?**

Only the ethmoid and the maxillary.

☐☐   **Differentiate between transudate and exudate.**

1) Transudate: Serum protein is < 0.5 and LDH is < 0.6. Most common with CHF, renal disease, and liver disease.

2) Exudate: Serum protein > 0.5, LDH > 0.6. Most common with infections, malignancy, and trauma.

☐☐   **Is a URI accompanied by a high fever usually caused by a bacterial or a viral source?**

Bacterial. However, most URI's are viral in origin.

❏❏   **A patient presents with cough, lethargy, dyspnea, conjunctivitis, glomerulonephritis, fever, and purulent sinusitis. What is the diagnosis?**

Wegener's granulomatosis. This is a necrotizing vasculitis and pulmonary granulomatosis that attacks the small arteries and veins. Treatment is with corticosteroids and cyclophosphamide.

❏❏   **What serological test is diagnostic for Wegener's granulomatosis?**

c-ANCA in association with appropriate clinical evidence. A renal, lung, or sinus biopsy may also be helpful in making the diagnosis.

❏❏   **Are sedatives beneficial for anxious asthmatic patients?**

Only if you are trying to kill them. However, sedatives are appropriate for use during Rapid Sequence Intubation (RSI).

❏❏   **What is the effect of macrolide antibiotics (erythromycin, clarithromycin) on mucus hypersecretion?**

Some macrolide antibiotics have the ability to down regulate mucus secretion by an unknown mechanism. This is thought to be due to an anti-inflammatory activity.

❏❏   **Is foreign body aspiration more common in children or adults?**

Children. In adults it is more common from the fourth decade onwards. It is more likely when food is poorly chewed and when alcohol or sedative drugs are taken.

❏❏   **What are the signs of a large obstructing foreign body in the larynx or trachea?**

Respiratory distress, stridor, inability to speak, cyanosis, loss of consciousness, death.

❏❏   **What are the symptoms of a smaller (distally lodged) foreign body?**

Cough, dyspnea, wheezing, chest pain, fever.

❏❏   **What are the complications of the Heimlich maneuver?**

Rib fractures, ruptured viscera, pneumomediastinum, regurgitation (and aspiration), and retinal detachment.

❏❏   **What is the procedure of choice for foreign body removal?**

Rigid bronchoscopy. Fiberoptic bronchoscopy is an alternate procedure in adults, not in children. If bronchoscopy fails, thoracotomy may be required.

❏❏   **What are the common radiographic findings in foreign body aspiration?**

Normal film, atelectasis, pneumonia, contralateral mediastinal shift (more marked during expiration), and visualization of the foreign body

❏❏   **What is the antibiotic choice for gastric acid aspiration?**

None.

❏❏   **What is the role of corticosteroids in gastric acid aspiration?**

None.

❏❏   **What is the main priority in treating gastric acid aspiration?**

Maintenance of oxygenation. Intubation, ventilation, and PEEP (positive end expiratory pressure) may be required.

❏❏   **What are the radiographic manifestations of acid aspiration?**

Varied, may be bilateral diffuse infiltrates, irregular "patchy" infiltrates, or lobar infiltrates.

❏❏   **What is the usual source of infected aspirated material?**

The oropharynx.

❏❏   **What pleuropulmonary infections may occur after aspirating infected oropharyngeal material?**

Necrotizing pneumonia, lung abscess, "typical" pneumonia, empyema.

❏❏   **What is the predominant oropharyngeal flora in outpatients?**

Anaerobes. Community acquired aspiration is usually anaerobic. The most common aerobes involved are streptococcus species.

❏❏   **How long after aspiration is lung abscess usually detected?**

2 weeks or more.

❏❏   **What is the duration of treatment for lung abscess?**

Until radiographic resolution or stabilization with a small residual scar or cyst. This may take 6 weeks or more.

❏❏   **What are the consequences of aspirating small (non-obstructing) food particles?**

Inflammation and hypoxemia, may result in chronic bronchiolitis or granulomatosis.

❏❏   **Lipoid pneumonia is associated with chronic aspiration of what?**

Mineral oil, also animal or vegetable oils, oil-based nose drops.

❏❏   **What is the annual U.S. mortality from drowning?**

9000. There are 500 near drownings for each drowning.

❏❏   **What is the definition of drowning?**

Death due to suffocation by submersion in water.

❏❏   **Can drowning occur without aspiration of water?**

Yes. 10% of victims die from intense laryngospasm.

❏❏   **How much fluid can be drained from the lungs after drowning in fresh water?**

Little, as hypotonic fresh water is rapidly absorbed from the lung, unlike salt water which is hypertonic and is retained. There is no difference in outcome.

❏❏   **What is the priority in treatment of near drowning?**

Maintenance of oxygenation.

❏❏   **When is the Heimlich maneuver applied directly after a near drowning?**

When foreign body aspiration is suspected.

❏❏   **What are the indications for intubation and ventilation after near drowning?**

Apnea, pulselessness, altered mental status, severe hypoxemia, respiratory acidosis.

GASTROINTESTINAL

"Medicine is not only a science; it is also an art. It does not consist of compounding pills and plasters; it deals with the very processes of life, which must be understood before they may be guided"
–Paracelsus (1493-1541)

☐☐　　**What is the typical profile of a patient with anorexia nervosa?**

Female, adolescent, upper class, perfectionist.

☐☐　　**What are some common conditions that mimic acute appendicitis?**

Mesenteric lymphadenitis, PID, Mittleschmertz, gastroenteritis, and Crohn's disease.

☐☐　　**What conditions are associated with an atypical presentation of acute appendicitis?**

Situs inversus viscerum, malrotation, hypermobile cecum, long pelvic appendix; retrocecal appendix, and pregnancy (1/2200).

☐☐　　**What are the most frequent symptoms of acute appendicitis?**

Anorexia and pain. The classical presentations of anorexia and periumbilical pain with progression to constant RLQ pain are present in only 60% of the cases.

☐☐　　**What percentage of acute appendicitis cases have an elevated WBC count?**

An elevated leukocyte count and an elevated absolute neutrophil count are present in 86% and 89% of the cases, respectively.

☐☐　　**What intraabdominal pathology should be assumed in a pregnant female with right upper quadrant pain until proven otherwise?**

Acute appendicitis.

☐☐　　**What does an ultrasound show in acute appendicitis?**

A fixed, tender, non-compressible mass, but only in 75-90% of these cases.

☐☐　　**What does abdominal CT scanning show in acute appendicitis?**

Not much in early appendicitis. However, the study is useful to determine the causes of a right lower quadrant mass, such as late appendicitis, perforation/abscess, carcinoma, and pseudomyxoma.

☐☐　　**What does laparoscopy show in acute appendicitis?**

Appendicitis, if you're lucky. Unfortunately, determining that the appendix is inflamed does not prove appendicitis. However, finding another cause of the abdominal pain does not rule out appendicitis either.

☐☐　　**Which method is more sensitive for locating the source of GI bleeding, a radioactive Tc-labeled red cell scan or an angiography?**

A bleeding scan can detect a site bleeding at a rate as low as 0.12 mL/minute, while angiography requires rapid bleeding (i.e., greater than 0.5 mL/min).

☐☐　　**Repeated violent bouts of vomiting can result in both Mallory-Weiss tears and Boerhaave's syndrome. Differentiate between the two.**

1) Mallory-Weiss tears involve the submucosa and mucosa, typically in the right posterolateral wall of the GE junction.

2) Boerhaave syndrome is a full-thickness tear, usually in the unsupported left posterolateral wall of the abdominal esophagus.

❑❑   **A 6-month-old infant is constipated, flaccid, and only stares straight ahead. He is not running a fever. However, his mother is especially worried because he won't take his bottle — not even for her "honey on the tip of the bottle" trick. Diagnosis?**

Infantile botulism. Infants ingest spores that are in the environment, most commonly in honey. The spores then grow and produce toxins within the host.

❑❑   **How does infantile botulism differ from food-borne botulism?**

Infantile botulism is caused by the spores of *C. botulinum* while adult food-borne botulism arises from the ingestion of *C. botulinum* neurotoxins.

❑❑   **What is the antidote for botulism poisoning?**

Trivalent A-B-E antitoxin. This antidote is not required for infantile botulism.

❑❑   **What is the most frequent complication of choledocholithiasis?**

Cholangitis (60%). Other complications are bile duct obstruction, pancreatitis, biliary enteric fistula, and hemobilia.

❑❑   **Gallbladder stones are generally formed of what substance?**

Cholesterol. The diagnostic test of choice is ultrasound. This technique may show stones, sludge, bile plugging, or dilated bile ducts.

❑❑   **A patient with a history of gallstones presents with an acute, postprandial right upper quadrant pain. What's the KUB likely to show?**

Nothing specific. Only around 10% of gallstones are radiopaque. Complications of cholelithiasis, such as emphysematous cholecystitis, perforation, and pneumobilia are uncommon but useful findings.

❑❑   **A child with sickle-cell disease presents with fever, shaking chills, and jaundice. What is the diagnosis?**

Charcot's triad suggests ascending cholangitis. The precipitating cause is probably pigment stones resulting from chronic hemolysis.

❑❑   **Name two findings in acute cholecystitis that mandate an emergent laparotomy.**

Emphysematous cholecystitis and perforation. Otherwise, timing of surgery is somewhat dependent upon the institution and surgeon.

❑❑   **A 12-year-old male complains of 2 days of rice-water stools, muscle cramps and extreme fatigue. He looks pale, dehydrated, and very ill. The patient states that he has just returned from India. What is the diagnosis?**

Cholera. The incidence of cholera in the U.S. is 1/10,000,000. Cholera usually develops in travelers returning from endemic areas, such as India, Africa, southeast Asia, southern Europe, Central and South America, and the Middle East. This disease can be prevented if the water ingested during the trip is purified and raw, and unpeeled fruits/vegetables and seafood are avoided altogether.

❑❑   **How does the pathology of Crohn's disease differ from that of ulcerative colitis?**

Crohn's is a trans-mucosal, segmental, granulomatous process, while ulcerative colitis is a mucosal, juxtapositioned, ulcerative process.

❏❏   **A young man with atraumatic chronic back pain, eye trouble, and painful red lumps on his shins develops <u>bloody</u> <u>diarrhea</u>. What is the point of this question?**

To remind you of the extraintestinal manifestations of inflammatory bowel disease, such as ankylosing spondylitis, uveitis, and erythema nodosum, not to mention kidney stones.

❏❏   **At least one-third of the patients with Crohn's disease develop kidney stones. Why?**

Dietary oxalate is usually bound to calcium and excreted. When terminal ileal disease leads to decreased bile salt absorption, the resulting fattier intestinal contents bind calcium by saponification. Free oxalate is "hyper-absorbed" in the colon, resulting in hyperoxaluria and calcium oxalate nephrolithiasis.

❏❏   **Complications of Crohn's include perirectal abscesses, anal fissures, rectovaginal fistulas, and rectal prolapse. What percentage of patients with Crohn's disease have perirectal involvement?**

Approximately 90%.

❏❏   **What are the odds that a patient with severe ileal disease will be cured by surgery?**

Virtually zero. Crohn's invariably recurs in the remaining GI tract. In contrast, total proctocolectomy with ileostomy is a curative procedure for ulcerative colitis.

❏❏   **What stool studies are crucial for evaluating acute diarrhea?**

Statistically speaking, acute diarrhea is so common and typically self-limited that most cases require no testing, just oral rehydration. In sick patients or those at risk for complications, (i.e., at the extremes of age, recently hospitalized, or the immunocompromised), enteroinvasive infection should be ruled out with a stool guaiac and test for fecal leukocytes. Gram's or methylene blue stains are comparable. Also consider checking for ova and parasites.

❏❏   **Which diarrheal illnesses cause fecal leukocytes?**

The usual culprits are *Shigella, Campylobacter*, and enteroinvasive *E. coli*. Others include *Salmonella, Yersinia, Vibrio parahaemolyticus*, and *C. difficile*. Fecal WBCs are absent in toxigenic and enteropathogenic infection, even with such a virulent organism as *Vibrio cholera*. Viral and parasitic infections rarely produce fecal WBCs.

❏❏   **Name the most probable cause of diarrhea in a 6-month-old in day-care.**

Viral diarrhea caused by *Rotavirus* is the most common. Also test for *Giardia* and *Cryptosporidia* because these agents have recently been added to the list of day-care-associated diarrheal illnesses.

❏❏   **What is the <u>most</u> <u>common</u> cause of bacterial diarrhea?**

E. coli (enteroinvasive, enteropathogenic, enterotoxigenic).

❏❏   **Which is the <u>most</u> <u>common</u> form of acute diarrhea?**

Viral diarrhea. It is generally self limited, lasting only 1- 3 days.

❏❏   **Diarrhea that develops within 12 hours of a meal is most probably caused by what?**

An ingested pre-formed toxin.

❏❏   **When does traveler's diarrhea typically occur?**

3-7 days after arrival in a foreign land.

❏❏   **What is the treatment for traveler's diarrhea?**

Traveler's diarrhea is caused by *E. Coli*; the preferable treatment is with Bactrim.

❏❏   **What is the definition of chronic diarrhea?**

Passage of greater than 200 g of loose stool per day for over 3 weeks.

❑❑   **Radiographs should be performed on all patients suspected of swallowing coins to determine the presence and location of the foreign body. How will the coin appear on a x-ray in the AP view?**

Coins in the esophagus lie in the frontal plane. Coins in the trachea lie in the sagittal plane.

❑❑   **What is the management of button batteries that have passed the esophagus?**

In the asymptomatic patient, repeat radiographs. The symptomatic patient and patients in whom the battery has not passed the pylorus after 48 hours require an endoscopic retrieval.

❑❑   **X-rays are crucial for finding suspected swallowed foreign bodies. In kids, what physical findings can tip you off?**

Besides the child's distress, a red or scratched oropharynx, dysphagia, a high fever, or peritoneal signs may be evident. In addition, subcutaneous air suggests perforation.

❑❑   **Most objects, even sharp ones, pass through the GI tract without incident. What objects should be removed?**

Any object that obstructs or perforates, that is > 5 cm long and > 2 cm wide, or that is toxic (such as a battery) should be removed, either endoscopically or surgically. Sharp or pointed objects, including sewing needles and razor blades, should be removed if they haven't passed the pylorus.

❑❑   **Which type of hepatitis is usually contracted through blood transfusion?**

Hepatitis C. Eighty five percent of post transfusion hepatitis is caused by hepatitis C.

❑❑   **A poor prognosis is associated with which two LFTs in acute viral hepatitis?**

A total bilirubin > 20 mg/dL and a prolongation of the prothrombin time > 3 seconds. The extent of transaminase elevation is not a useful marker.

❑❑   **Match the following hepatitis serologies with the correct clinical description.**

1) HBsAg (-), and antiHBs (+)
2) IgM HBcAb (+), antiHBs (-)
3) IgG HBcAb (+), antiHBs (-)
4) HBeAg (+)

a) Ongoing viral replication, highly infectious.
b) Remote infection, not infectious.
c) Recent or ongoing infection; a high titer means high infectivity, while a low titer suggests chronic, active infection.
d) Prior infection or vaccination, not infectious.

Answers: (1) d, (2) c, (3) b, and (4) a.

HBeAg (+):   "e"   = "Eeek! I'm infectious!" for e ANTIGEN, anti-HBe implies decreased infectivity.
IgG HBcAb (+):   "G"   = Gone.
IgM HBcAb (+):   "M"   = Might be contagious still.
ANTIHBs (+):   "s"   = Stopped. Patient has antibodies to surface antigen.

Warning! You must specify whether the antigen or the antibody is present when learning these letter codes; otherwise you will learn these the wrong way around! Go over it ten times in your text of choice so it will make sense. Then, remembering the letters won't be necessary.

❑❑   **T/F: The "δ-agent" can cause hepatitis D in a patient without active hepatitis B.**

False. The d-agent is an incomplete, "defective" RNA virus that is responsible for hepatitis D. It is an obligate covirus and requires hepatitis B for replication.

❑❑   **You stick yourself with a needle from a chronic hepatitis B carrier. You've been vaccinated, but have never had your antibody status checked. What is the appropriate post exposure prophylaxis?**

Measure your anti-HBs titer. If it's adequate (> 10 mIU), treatment is not required. If it is inadequate, you need a single dose of HBIG as soon as possible and a vaccine booster.

❏❏   **Which is more dangerous, a small hernia or a large one?**

Incarceration is more likely with small hernias.

❏❏   **Which hernia is the most common in females, inguinal or femoral?**

Inguinal, not femoral. Although it's true that femoral hernias are more common in females than in males, inguinal hernias still remain the most common hernia in females.

❏❏   **Distinguish between a groin hernia, a hydrocele, and a lymph node.**

Hydroceles transilluminate and are non-tender. Lymph nodes are freely moving and firm. Hernias don't transilluminate and may produce bowel sounds.

❏❏   **A patient tells you that 2 days ago his groin bulged. He then developed severe pain with progressive nausea and vomiting. He also has a tender mass in his groin. What shouldn't you do?**

Don't try to reduce a long-standing, tender, incarcerated hernia! The abdomen is no place for dead bowel.

❏❏   **In addition to conjugated hyperbilirubinemia, what liver function abnormalities suggest biliary tract disease?**

Elevated alkaline phosphatase out of proportion to transaminases.

❏❏   **Currant jelly stool in a child is indicative of what?**

Intussusception.

❏❏   **What is the most common cause of bowel obstruction in children under 2?**

Intussusception. Usually the terminal ileum will slide into the right colon. The cause is unknown but suspected to be due to hypertrophied lymph nodes at the junction of the ileum and colon.

❏❏   **What is the treatment for intussusception?**

A barium enema is both a diagnostic tool and curative (i.e., by reducing the intussusception). If the barium enema is unsuccessful, surgical reduction may be required.

❏❏   **Crampy abdominal pain with mucus in the stool is indicative of what syndrome?**

The irritable bowel syndrome. Patients are afebrile and often improve after passing flatus.

❏❏   **List 4 contraindications to the introduction of a nasogastric tube.**

1) Suspected esophageal laceration or perforation.
2) Near obstruction due to stricture.
3) Esophageal foreign body.
4) Severe head trauma with rhinorrhea.

❏❏   **What is the hallmark sign of a perforated viscus?**

Abdominal pain.

❏❏   **Burning epigastric pain shooting to the back, hypovolemic shock, and a high amylase suggest:**

A posterior perforation of a duodenal ulcer.

❏❏   **What percentage of patients with a perforated viscus also have radiographic evidence of a pneumoperitoneum?**

60-70%. Therefore, one-third of patients will not have this sign. Keep the patient in either the upright or left lateral decubitus position for at least 10 minutes prior to performing x-rays.

❑❑   **Peptic ulcer disease is more common in which sex?**

The male sex by a ratio of 3:1.

❑❑   **What percentage of PUD patients are afflicted with duodenal ulcers? Gastric ulcers?**

Seventy five percent of patients with PUD have duodenal ulcers; 25% have gastric ulcers.

❑❑   **Are patients with duodenal PUD usually younger or older?**

Younger. Duodenal PUD is more often associated with *H. pylori*. Older people tend to develop gastric ulcers due to NSAID use.

❑❑   **What are some indications for surgery in a bleeding ulcer?**

A visible vessel in the ulcer bed, more than 6 units of blood transfused in 24 hours, or more than 3-4 units per day in three days.

❑❑   **Which type of ulcer heals faster, gastric or duodenal?**

Duodenal.

❑❑   **Where is the most common location of a perforated peptic ulcer?**

The anterior surface of the duodenum or pylorus and the lesser curvature of the stomach.

❑❑   **Is a person with massive upper GI bleeding likely to have a perforated ulcer?**

No.

❑❑   **After the fluid and blood resuscitation of a patient with a bleeding ulcer, what is the most useful diagnostic test?**

Endoscopy, which can also be therapeutic, with cryo- or electrocautery of an arterial bleeder.

❑❑   **Name two endocrine problems that cause peptic ulcer.**

Zollinger-Ellison syndrome and hyperparathyroidism (hypercalcemia).

❑❑   **A postprandial midabdominal pain is indicative of what ectopic syndrome?**

Peptic ulcer in a Meckel's diverticulum.

❑❑   **In adults, pruritus ani develops because of dietary factors contributing to liquid stool, such as caffeine and mineral oil, sexually transmitted infections, fecal contamination, overzealous hygiene, and vitamin deficiencies. What is the most common cause in children?**

Enterobius vermicularis, or pinworm. Test for pinworms by applying a piece of scotch tape, sticky-side down, to the perineal area, and than smooth the tape out on a glass slide using a cotton swab. Examine the slide for eggs with a microscope set on low power. Treat the pediatric patient with mebendazole, 100 mg in a single dose, repeated in 2 weeks if necessary.

❑❑   **A patient with chronic and occasionally bloody diarrhea develops severe diarrhea and abdominal pain with marked distention. What "can't-miss" diagnosis is confirmed by these signs?**

Toxic megacolon. This condition is a life-threatening complication of ulcerative colitis.

❑❑   **What are the peak ages for the onset of ulcerative colitis?**

15-35 years with a smaller incident rate in the seventh decade.

❑❑ **What percentage of ulcerative colitis cases have rectal involvement?**

95%. The inflammation extends proximally and continuously.

❑❑ **A double bubble on x-ray or a "bird's beak" and dilated colon on a barium enema are indicative of what?**

Volvulus.

❑❑ **A patient presents with tremor, ataxia, dementia, cirrhosis, and grey-green rings around the edge of his cornea. What is the diagnosis?**

Wilson's disease. Kaiser Fleischer rings (i.e., golden brown or gray green pigmentation around the cornea), CNS disturbances, chronic hepatitis, and cirrhosis are all caused by copper retention as a result of impaired copper excretion.

❑❑ **In Wilson's disease, are the levels of copper low or high in both urine and serum?**

Serum copper levels are low because there is a deficiency in the copper-binding protein, ceruloplasmin. However, urine copper is high. Treatment for this disease is penicillamine, which chelates copper and thereby reverses the disease.

❑❑ **What are potential gastro-intestinal causes of apnea and bradycardia in neonates?**

Oral feeding, bowel movement, G.E. Reflux, esophagitis and intestinal perforation.

❑❑ **What substances can mimic upper GI bleeding?**

Red food coloring in cereals, Jell-O, drinks such as Kool-Aid and fruit juices and natural coloring in beets.

❑❑ **What substance can mimic melena?**

Iron supplements, dark chocolate, spinach, cranberries, grape juice, bismuth, blueberries.

❑❑ **Name the infectious causes of hematochezia.**

Salmonella, Shigella, Yersinia enterocolitica, Campylobacter jejuni, Escherichia coli, Clostridium difficile, Aeromonas hydrophilia and Entamoeba histolytica.

❑❑ **A 10-year-old child presents with a 3-day history of episodic abdominal pain and hematochezia. Examination reveals a palpable purpuric rash mostly on the lower limbs. Platelet count is normal. What is the most likely cause?**

Henoch-Schonlein Purpura (Anaphylactoid purpura).

❑❑ **What are the 3 most common causes of upper gastrointestinal bleeding in neonates?**

Swallowed maternal blood, gastritis, duodenitis.

❑❑ **What test can differentiate neonatal from swallowed maternal blood?**

Apt test – which is based on the conversion of oxyhemoglobin to hematin when mixed with alkali. Fetal hemoglobin is resistant to alkali (pink reaction) while maternal hemoglobin is denatured (dirty brown).

❑❑ **What test can be used to detect neonatal blood in the mothers' circulation?**

Kleiheuer-Betke test. Can be used quantitatively if you are worried about abruption.

❑❑ **Name the more common prescription drugs associated with gastric ulcers in children.**

Salicylates, Nonsteroidal anti-inflammatory agents, Aminophylline, Anticoagulants, and Antimetabolites.

❑❑ **Is there an increased risk for GI bleeding in patients with Turner Syndrome?**

Yes. Turner syndrome is associate with GI vascular malformations and Inflammatory bowel disease.

❏❏   **What is the comparative usefulness of endoscopy as opposed to an upper GI series in identifying bleeding sources?**

A diagnosis can be made in 90% of cases by using endoscopy, but less than 50% of cases by upper GI series.

❏❏   **At what age does intussusception most commonly occur?**

60% of all cases occur by 12 months of age, and 80% by 24 months.

❏❏   **What are common types of injuries to peridontal structures?**

Concussion, subluxation, intrusive luxation - most common injury to primary dentition, extrusive luxation, and evulsion.

❏❏   **How common is infantile hypertrophic pyloric stenosis?**

Affects approximately 1:150 males and 1:750 females, and is more common in first born males.

❏❏   **Name the three areas of physiologic narrowing in the esophagus, where an ingested coin is likely to lodge.**

Below the cricopharyngeal muscle, at the level of the aortic arch, and just below the diaphragm.

❏❏   **What is the classical metabolic picture in infants with pyloric stenosis?**

Hypochloremic alkalosis.

❏❏   **When does midgut volvulus usually present?**

50% of cases in the 1st week of life and 80% within the first month.

❏❏   **Do infants with malrotation always present with bilious vomiting?**

No. About 25% of infants under 2 months present with nonbilious emesis.

❏❏   **What is the incidence of meconium ileus in newborn infants with cystic fibrosis?**

Meconium ileus is most commonly seen in infants with cystic fibrosis, but less than 10% of infants with cystic fibrosis have meconium ileus.

❏❏   **What are the typical radiographic findings in meconium ileus?**

Lack of air in the distal colon; distended loops of small bowel associated with bubbles of stool and air- described as a ground-glass appearance or Neuhauser's sign.

❏❏   **How common is diabetes mellitus in patients with cystic fibrosis?**

It is 40-200 times higher than in the general pediatric population, but is relatively mild, resulting infrequently in ketosis.

❏❏   **How common is rectal prolapse in children with cystic fibrosis?**

It occurs in almost 20% of patients and is the presenting sign of CF in half of these.

❏❏   **What could happen to patients with cystic fibrosis during periods of increased physical activity and heat stress?**

Hyponatremic dehydration due to the high losses of sodium in sweat.

❏❏   **Name the 3 leading causes of acute pancreatitis in children.**

Viral infections, drugs and trauma.

❏❏   **What is the most common clinical finding in children with acute pancreatitis?**

Epigastric tenderness with decreased bowel sounds.

❏❏ **What is the age of patients when ulcerative colitis in childhood is usually diagnosed?**

5-16 years.

❏❏ **What are the most common presenting signs and symptoms of ulcerative colitis?**

Stool mixed with mucus and blood; lower abdominal cramping which is most intense during defecation.

❏❏ **How common is retrocecal appendix?**

19-20%, according to most recent reviews

❏❏ **Name the most common non-infectious causes of chronic diarrhea in children.**

Food allergy, food intolerance, chronic nonspecific diarrhea (CNSD), lactase deficiency, irritable colon, encopresis, metabolic/malabsorption disease, ulcerative colitis, regional enteritis, and Hirschsprung's disease.

❏❏ **When you suspect that a child has CNSD, what are the "four Fs" to which you should pay special attention?**

Fiber, Fluid, Fat, and Fruit juices.

❏❏ **Pedialyte is frequently used for oral hydration in infants. What is the composition of this solution?**

Na	-	45meq/L
K	-	20meq/L
Cl	-	35 meq/L
HCO3	-	30 meq/L
Glucose	-	25 meq/L

❏❏ **Is this oral solution appropriate for rehydration?**

The American Academy of Pediatrics recommends a solution containing at least 75-90m Eq Na per liter for rehydration. REHYDRALITE and the WHO solution are two such solutions.

❏❏ **What is the most common reason for "spitting up" in young infants?**

Overfeeding! Parents frequently report that the child is vomiting.

❏❏ **A 2-week-old male infant presents with persistent emesis and dehydration. Blood electrolytes reveal significant hyperkalemia. What potential lesion must be ruled out?**

Congenital adrenal hyperplasia (CAH)

❏❏ **What anti-emetic is recommended in the infant who presents with emesis?**

Trick question! Antiemetics are strongly discouraged because of the incidence of side effects.

❏❏ **Two children from the same family present with severe nausea and vomiting about 4-6 hours after eating. What are the most likely causes?**

S. aureus toxins, *Bacillus cereus*, heavy metals.

❏❏ **Two children from another family develop parasthesias a few hours after eating. What causes should you consider?**

Fish (scombroid and ciguatera poisoning), shellfish (neurotoxic & domoic acid poisoning), and monosodium glutamate (Chinese Restaurant Syndrome).

❏❏ **What is a common G.I. complication of nephrotic syndrome?**

Spontaneous bacterial peritonitis

❏❏   **Is perforation following appendicitis more common in children than in adults?**

Yes, because localization of abdominal pain is more difficult. Also, the omentum is not as well developed and cannot wall off the inflamed appendix.

❏❏   **Give the DDX of an inguino-scrotal mass.**

Inguinal hernia, hydrocele, hydrocele of a cord, and retractile testes

❏❏   **What are the common causes of unconjugated hyperbilirubinemia in the neonatal age group?**

Physiological jaundice, blood group incompatibility, and breast-milk jaundice.

❏❏   **At what level of serum bilirubin will a newborn appear icteric?**

5-7 mg/dl

❏❏   **In older children?**

2-3 mg/dl

❏❏   **What are the most common causes of unconjugated hyperbilirubinemia in childhood?**

Sickle cell anemia and other hemolytic disorders, i.e., hereditary spherocytosis, hereditary elliptocytosis.

❏❏   **What clinical investigations would you consider for the initial work-up of a case of unconjugated hyperbilirubinemia?**

Serum bilirubin and direct fraction, Coombs' test, Hematocrit, and RBC morphology/Retic count.

❏❏   **What pathognomonic eye-sign is noted in all patients of Wilson's disease with neurological symptoms?**

Kayser-Fleisher rings.

❏❏   **What is the best screening test for Wilson's disease?**

Serum Ceruloplasmin level (decreased).

❏❏   **What agent is commonly used in the treatment of Wilson's disease?**

D-Penicillamine (chelates copper).

❏❏   **The consumption of what agent has been implicated in the incidence of Reye's syndrome in children with an influenza-like illness?**

Aspirin.

❏❏   **What age group is Reye's syndrome seen most commonly?**

4-12 years.

❏❏   **What is the major lethal factor in children with Reye's syndrome?**

Increased intracranial pressure secondary to cerebral edema.

❏❏   **What is the most common indication for pediatric liver transplantation?**

Hepatic bililary atresia, after a failed portoenterostomy (Kasai procedure).

❏❏   **What is the most important pre-liver transplantation management for a patient?**

Ensure adequate nutritional status, with regard to caloric intake, vitamins, and mineral supplementation.

☐☐ **What percent of liver transplant patients will become infected with cytomegalovirus if prophylaxis is not given?**

50%.

☐☐ **What are some common types of early infection in liver transplant patients?**

Gram negative enteric pneumonia, cholangitis, soft tissue wound infections, intraabdominal abscess, peritonitis, disseminated candidiasis.

☐☐ **During the first six months, post liver transplant patients have a 15% chance of developing what type of hepatitis?**

CMV Hepatitis.

☐☐ **Name some drugs associated with hepatic injury in children?**

Acetaminophen, Sulfonamide, Erythromycin, Ceftriaxone, INH, Valproic acid, Phenytoin.

☐☐ **What are some causes of fulminant hepatic failure?**

Viral hepatitis.
Hepatotoxic drugs and chemicals.
Circulatory shock.
Metabolic liver diseases like Wilson's or galactosemia.

☐☐ **What are the common causes of biliary colic?**

Gall stones caused by hemolytic diseases like spherocytosis, infections like Salmonellosis, and parasitic infestations like ascariasis biliary atresia.

☐☐ **What metabolic condition manifests with jaundice, hypoglycemia, convulsions, cataracts, and mental retardation?**

Galactosemia.

☐☐ **Do the levels of liver-dependent coagulation factors decrease after birth?**

Yes, they fall 48 - 72 hours after birth, and return to birth levels only by 7 to 10 days of life.

☐☐ **Can a newborn manifest Vitamin K deficiency induced bleeding within the first 24 hours of life?**

Yes, if the mother has been on Phenobarbital or Phenytoin. Classic Hemorrhagic Disease of the Newborn is seen between 2-7 days of life.

☐☐ **What is the most commonly occurring malignant liver neoplasm in the pediatric age group?**

Hepatoblastoma.

☐☐ **Of the hepatitis viruses A through E, which are transmitted by the feco-oral route?**

Hepatitis A and E.

☐☐ **What recommendations would you make regarding the immunization of a full-term newborn, the HbsAg status of whose mother is not known?**

Administration of HBIg and Hepatitis B vaccine simultaneously, at two different sites.

☐☐ **How long can you defer giving HBIg to a newborn infant?**

12 hours after birth.

❑❑   **Has the American Academy of Pediatrics recommended universal administration of Hepatitis A vaccine?**

No, it is used only in high-risk children, and in those considering travel to Hepatitis A-endemic areas.

❑❑   **What is the chief sequela of untreated perinatal acquired Hepatitis B?**

Chronic infection, which might occur in close to 70-90 % of the cases.

❑❑   **What is breast-feeding jaundice?**

Elevated levels of serum bilirubin, approaching 15-20 mg/dl, seen in the second or third week of life in breast-fed infants who are otherwise healthy.

❑❑   **What effect is encountered in an infant with conjugated hyperbilirubinemia who is subjected to phototherapy?**

"Bronze baby syndrome," caused by an unusual bronzing of the skin by bilirubin breakdown pigments. This is reversible.

❑❑   **An infant with biliary atresia is noted on follow-up to be of short-stature, and has round, bony prominences at the costochondral junctions. What is the pathology you suspect?**

Vitamin D deficiency, leading to rickets.

❑❑   **You see a 10-year-old boy in the ED, with ear ache, and diagnose him as having otitis media. The boy is clearly jaundiced, and his mother informs you that he has the Dubin-Johnson syndrome. What management would you like to offer for his jaundice?**

Nothing, the condition is benign. However, drugs capable of aggravating jaundice should be avoided.

❑❑   **An 11-year-old girl with cystic fibrosis presents with a 1-day history of fever. On examination she is noted to have equal breath sounds on both sides. She has right upper abdominal quadrant pain. Labs reveal leukocytosis, with an increase in serum bilirubin. What do you suspect?**

Acute calculous cholecystitis, seen in up to 4% of patients with cystic fibrosis.

❑❑   **What are some poor prognostic factors for survival in a patient with hepatic encephalopathy?**

Jaundice for more than 7 days before the onset of encephalopathy; a prothrombin time more than 50 sec; a serum bilirubin level more than 17.5 mg/dl.

❑❑   **In what percentage of the population is the gall bladder congenitally absent?**

0.1%

❑❑   **What is Charcot's triad?**

The triad of right upper quadrant abdominal pain, shaking chills, and spiking fever, when seen with jaundice - leading to the suspicion of cholangitis.

❑❑   **Enumerate some steps in the emergency management of a case of suspected cholangitis.**

Discontinue oral intake, Start IV fluids.
Lab tests (CBC, Liver function tests, Abdominal/Chest x-ray, and amylase).
Withhold antibiotics until a liver biopsy and culture can be done. However, in a clinically septic child, a cephalosporin and gentamicin may be started after a blood culture.
Withhold narcotics until a tentative decision regarding surgery is made.

CRITICAL CARE

The great secret, known to internists and learned very early in marriage by their wives [and husbands], but still hidden from the general public, is that most things get better by themselves. Most things, in fact, are better by morning."
- Lewis Thomas

☐☐　**Acute renal failure, Coomb's negative hemolytic anemia, and thrombocytopenia comprise the triad for which syndrome?**

Hemolytic-Uremic Syndrome (HUS).

☐☐　**Aplastic crisis in sickle cell disease is associated with what condition?**

Parvo virus. Primary erythropoietic failure can result in life-threatening anemia in a patient with a significantly decreased RBC life span.

☐☐　**Primary or spontaneous bacterial peritonitis is more frequently seen with patients who have which underlying conditions?**

Nephrotic syndrome, chronic liver disease, and systemic lupus erythematosus.

☐☐　**What are the features required to diagnose Guillain-Barre Syndrome?**

Progressive motor weakness and areflexia.

☐☐　**What is the hallmark in cerebrospinal fluid which indicate that the patient might have Guillain-Barre Syndrome?**

Albumino-cytologic dissociation, which is found as early as the third day into the illness, but may occur as late as the second or third week.

☐☐　**What is the most common cause of fulminant hepatic failure in the U.S.?**

Acute viral hepatitis.

☐☐　**The liver dysfunction in fulminant hepatic failure is evidenced by what condition?**

Uncorrectable coagulopathy, jaundice and encephalopathy. All three occur together in an illness of less than eight weeks duration.

☐☐　**What is the most potent therapy for the temporary treatment of hyperkalemia?**

Insulin, plus hypertonic dextrose.

☐☐　**Decompensated shock is characterized by what conditions?**

Hypotension and low cardiac output.

☐☐　**What is often the first objective sign that a child is about to go into shock?**

Tachycardia

☐☐　**Why shouldn't blind finger sweeps of the mouth be performed for manual removal of a foreign body?**

Because the foreign body may be pushed back into the airway, resulting in further obstruction.

❑❑   **Resistance to airflow in the airway is inversely proportional to what?**

The fourth power of the airway radius.

❑❑   **When should atropine be used to treat bradycardia?**

Only after adequate ventilation and oxygenation have been established, since hypoxemia is a common cause of bradycardia.

❑❑   **What are the three inotropic agents commonly used in the post-arrest setting?**

Dopamine, dobutamine and epinephrine.

❑❑   **Name some complications associated with intraosseous cannulation and infusion.**

Tibia fracture, compartment syndrome, skin necrosis and osteomyelitis. This has been reported in less than 1 % of patients.

❑❑   **What are the most common causes for deterioration of ventilatory status in a stable, intubated patient?**

Endotracheal tube dislodgment, occlusion, pneumothorax and equipment failure.

❑❑   **Hypoxemia with a normal alveolar-arterial oxygen difference is the result of what?**

Hypoventilation.

❑❑   **What is the major therapeutic priority in the management of status epilepticus?**

Maintenance of oxygenation, adequate ventilation, and the prevention of hypoxia.

❑❑   **Transplant patient on chronic immunosuppressive agents presents with two week history of persistent, severe headache without fever. What is your diagnostic management?**

Neurological exam, CT scan, MRI, and an lumbar puncture unless contraindicated by evidence increased intracranial pressure.

❑❑   **What is the major complication in the treatment for diabetic ketoacidosis?**

Cerebral edema.

❑❑   **When cerebral edema is clinically evident, management should include what?**

Administration of Mannitol, reduce the rate of fluid infusion and hyperventilation.

❑❑   **What is the treatment of choice for a brain tumor edema?**

Dexamethasone.

❑❑   **Cardiac index is calculated by using which parameters?**

Cardiac output/ body surface area.

❑❑   **A 12 year-old child was involved in a motor vehicle accident. He was unconscious at the scene, and arrived at the emergency room via ambulance with a Glasgow coma scale of 15, only to have a rapid deterioration of the mental status. What is your diagnosis?**

An epidural hematoma.

❑❑   **What are the two symptoms which characterize heat stroke?**

An altered mental status, and a rectal temperature of > 40 C.

❏❏ **A sixteen-year-old sickle cell patient presents with pallor, weakness, tachycardia and abdominal fullness. What should you suspect?**

Acute splenic sequestration.

❏❏ **How should you treat the patient characterized in the previous question?**

Colloid and whole blood transfusions for correction of hypovolemia, anemia and prevention of circulatory failure.

❏❏ **How may subsequent episodes of acute splenic sequestration be avoided?**

Splenectomy or chronic transfusions.

❏❏ **Which cardiac anomalies are associated with congenital Rubella?**

Pulmonic stenosis and PDA.

❏❏ **Which infectious agents are commonly associated with necrotizing enterocolitis?**

Gram negative enteric bacilli, *E. coli*, Klebsiella pneumonia, and Enterococcus.

❏❏ **Name some conditions in which both intracranial calcifications and skin lesions are present.**

Toxoplasmosis, Cytomegalovirus and Sturge-Weber Syndrome.

❏❏ **What is the narrowest part of the respiratory tract in children?**

The inferior ring portion of the cricoid cartilage.

❏❏ **In what phase of respiration is stridor observed?**

Inspiratory.

❏❏ **What causes stridor?**

With extrathoracic airway obstruction, the pressure inside the extrathoracic part of the airway is negative relative to the level of atmospheric pressure. This results in further narrowing of the larynx during inspiration and therefore, stridor.

❏❏ **Grunting is observed during what phase of respiration?**

Expiratory - exhalation against a closed glottis.

❏❏ **What is the most common etiologic agent isolated from blood cultures taken from children with epiglottitis?**

H. influenzae, type B.

❏❏ **What is the most common etiology of croup or laryngotracheobronchitis?**

Parainfluenza virus.

❏❏ **What is the most common organism isolated from patients with bacterial tracheitis?**

Staphyloccocus aureus.

❏❏ **How do retropharyngeal abscesses arise?**

Lymphatic spread of infections in the nasopharynx, oropharynx, or external auditory canal.

❏❏ **What is the most common type of tracheo-esophageal fistula?**

Blind esophageal pouch with a fistulous connection of the trachea to the distal esophagus.

❑❑   The croup score is used to assess the degree of respiratory distress accompanying an illness. Which symptoms are evaluated in the score?

Stridor, cough, air entry, flaring/retractions, and color.

❑❑   Why does a newborn with bilateral choanal atresia present with severe respiratory distress that is relieved by the insertion of an oral airway?

Because the newborn is an obligatory nose breather.

❑❑   The funnel-shaped narrowing of the glottis and subglottic airway, commonly known as "steeple sign", is observed in what type of extrathoracic airway obstruction?

Croup or laryngotracheobronchitis.

❑❑   Name one of the conditions which makes a child a likely candidate for tonsillectomy.

Recurrent tonsillar abscesses.

❑❑   A six-year old male complains of dysphagia and fever. Tonsillar exudates and anterior cervical adenitis are noted. What sign differentiates Group A strep from other causes of pharyngitis?

A sandpaper-like rash.

❑❑   A 4-year old child has high fever, hoarseness, and increased stridor of 3 hours duration. He has a low fever and sore throat earlier in the day. He is ill appearing, with a temperature of 40°C, inspiratory stridor, drooling and mild intercostal retractions. He prefers to sit up. What is the most likely diagnosis?

Epiglottitis.

❑❑   An 11-month old male presents with rhinorrhea, cough and increasing respiratory distress. Treatment with bronchodilators have produced equivical results. He is now in obvious distress with retractions, grunting, prolonged expiratory time, inspiratory and expiratory wheezes. Chest x-ray shows a tracheal shift to the left and hyperexpansion of the right chest. What is the most likely diagnosis?

Foreign body aspiration.

❑❑   A neonate has Apgar scores of 8 and 8. He is actively crying, but cyanosis and retractions appear when he is quiet. What is the most likely diagnosis?

Choanal atresia.

❑❑   Cor pulmonale resulting from chronic airway obstruction is thought to be due to what?

Chronic alveolar hypoventilation and the resulting increase in pulmonary vascular resistance.

❑❑   The total work of breathing is divided into two parts. Name them.

1) To overcome lung and chest wall compliance.
2) To overcome airway and tissue resistance.

❑❑   Total work of breathing in neonates and infants is lowest at what respiratory rate?

35-40/minute.

❑❑   Why are infants more susceptible to inflammatory changes in the airway?

Because the airway in infants is smaller, and is also much more compliant.

❑❑   Grunting is usually more prominent in what type of respiratory pathology?

Typically in smaller airway disease such as bronchiolitis, or in diseases with loss of functional residual capacity such as pneumonia or pulmonary edema because grunting is an effort to maintain positive airway pressure during expiration.

❏❏   **Which drugs can be administered through the endotracheal tube?**

Lidocaine, Atropine, Naloxone and Epinephrine.

❏❏   **What is the most common cause of cardiac arrest in children?**

Hypoxia.

❏❏   **What are the most common arrhythmias in pediatric patients?**

Sinus bradycardia or asystole.

❏❏   **What is the drug of choice in the treatment of supraventricular tachycardia?**

Adenosine, at a dose of 0.1 mg/kg. Propanolol, digoxin, and verapamil are also indicated. Verapamil, however, is not indicated in patients less than one year of age because it can cause profound hypotension.

❏❏   **Why must adenosine be given as a rapid intravenous bolus?**

Its half-life is less than 10 seconds.

❏❏   **What are the most common causes of pulseless electrical activity (PEA)?**

Pneumothorax, Pericardial tamponade, Hypoxemia, Acidosis, Hypovolemia.

❏❏   **To achieve more than 90% FiO2 in a non-intubated patient, which oxygen device should be used?**

Non-rebreather mask.

❏❏   **Name some acceptable modes of intravascular access.**

Intraosseus, peripheral veins, central veins, surgical cut-down.

❏❏   **What are the acceptable routes for central venous access?**

External jugular, internal jugular, subclavian, umbilical (newborns less than 2 weeks of age), and femoral veins.

❏❏   **Is the femoral vein lateral or medial to the femoral artery?**

Medial (if you didn't know this, you might now understand why your patients complain of paresthesias down their leg).

❏❏   **Name some skin manifestations of shock/hypoxemia.**

Circumoral pallor/cyanosis, Mottled skin, Distal cyanosis, Prolonged capillary refill, Diminished distal pulses.

❏❏   **What are the signs and symptoms of central nervous system hypoxia?**

Irritability, Diminished response to pain, Seizures, and Lethargy.

❏❏   **A three year old presents with signs/symptoms of epiglottitis. Should intravenous access be a priority?**

No. Intravenous access is an absolute contraindication in suspected epiglottitis. The procedure is to put the patient in a comfortable position with supplemental oxygen and minimize the level of anxiety in the patient. All invasive procedures are to be done in the operating room.

❏❏   In a child who is hypoglycemic and hypotensive, is it appropriate to use a solution containing dextrose for fluid resuscitation?

No. The use of a glucose containing solution for fluid resuscitation will result in an osmotic diuresis secondary to hyperglycemia.

❏❏   What is the appropriate treatment for a hypoglycemic child?

D50W, 1.0 ml/kg through a central line, or D25W, 2.0 ml/kg through a central or peripheral line.

❏❏   What fluids are suitable for the initial treatment of hypotension?

Normal saline. The dose is 10-20 ml/kg IV bolus.

❏❏   What are the relative contraindications to the use of a nasopharyngeal airway?

Suspected airway trauma, adenoidal hypertrophy, and bleeding diatheses.

❏❏   After intubating a 1 month old baby for respiratory failure, you confirm appropriate tube placement by auscultation. However, CXR reveals the tube is in the right mainstem bronchus. Why were you able to hear breath sounds bilaterally?

In small infants, it is not uncommon to hear transmitted breath sounds. In these patients, the physician is advised not only to auscultate, but also to visualize adequate chest rise bilaterally.

❏❏   What is the amount of FiO2 each device can deliver?

Nasal cannula: 30-40%
Oxygen hood/tent: up to 80-90%
Simple mask: up to 40%
Partial rebreathing mask: up to 60%
Nonrebreathing mask: 100%

❏❏   What is the rate of chest compressions in an infant?

100-120 times per minute.

❏❏   What is the time-frame for a normal capillary refill?

Two to three seconds. When assessing capillary refill, make sure the skin is warm. Cold ambient temperature will cause prolonged capillary refill, and can be misleading in the assessment of the circulatory system.

❏❏   Renal output is a good indicator of adequate cardiac output. What can the physician do to assess recent urinary output in a patient brought to the ER?

Assessment of simple things, like the color of the urine (dark color indicating concentrated urine) and the number of wet diapers can provide the physician with a general idea of recent urinary output.

❏❏   What are the complications associated with subclavian vein cannulation?

Hemothorax, pneumothorax, and trauma to the subclavian artery.

❏❏   When is sodium bicarbonate indicated in cardiac resuscitation?

The use of sodium bicarbonate in cardiac arrest is controversial. Current thinking is to use it if there is a documented metabolic acidosis with pH < 7.00.

❏❏   A term newborn is delivered in your office. You check the heart rate and it is approximately 80-120 beats/min. After drying, suctioning, and stimulation, the heart rate remains low. What should the next step be?

100% oxygen should be given by hood or face mask. Most babies with bradycardia will respond to stimulation or administration of oxygen. Infants that remain bradycardic will need endotracheal intubation, hand-bagging with 100% oxygen, and chest compressions.

☐☐   **What are some major complications of endotracheal intubation?**

Esophageal intubation/perforation, trauma to the teeth, emesis and aspiration, and bradycardia. It is recommended that the physician has atropine ready for administration when intubating an infant or child, because they can develop reflective (vasovagal) bradycardia.

☐☐   **What are the major side effects of lidocaine?**

Lidocaine is used in the treatment of ventricular tachycardia and fibrillation. The recommended dose is 1 mg/kg, followed by a constant infusion of 20-50 micrograms/kg/min. The major side effect is hypotension, therefore, it should be used with caution in patients with myocardial depression. Lidocaine is also used as a sedative prior to intubation in patients with suspected increased intracranial pressure.

☐☐   **A 2 year old boy presents to the emergency room with SVT. Blood pressure is 50 systolic, and he is unresponsive. Should the physician use synchronized or unsynchronized cardioversion?**

In patients with unstable SVT or unstable ventricular tachycardia, the physician should use unsynchronized cardioversion.

☐☐   **What are the indications for the use of calcium?**

Suspected hypocalcemia, hyperkalemia, hypermagnesemia, and calcium channel blocker overdose. Calcium is no longer indicated in the treatment of asystole or electromechanical dissociation.

☐☐   **Is there a difference between calcium chloride and calcium gluconate, in an emergency situation?**

Yes. The liver must first metabolize calcium gluconate before elemental calcium is available. Therefore, calcium chloride is the preferred drug during an emergency. The dose should be 10 mg/kg. If a peripheral route is used, the drug should be given slowly. Extravasation of calcium can lead to tissue damage and necrosis.

☐☐   **What is the catecholamine of choice when treating small infants with heart failure?**

Dopamine. In small infants, cardiac output is more dependent on heart rate than stroke volume. Dopamine is an excellent chronotrope, and will have a profound effect on blood pressure and cardiac output by increasing the heart rate. However, dopamine can cause tachyarrhythmias, so its use should be carefully monitored. Unlike adults, dopamine causes little renal vasoconstriction or vasodilatation in pediatric patients.

☐☐   **When inserting an intraosseous needle into the tibia, in which direction should the needle be placed?**

Caudal, away from the epiphysial plate. This will avoid damage to the growth plate of the tibia.

☐☐   **When is isoproterenol indicated?**

Isoproterenol is ideal for the treatment of bradyarrhythmias and heart block. It can also be used in small infants with heart failure, because of its chronotropic properties. Adverse reactions include tachyarrhythmias and hypotension.

☐☐   **What are the steps in the initial resuscitation of a newborn?**

Airway, breathing, circulation, and temperature control. Newborns are very sensitive to heat loss, so they should be dried immediately after birth, and placed under a radiant warmer to prevent heat loss through the skin. Excessive hypothermia can lead to acidosis and hypoxemia.

☐☐   **What are some of the high-risk factors a physician should be aware of when assisting a mother during an emergency delivery?**

Multiparity, lack of prenatal care, teenage pregnancy, placental abruption, trauma-induced labor, history of drug abuse, and meconium stained amniotic fluid. Although in an emergency delivery it is hard to obtain a good medical history, the physician should try to determine the presence or absence of any of the aforementioned factors.

☐☐   **What is the acceptable heart rate for a newborn?**

120 beats/min or higher.

☐☐   **List the equipment necessary for intubation.**

Oxygen source, bag and mask, endotracheal tube, suction device, stylet, laryngoscope and blade, pulse oximeter, adhesive tape, appropriate sedative and muscle relaxant, resuscitation medications.

☐☐   **What is the best place to assess heart rate in a newborn?**

The umbilical cord.

☐☐   **You are asked to assist in a precipitous delivery. The newborn is lethargic and unresponsive to tactile stimulation. The mother admits to recent heroin use. How should you proceed?**

The infant is most likely suffering from narcotic induced respiratory depression. Treatment is naloxone hydrochloride given either intravenously, intratracheally, intraosseously, subcutaneously, or intramuscularly, at a dose of 0.1 mg/kg,. The first two methods are the routes of choice.

☐☐   **What are the most common causes of bradycardia in a newborn?**

Hypoxemia, hypoglycemia, hypothermia, exposure to narcotics, and sepsis.

☐☐   **A seven day old baby is cyanotic. Physical exam reveals a holosystolic murmur. He remains cyanotic after treatment with 100% oxygen. What is the possible diagnosis and subsequent treatment of choice?**

The patient has a ductus-dependent cyanotic congenital heart defect. The treatment of choice is prostaglandin E1.

☐☐   **While hand-bagging a patient, his oxygen saturation drops acutely. What are some of the possible causes?**

Dislodgment of the endotracheal tube, obstruction of the endotracheal tube, pneumothorax, or equipment failure (i.e., bag disconnected from the oxygen, etc.).

☐☐   **While hand-bagging a 14 year old patient, you notice the stomach is getting distended. What steps should you take to remedy the situation?**

Apply gentle cricoid pressure to occlude the esophagus. Insertion of a nasogastric or orogastric tube can also be used to decompress the stomach. It is imperative that pressure not be applied to the stomach for decompression, as this can lead to emesis and aspiration.

☐☐   **Where is the best location to palpate the pulse in an infant?**

The brachial or femoral artery.

☐☐   **What complications are associated with chest compression in the newborn?**

Broken ribs, laceration of the liver, pneumothorax, cardiac contusion, pericardial tamponade.

❐❐ **What is the rate for chest compressions and the administration of ventilation during resuscitation of a neonate?**

100-120 chest compressions per minute and 30 breaths per minute.

❐❐ **What is the normal systolic pressure in a neonate?**

Greater than 60 mm Hg.

❐❐ **When treating a patient with suspected facial trauma, which route should you use to place a gastric tube?**

The orogastric route. With suspected facial trauma, the use of a nasogastric tube (a.k.a. nasal intubation) is contraindicated.

❐❐ **Which fluids are indicated in the resuscitation of a newborn?**

Normal saline, 5% albumin; ringer's lactate; and whole blood, which can be obtained from the placenta.

❐❐ **What are the complications of intraosseous cannulation?**

Fracture of the tibia, tissue infiltration, skin necrosis, osteomyelitis.

❐❐ **What are the signs of hypovolemia in a newborn?**

Poor response to resuscitation, Persistent pallor after appropriate oxygenation, Weak pulses, Hypotension.

❐❐ **Which actions are appropriate to provide tactile stimulation on a newborn in order to encourage the patient to cry?**

Flick or slap the sole of foot, or rub the back (preferably with a towel while drying the baby).

❐❐ **When is cardioversion indicated?**

During SVT, ventricular fibrillation, ventricular tachycardia (VT). For SVT and VT, use synchronized cardioversion. However, if the arrhythmia is associated with hypotension and/or shock, use unsynchronized cardioversion.

❐❐ **What is the age limit for the use of the intraosseous technique?**

6.

❐❐ **A five year old takes several KCL tablets. An EKG shows peaked T-waves, and the presence of U-waves. What is the indicated therapy?**

Calcium chloride, 10 mg/kg IV; sodium bicarbonate, 0.5-1.0 mEq/kg IV; glucose and insulin intravenous drip; sodium polysterene sulfonate (Kayexalate), 1 gm/kg/dose Q2-6 hours PR.

❐❐ **What three signs suggest that a newborn is responding to resuscitation?**

Increasing heart rate, spontaneous respirations, improving color.

❐❐ **A 5 year old boy arrives at the emergency room in a coma. What is the differential diagnosis?**

Hypoxemia, hypoglycemia, hypotension, drug overdose, postictal state after a seizure, and/or toxin ingestion.

❐❐ **What are the initial steps in neonatal resuscitation?**

Positioning, suctioning, tactile stimulation, ventilation.

□□ **What is the compression/ventilation ratio during cardiopulmonary resuscitation when treating pediatric patients who are older than newborns?**

5:1

□□ **Failure to respond to cardioversion is due to what?**

Hypothermia, hypoglycemia, acidosis, hypoxia.

□□ **What complications may occur as a result of central venous catheterization?**

Infection, air embolism, hemorrhage, injury to the adjacent nerve or artery, and pneumothorax in subclavian and internal jugular catheterization.

□□ **After a few minutes, the patient described in the previous question becomes unconscious. What should be the next step?**

Administer 5 back blows, followed by 5 abdominal thrusts until object is dislodged. When treating infants, administer 5 back blows, followed by 5 chest thrusts.

□□ **Which site is used to evacuate a pneumothorax by using needle thoracentesis?**

The second intercostal space at the midclavicular line, or the fourth intercostal space at the anterior or midaxillary line.

□□ **What the best place to palpate the pulse in children?**

The carotid artery.

□□ **What are the indications for endotracheal intubation?**

Oxygenation and ventilation, airway protection, removal of airway secretions, hyperventilation (when increased intracranial pressure is suspected), and cardiovascular instability.

□□ **Which laboratory studies can be obtained through an intraosseous needle?**

Electrolytes and blood cultures.

□□ **What is the APGAR score?**

A scoring system which measures five physiological variables [**A**ppearance/color, **P**ulse, **G**rimace (reflex irritability), **A**ctivity (muscle tone), and **R**espirations], enabling a rapid evaluation of a newborn's physiological status. It was named after Virginia Apgar, who came up with the scale to assess newborns.

□□ **Are there any differences in the "ABC" approach to cardiopulmonary arrest in children (as compared to adults)?**

Only one. The airway and breathing are relatively more stressed in children than is circulation. Except in the child with congenital cardiovascular anomalies, there are few purely cardiac causes of cardiopulmonary arrest. The basic "ABC" algorithm remains sound.

□□ **What anatomic site is preferred for IO infusion?**

The preferred IO site is on the anteromedial surface of the tibia, one or two centimeters below the palpable tubercle. This area is relatively flat and easy to locate.

□□ **Why is hypothermia a particular concern in the field treatment of small children?**

Children have poorly developed heat regulation mechanisms (e.g. poor shivering), and a relatively larger surface area to volume ratio than adults. Accordingly, infants and small children are more likely to become hypothermic if exposed to the cold for prolonged periods, as may occur during extrication from a motor vehicle crash.

METABOLIC, ENDOCRINE AND NUTRITION

"Once we have recognized that disease is naught else than the process of life under altered conditions, the concept of healing expands to imply the maintenance or re-establishment of the normal conditions of existence."
- Rudolf Virchow

☐☐ **What are the causes of factitious hyponatremia?**

Hyperglycemia, hyperlipidemia, or hyperproteinemia.

☐☐ **How does hyperglycemia lead to hyponatremia?**

Because glucose stays in the extracellular fluid, hyperglycemia draws water out of the cell into the extracellular fluid. Each 100 mg/dL increase in plasma glucose decreases the serum sodium by 1.6 to 1.8 mEq/L.

☐☐ **What is the <u>most</u> <u>common</u> cause of hypovolemic hyponatremia in children?**

Viral gastroenteritis. Vomiting and/or diarrhea occurs with this condition.

☐☐ **What is the <u>most</u> <u>common</u> cause of euvolemic hyponatremia in children?**

Syndrome of inappropriate secretion of antidiuretic hormone (SIADH). Causes include CNS disorders, medications, tumors, and pulmonary disorders.

☐☐ **What are the signs and symptoms of hyponatremia?**

Weakness, nausea, anorexia, vomiting, confusion, lethargy, seizures, and coma.

☐☐ **What are the <u>most</u> <u>common</u> causes of hypotonic fluid loss leading to hypernatremia?**

Diarrhea, vomiting, hyperpyrexia, and excessive sweating.

☐☐ **What are the signs and symptoms of hypernatremia?**

Confusion, muscle irritability, seizures, respiratory paralysis, and coma.

☐☐ **What is the quickest way to treat hyperkalemia?**

Administration of calcium gluconate (10%) 10-20 mL, IV with an onset of action of 1-3 minutes.

☐☐ **What are the causes of hyperkalemia?**

Acidosis, tissue necrosis, hemolysis, blood transfusions, GI bleed, renal failure, Addison's disease, primary hypoaldosteronism, excess po K+ intake, RTA type IV, and medications (such as high dose penicillin).

☐☐ **What are the causes of hypocalcemia?**

Shock, sepsis, multiple blood transfusions, hypoparathyroidism, vitamin D deficiency, pancreatitis, hypomagnesemia, alkalosis, fat embolism syndrome, phosphate overload, chronic renal failure, hypoalbuminemia, , and medications, such as Dilantin, phenobarbital, heparin, theophylline, cimetidine, and gentamicin.

❑❑ **What is the <u>most</u> <u>common</u> cause of hyperkalemia?**

Lab error. Chronic renal failure is the most common cause of "true hyperkalemia."

❑❑ **What are the <u>most</u> <u>common</u> causes of hypercalcemia?**

In descending order, malignancy, primary hyperparathyroidism, and thiazide diuretics.

❑❑ **What are the signs and symptoms of hypercalcemia?**

The most common gastrointestinal symptoms are anorexia and constipation. A classic mnemonic can be used to remember them:

Stones: renal calculi.
Bones: osteolysis.
Abdominal groans: peptic ulcer disease and pancreatitis.
Psychic overtones: psychiatric disorders.

❑❑ **What is the initial treatment for hypercalcemia?**

Patients with hypercalcemia are dehydrated because high calcium levels interfere with ADH and the ability of the kidney to concentrate urine. Therefore, the initial treatment is restoration of the extracellular fluid with 5 to 10 L of normal saline within 24 hours. After the patient is rehydrated, administer furosemide in doses of 1 to 3 mg/kg.

❑❑ **What is the <u>most</u> <u>common</u> cause of hyperphosphatemia?**

Acute and chronic renal failure.

❑❑ **What are the two primary causes of primary adrenal insufficiency?**

Tuberculosis and autoimmune destruction account for 90% of the cases.

❑❑ **What are the signs and symptoms of primary adrenal insufficiency?**

Fatigue, weakness, weight loss, anorexia, hyperpigmentation, nausea, vomiting, abdominal pain, diarrhea, and orthostatic hypotension.

❑❑ **What characteristic lab findings are associated with primary adrenal insufficiency?**

Hyperkalemia, hyponatremia, hypoglycemia, azotemia (if volume depletion is present), and a mild metabolic acidosis.

❑❑ **How should acute adrenal insufficiency be treated?**

Administration of hydrocortisone, 100 mg IV, and crystalloid fluids containing dextrose.

❑❑ **What are the main causes of death during an adrenal crisis?**

Circulatory collapse and hyperkalemia-induced arrhythmias.

❑❑ **What are the causes of acute adrenal crisis?**

It occurs secondary to a major stress, such as surgery, severe injury, myocardial infarction, or any other illness in a patient with primary or secondary adrenal insufficiency.

❑❑ **What is thyrotoxicosis, and what are the causes?**

A hypermetabolic state that occurs secondary to excess circulating thyroid hormone caused by thyroid hormone overdose, thyroid hyperfunction, or thyroid inflammation.

❑❑   **What are the hallmark clinical features of myxedema coma?**

Hypothermia (75%) and coma.

❑❑   **What is the <u>most</u> <u>common</u> cause of hypoglycemia seen in the ED.**

An insulin reaction in a diabetic patient.

❑❑   **What is the role of phosphate replacement during the treatment of DKA?**

Phosphate supplementation is not indicated until a serum concentration is below 1.0 mEq/dL.

❑❑   **What is the most important "initial" step for the treatment of DKA?**

Rapid fluid administration.

❑❑   **In the first two years of life, what is the <u>most</u> <u>common</u> cause of drug-induced hypoglycemia?**

Salicylates. Between 2 and 8, alcohol is the most likely cause, and between 11 and 30, insulin and sulfonylureas are the culprits.

❑❑   **Which principle hormone protects the human body from hypoglycemia?**

Glucagon.

❑❑   **What is the <u>most</u> <u>common</u> type of hypoglycemia in a child?**

Ketotic hypoglycemia. Attacks usually occur when the child is stressed by caloric deprivation. This condition usually develops in boys between 18 months and 5 years of age. Attacks may be episodic and are more frequent in the morning or during periods of illness.

❑❑   **What are the neurologic signs and symptoms of hypoglycemia?**

Hypoglycemia may produce mental and neurologic dysfunction. Neurologic manifestations can include paresthesias, cranial nerve palsies, transient hemiplegia, diplopia, decerebrate posturing, and clonus.

❑❑   **What lab findings are expected with diabetic ketoacidosis?**

Elevated ß-hydroxybutyrate, acetoacetate, acetone, and glucose. Ketonuria and glucosuria are present. Serum bicarbonate levels, pCO_2, and pH are decreased. Potassium may be initially elevated but falls when the acidosis is corrected.

❑❑   **Outline the basic treatment for DKA.**

Administer fluids. Start with normal saline (the total deficit may be 5-10 L), followed by potassium (100-200 mEq in the first 12-24 hours). Prescribe insulin, 20 units bolus followed by 5-10 units/hour. (Ed. Note: Many physicians no longer give bolus.) Add glucose to the IV fluid when the glucose levels fall below 250 mg/dL and give the patient a phosphate supplement when the levels drop below 1.0 mg/dL.

For pediatric patients, administer NS (20 mL/kg/hour for 1-2 hours) and insulin (0.1 units/kg bolus followed by 0.1 units/kg/hour drip).

❑❑   **A 14 year old female presents with a history of palpitations, sweating, diplopia, blurred vision, and weakness. The family indicates she has been confused and the symptoms usually occur before breakfast. What is the diagnosis?**

Islet cell tumor of the pancreas can result in fasting hypoglycemia. Of course, it could be initial presentation of diabetes (never forget to look past the zebras)

❑❑   **Distinguish between type A and type B lactic acidosis.**

Type A lactic acidosis is often seen in the ED. The onset of this condition usually occurs because of shock. Type A lactic acidosis is associated with inadequate tissue perfusion and resultant anoxia, and with subsequent lactate and hydrogen ion accumulation. Type B lactic acidosis includes all forms of acidosis in which there are no evidence of tissue anoxia.

❑❑ **What pathognomonic findings and confirmatory lab tests are diagnostic of thyroid storm?**

Trick question. Thyroid storm is based on a clinical impression. There are no findings or confirmatory tests available.

❑❑ **What is the most common precipitant of thyroid storm?**

Pulmonary infections.

❑❑ **What clinical clues are helpful for diagnosing thyroid storm?**

Eye signs of Graves' disease, a history of hyperthyroidism, widened pulse pressure, hypertension, and a palpable goiter.

❑❑ **What are the diagnostic criteria for thyroid storm?**

Tachycardia, CNS dysfunction, cardiovascular dysfunction, GI system dysfunction, and a temperature greater than 37.8°C (100°F).

❑❑ **What are the signs and symptoms of thyroid storm?**

Tachycardia, fever, diaphoresis, increased CNS activity, emotional lability, heart failure, coma, and death.

❑❑ **What are the complications of bicarbonate therapy in DKA?**

Paradoxical CSF acidosis, cardiac arrhythmias, decreased oxygen delivery to tissue, and fluid and sodium overload.

❑❑ **What is the overall mortality of nonketotic hyperosmolar coma?**

Approximately 50%.

❑❑ **What is the most common cause of secondary adrenal insufficiency and adrenal crisis?**

Iatrogenic adrenal suppression from prolonged steroid use. Rapid withdrawal of steroids may lead to collapse and death.

❑❑ **An increase of pCO_2 of 10 mm Hg leads to an expected decrease in pH of about:**

0.08.

❑❑ **A decrease of pCO_2 of 10 mm Hg leads to an expected increase in pH of about:**

0.13.

❑❑ **What expected increase in pH is associated with a rise in HCO_3 of 5.0 mEq/L?**

0.08.

❑❑ **What expected decrease in pH is associated with a decrease in HCO_3 of 5.0 mEq/L?**

0.10.

❑❑ **How is the anion gap calculated from electrolyte values?**

Anion gap = $Na - Cl - CO_2$. The normal gap is 12 ± 4 mEq/L.

❑❑ **Acidosis is closely related to anion gap measurement. Name the causes of an increased anion gap acidosis.**

A MUDPILE CAT

A   = alcohol,

M   = methanol,
U   = uremia,
D   = DKA,
P   = paraldehyde,
I   = iron and isoniazid,
L   = lactic acidosis,
E   = ethylene glycol,

C   = carbon monoxide,
A   = aspirin,
T   = toluene.

❏❏   **That's a pretty big differential. Obtaining a history and performing a physical can go a long way in narrowing down this list. The magnitude of the anion gap can also be useful. Why?**

Anion gap > 35 mEq/L is usually caused by ethylene glycol, methanol, or lactic acidosis.
Anion gap 23-30 mEq/L also occurs because of an increase in organic acids.
Anion gap 16-22 mEq/L may be due to uremia, which must be quite advanced before it causes an increased gap.

❏❏   **What is the most common endocrine disorder of childhood and adolescence?**

Diabetes mellitus (DM).

❏❏   **How is the etiology of type I DM different from type II DM?**

Type I DM is associated with Human Leucocyte Antigens (HLA), autoimmunity, and or islet cell antibodies. Type II DM usually involves a genetic mutation resulting in inactive pancreatic and liver enzymes as well as insulin receptor defects.

❏❏   **What are the causes of an oxygen saturation curve's shift to the right?**

A shift to the right delivers more O_2 to the tissue.

The mnemonic "CADET! Right face!" helps in remembering causes of an O_2 shift to the right.
<u>R</u>ight =	<u>R</u>elease to tissues.
Hyper	<u>C</u>arbia.
	<u>A</u>cidemia.
2,3	<u>D</u>PG.
	<u>E</u>xercise.
Increased	<u>T</u>emperature.

❏❏   **When body waste materials, urine and stool, are enterally recycled, they can cause a <u>normal anion gap</u> metabolic acidosis. Remember:**

U   = ureteroenterostomy,
S   = small bowel fistula,
E   = extra chloride (NH_4Cl or amino acid chlorides 2° TPN),
D   = diarrhea.

C   = carbonic anhydrase inhibitors,
R   = renal tubular acidosis,
A   = adrenal insufficiency,
P   = pancreatic fistula

❏❏   **What are the two primary causes of metabolic alkalosis?**

Loss of hydrogen and chloride from the stomach (i.e. vomiting) and overzealous diuresis with loss of hydrogen, potassium, and chloride.

❏❏ **What is central pontine myelinolysis (osmotic demyelination syndrome)?**

The complication of brain dehydration following the "rapid" correction of severe hyponatremia. Correct hyponatremia slowly (i.e., < 12 mEq/day for chronic hyponatremia).

❏❏ **What etiologies are responsible for secondary DM?**

Exocrine pancreatic diseases like cystic fibrosis, pancreatic cancer and Cushing's disease.

❏❏ **What are the peak age groups in children who develop IDDM?**

Between the ages of 5 and 7 and at puberty.

❏❏ **What is the renal threshold for serum glucose before glucosuria develops?**

Approximately 180 mg/dL.

❏❏ **What is the equation for determining serum osmolarity?**

Osm_{serum} = serum Na+(mEq/L) x 2 + [glucose(mg/dL) /18 + BUN(mg/dL)/ 3].

❏❏ **What condition should be suspected in a child who presents with lethargy, weight loss, and new onset enuresis in a previously toilet trained child?**

New onset DM.

❏❏ **How does a child with DKA present?**

The child will present with vomiting, polyuria, dehydration, Kussmaul breathing and abdominal pain.

❏❏ **What conditions should be considered in the differential diagnosis of metabolic acidosis in children?**

DKA, uremia, gastroenteritis with dehydration, lactic acidosis, salicylate poisoning, and encephalitis (remember MUD PILES).

❏❏ **What condition should be suspected in a child with a serum glucose of 642 mg/dL, mild ketonuria, depressed sensorium and positive Babinski sign?**

Non-ketotic hyperosmolar coma (NKHC).

❏❏ **How do you treat NKHC?**

Dehydration should be corrected using .45%NS with 50% of the deficit being corrected in the first 12 hrs and the remainder corrected in the following 24 hrs. When the BGL approaches 300 mg/dL the fluid should be changed to 5% dextrose in .2% NS with 20 mEq of K+ added to each liter. Insulin therapy should be initiated in the second hour with a loading dose of .05 U/kg of regular insulin followed by .05 U/kg/hr.

❏❏ **How is the insulin requirement different between DKA and NKHC?**

In DKA the rate of insulin infusion is .1 U/kg/hr while in NKHC it is .05 U/kg/hr. The lower dose of insulin in NKHC is due to the dramatic decrease in glucose levels due to rehydration alone.

❏❏ **What are the dangers of administering HCO3- to a child with DKA?**

Alkalosis shifts the oxygen distribution curve to the left ultimately diminishing the release of oxygen to peripheral tissue. Also, use of HCO3- can result in a paradoxical acidosis.

❏❏ **What is paradoxical acidosis?**

When exogenous HCO_3^- combines with H^+, H_2O and CO_2 are formed. The blood brain barrier is more permeable to CO_2 that to HCO_3^- thus CO_2 accumulates in the CNS. Therefore, a CNS acidosis will be created while the systemic acidosis is being treated.

☐☐   **What is the primary life threatening complication in the aggressive treatment of DKA?**

Cerebral edema.

☐☐   **What signs and symptoms should a physician look for when considering cerebral edema in a patient being treated for DKA?**

Change in mental status, "delirious outbursts", bradycardia, vomiting, decreased reflexes, and changes in pupillary response.

☐☐   **What is the appropriate mixture of regular and intermediate acting insulin in a single daily insulin injection regimen?**

2/3 of the total dose should be intermediate acting with 1/3 being regular insulin. The single injection should be given 30 minutes prior to breakfast.

☐☐   **What is the appropriate mixture of regular and intermediate acting insulin in a twice daily insulin injection regimen?**

2/3 of the dose should be given 30 minutes prior to breakfast and the remaining one third should be given 30 minutes prior to dinner. Both injections should be 2/3 intermediate acting and 1/3 short acting insulin.

☐☐   **How should insulin be administered to children?**

The injection is given subcutaneously in a rotating pattern utilizing the thighs, buttocks, and abdomen. Parents should administer insulin for children younger than 10-12 years of age.

☐☐   **How should parents of a diabetic child monitor BGLs once discharged from the hospital?**

Blood glucose testing should be done at least two times a week. On all other days urine glucose should be monitored prior to each of the major meals as well as prior to the evening snack.

☐☐   **What is the ideal BGL range in a diabetic child?**

Ideally the BGL should be maintained between 80 - 140 mg/dL. BGLs between 60 - 240 mg/dL are acceptable in children.

☐☐   **What is the significance of the HbA1C?**

It represents the fraction of hemoglobin that has been nonenzymatically glycosolated. It provides an accurate estimation of the relative BGL over the preceding two to three months.

☐☐   **What is an acceptable HbA1C in a diabetic child?**

6 - 9% represents good control, 9 - 12% is fair control, above 12% is poor control.

☐☐   **What does the "honeymoon period" refer to in a newly diagnosed diabetic?**

After a newly diagnosed diabetic is stabilized more than three quarters will experience a significant reduction in insulin requirement as the pancreas makes a final effort to produce insulin.

☐☐   **What is meant by the term "brittle diabetic"?**

A brittle diabetic refers to a patient who has poor blood glucose control with wide fluctuations in BGLs that require frequent alterations in insulin requirements.

☐☐   **What percent of pediatric patients have DKA at their first hospital presentation?**

DKA is present at 30% of initial presentations of newly diagnosed juvenile onset diabetics.

□□ **What is the most serious immediate life threatening risk to a child with DKA?**

Dehydration. While patients may have hyperglycemia and metabolic acidosis, dehydration is the most serious life threatening condition.

□□ **When a child in DKA presents to the emergency department, The K+ will be increased, decreased, or normal?**

Total body K+ is depleted. Transcellular shifts during acidosis move K+ extracellular in exchange for H+ ions. The osmotic diuresis due to the hyperglycemia results in overall K+ loss. In addition, the dehydration stimulates aldosterone secretion which further contributes to K+ excretion.

□□ **How do established diabetics present differently than new onset diabetics?**

Established diabetics will have the prodrome of polydipsia, polyphagia, and polyurea for less than 24 hrs. New onset diabetics may be symptomatic for days to weeks prior to presentation.

□□ **What are the presenting symptoms of DKA in children?**

Abdominal pain, nausea, vomiting, listlessness, lethargy and anorexia.

□□ **Deep sighing respirations in a known diabetic are referred to as what?**

Kussmaul respirations.

□□ **How do you calculate the water deficit in a patient with DKA?**

The fluid deficit is estimated to be approximately 10% of the patient's weight in kilograms.

□□ **How should the fluid loss be replaced over the next 24 hours?**

TIME (hr) REPLACEMENT FLUIDAMOUNT REPLACED
First 8 hrs.9% normal saline 1/3 of the 24hr maintenance + 1/2 of the deficit
Next 16 hrs.45% normal saline 2/3 of the 24 hr maintenance + 1/2 of the deficit

□□ **What dose of insulin should be administered to a child in DKA?**

Regular insulin at a starting dose of .1 U/kg/hr IV drip. Once the BGL is less than 250 mg/dL the drip can be decreased to .02 - .05 U/kg/hr. (NOTE: the BGL should never decrease by more than 100 mg/dL/hr).

□□ **When should glucose be added to the IVF in the treatment of DKA?**

When the BGL reaches 300mg/dL the IVF should be changed to D5.45%NS.

□□ **How often should you monitor the serum K+ in a child with DKA?**

At 2, 4, and 24 hrs after the initiation of therapy.

□□ **Why do DKA patients experience changes in vision following the initiation of therapy?**

Rehydration in conjunction with the correction of hyperglycemia causes fluid shifts in the eyes with reversible lens distortion.

□□ **How is hypoglycemia defined?**

A BGL less than 50 mg/dL with or without symptoms.

□□ **What is the differential diagnosis for hypoglycemia?**

Malnutrition, acute diarrhea, glycogen storage disease, insulinoma, endogenous administration of insulin or oral hypoglycemics, Wilm's tumor, and sepsis.

□□ **What are the hormonal effects of insulin?**

Insulin promotes glucose uptake in muscle and fat while promoting glycogenesis in the liver. Insulin inhibits lipolysis and glycogenolysis.

❑❑   **What are the substances that oppose insulin's effects?**

Glucagon, cortisol, epinephrine, and growth hormone.

❑❑   **What are the signs and symptoms of hypoglycemia?**

They are nonspecific but may include seizures, tremulousness, confusion, palpitations, sweating, and irritability.

❑❑   **In patients where the diagnosis of hypoglycemia vs. hyperglycemia is uncertain, what should be the initial course of therapy?**

A glucose solution should be administered until a definitive diagnosis can be made. Temporary hypoglycemia can be fatal while temporary hyperglycemia is much less likely to significantly alter the prognosis of the patient.

❑❑   **What is the differential diagnosis in a child who presents with hypoglycemia without urine ketones?**

Hyperinsulinemia (exogenous or endogenous) or an enzymatic defect in the fatty acid oxidation pathway.

❑❑   **How is a child with hypoglycemia treated?**

Administer 2.5 ml/kg of 10% dextrose. If convulsions are present increase to 4 ml/kg of 10% dextrose. Maintain the BGL using 8 mg/kg/min of a 10% dextrose solution.

❑❑   **What is the most common cause for hypothyroidism in the neonate?**

Thyroid dysgenesis.

❑❑   **What is the most common thyroid anomoly in childhood?**

The thyroglossal duct cyst which is remnant of the thyroglossal duct.

❑❑   **Are infants born with complete thyroid agenesis symptomatic at birth?**

No. Transplacental T4 provides adequate thyroid hormone however the TSH level will still be elevated enough for detection of the abnormality.

❑❑   **Untreated hypothyroidism in a child leads to what condition?**

Cretinism.

❑❑   **What are the clinical manifestations of cretinism?**

Severe mental retardation, decreased physical growth leading to dwarfism, macroglossia and a protuberant abdomen.

❑❑   **A mass at the base of the tongue in a newborn with adequate T4 levels is suggestive of what disorder?**

A sublingual thyroid or a thryroglossal duct cyst.

❑❑   **What is a possible cause for transient congenital hypothyroidism?**

Maternal antibodies that inhibit TSH binding.

❑❑   **How many times stronger is T3 than T4?**

Approximately three to four times stronger.

❑❑   **What is the predominant protein that binds T4?**

Thyroxin binding globulin (TBG) binds 70% of thyroxine while the remainder is bound by transthryretin and albumin.

❑❑ **What percent of circulating thyroxine is "free"?**

Less than 1%.

❑❑ **What are the causes for elevated TBG levels?**

Pregnancy, newborn state, estrogens, and heroin.

❑❑ **What are the signs of neonatal hypothyroidism?**

Poor appetite, sluggishness, macroglossia, somnolence, large abdomen, hypothermia, mottled skin, constipation, edema and bradycardia.

❑❑ **What is the most common cause of acquired hypothyroidism?**

Lymphocytic thyroiditis.

❑❑ **What are the clinical manifestations of acquired hypothyroidism?**

Myxedema of the skin, cold intolerance, constipation, low pitched voice, menorrhagia, mental and physical slowing, dry skin, coarse brittle hair, and decreased energy level with increased need for sleep.

❑❑ **What percent of children with lymphocytic thyroiditis have antimicrosomal antibodies?**

Approximately 90%.

❑❑ **Is there a gender predominance in lymphocytic thyroiditis?**

Yes. Girls are affected 4 -7 times more frequently than boys.

❑❑ **What is the most common clinical manifestation of lymphocitic thyroiditis?**

The appearance of a goiter.

❑❑ **Patients with lymphocytic thyroiditis are usually hypothyroid, euthyroid, or hyperthyroid?**

The majority of patients will be euthyroid however, many will eventually become hypothyroid while only a few will clinically manifest the symptoms of hyperthyroidism.

❑❑ **What is DeQuervain's disease?**

It is a subacute nonsupporative thyroiditis. Clinical manifestations involve a tender thyroid, fever and chills usually remitting within several months.

❑❑ **What is the etiology of DeQuervain's thyroiditis?**

It is most likely due to a viral infection such as mumps or coxsackie virus.

❑❑ **What is the differential diagnosis of a congenital goiter?**

Antithyroid drugs or iodine containing medications used during pregnancy, hyperthyroid infants, iodine deficient infants and rarely congenital teratoma.

❑❑ **Which medications are commonly found to result in sporadic goiters?**

Lithium, amiodarone and iodide containing asthma inhalers.

❑❑ **What is a thyrotropin receptor-stimulating antibody?**

It is an antibody commonly found in Grave's disease which binds to the TSH receptor leading to thyroid stimulation and goiter production.

❑❑   **Is Grave's disease more common in boys or girls?**

Girls are affected five times as much as boys.

❑❑   **What are the classical signs and symptoms of Grave's disease?**

Emotional liability, autonomic hyperactivity, exopthalmos, tremor, increased appetite with no weight gain or weight loss, diarrhea, and a goiter in nearly all affected individuals.

❑❑   **How is Grave's disease confirmed by laboratory testing?**

One would find increased bound and free T3 and T4 with decreased TSH. Frequently there is a presence of thyroid peroxidase and TSH receptor stimulating antibodies.

❑❑   **What treatment options exist for children with Grave's disease? What treatment is recommended?**

Children can be managed medically with propylthiouracil (PTU) or methimazole, surgically with a subtotal thyroidectomy or with radioiodine therapy. Medical management is the treatment of choice.

❑❑   **How much time must pass before noticing a clinical response when using medical treatment for Grave's disease?**

2 - 3 weeks.

❑❑   **What medication is available to treat the autonomic hyperactivity associated with Grave's disease?**

Propranolol, a beta blocker dosed at .5 - 2.0 mg/kg/d divided T.I.D.

❑❑   **What are the three largest concerns with surgical management of Grave's disease?**

Hyper or hypothyroidism depending on the amount of tissue removed, hypoparathyroidism, and vocal cord paralysis.

❑❑   **What is the most common cause for congenital hyperthyroidism?**

Transplacental passage of thyroid receptor antibodies from a mother with Grave's disease.

❑❑   **What is the most common type of thyroid carcinoma in children?**

Papillary thyroid carcinoma. This type of cancer makes up greater than 80% of thyroid cancer in children.

❑❑   **What combination of medical illnesses account for multiple endocrine neoplasia (MEN) type IIA?**

Medullary carcinoma of the thyroid, adrenal medullary hyperplasia or pheochromocytoma, and parathyroid hyperplasia.

❑❑   **What is the mode of inheritance of MEN Type IIA?**

Autosomal dominant.

❑❑   **How is MEN Type IIA different from MEN Type IIB?**

Men Type IIB is associated with multiple neuromas. It, too. is autosomal dominant.

❑❑   **What are the symptoms of a child suffering from thyroid storm?**

Tachycardia, systolic hypertension, tremulousness, delirium and hyperthermia.

❑❑   **How do you manage acute thyrotoxicosis?**

Propranolol at 10 mg/kg IV over 10 - 15 minutes for hypertension and increased metabolic rate. Lugol's iodide, 5 drops PO every eight hrs or Na+ iodide 125 - 250 mg/d IV over 24 hrs will stop thyroxine production.

❏❏ **What measures can be taken to further reduce peripheral conversion of T4 to T3?**

Oral dexamethasone at .2 mg/kg or oral hydrocortisone 5 mg/kg.

❏❏ **What is the differential diagnosis of acute primary adrenal insufficiency?**

Congenital adrenal hypoplasia, autoimmunity, TB, infection, trauma, and adrenal hemorrhage.

❏❏ **What are the clinical manifestations of adrenocortical insufficiency?**

Low blood pressure, muscular weakness, weight loss, anorexia and salt craving.

❏❏ **What conditions have been implicated in precipitating adrenal crisis?**

Infection, trauma, fatigue, and various medications.

❏❏ **Which symptom is most commonly seen in children with Addison's disease?**

Hypoglycemia.

❏❏ **How is adrenal insufficiency diagnosed?**

Plasma levels of cortisol are measured before and after administration of ACTH.

❏❏ **What is the Waterhouse-Friderichsen Syndrome?**

Primary adrenal insufficiency due to adrenal hemorrhage. It is often secondary to meningococcemia induced shock.

❏❏ **Does the clinical presentation of adrenal insufficiency differ between primary and secondary causes?**

Yes. Primary causes involve the adrenals directly while secondary causes involve the hypothalamic-pituitary axis. Also, primary insufficiency involves both glucocorticoids and mineral corticoids while secondary insufficiency will only involve glucocorticoids.

❏❏ **How do you manage a child in acute adrenal insufficiency?**

The two mainstays of therapy include fluid replacement and exogenous glucocorticoids.

❏❏ **What is the dose of glucocorticoid to be administered to a child with acute adrenal insufficiency?**

Hydrocortisone 2 mg/kg/dose q6hr. Larger doses may be needed during high stress situations.

❏❏ **What is the most common cause of primary adrenal insufficiency?**

Autoimmune destruction of the adrenal glands.

❏❏ **What percent of children with primary adrenal insufficiency also have another autoimmune endocrinopathy?**

45%. Most involving the thyroid gland.

❏❏ **What is adrenoleukodystophy?**

It is an autosomal disorder involving defective peroxisomes leading to fatty infiltration of the adrenal glands with concomitant dysfunction. It is commonly associated with CNS abnormalities.

❏❏ **What two autosomal dominant diseases have a high prevelance of pheochromocytomas?**

Neurofibromatosis and Von Hippel-lindau disease.

🔲🔲   **What percent of pheochromocytomas in children are bilateral?**

Up to 30%.

🔲🔲   **What laboratory tests will help to make the diagnosis of pheochromocytoma?**

Look for increased total 24 hr urinary catecholamines and their metabolites (i.e., epinephrine, norepinephrine, metanephrine and VMA).

🔲🔲   **What are the classic signs and symptoms of pheochromocytomas?**

Paroxysmal hypertension, autonomic hyperactivity, headache, visual changes and weightloss.

🔲🔲   **Which class of antihypertensive drugs are recommended for the temporary treatment of pheochromocytoma associated hypertension?**

Alpha adrenergic blocking agents like phenoxybenzamine and prazosin.

🔲🔲   **What is a neuroblastoma?**

It is a malignant catecholamine producing tumor of early childhood. It is most commonly found in the adrenal medulla.

🔲🔲   **Where is ADH synthesized? Where is it stored?**

ADH is made in the supraoptic and paraventricular nuclei of the hypothalmus. Following production it is stored in the posterior pituitary.

🔲🔲   **What conditions stimulate the secretion of ADH?**

Increased serum osmolarity, hypernatremia, and decreased right atrial pressure due to hypovolemia or shock.

🔲🔲   **At what decreased Na+ concentration do children generally become symptomatic?**

When the serum Na+ is less than 120 mEq/L.

🔲🔲   **What are the six peptide hormones secreted from the anterior and posterior pituitary gland respectively?**

Anterior pituitary hormones include; growth hormone, prolactin, thryroid stimulating hormone, and corticotropin. Posterior pituitary hormones include oxytocin and vasopressin.

🔲🔲   **What is panhypopituitarism?**

A condition where growth hormone, TSH, ACTH, FSH and LH are all abnormally low due to a non functioning or absent pituitary gland.

🔲🔲   **What hormones need to be replaced in a patient with panhypopituitarism?**

Hydrocortisone, growth hormone, thyroid hormone, and estrogen or testosterone at puberty.

🔲🔲   **What syndrome is likely to be present in a 7 year old child who presents with nausea, vomiting, and a single seizure with laboratory results consistent with hyponatremia and increased urine osmolarity?**

The syndrome of inappropriate antidiuretic hormone (SIADH).

🔲🔲   **What is SIADH?**

It is a the syndrome of inappropriate ADH (antidiuretic hormone) secretion. It occurs when the plasma vasopressin levels are abnormally elevated for the corresponding plasma osmolarity.

❐❐   **What is the most common cause of SIADH in children?**

Infection. 50% of children with bacterial meningitis have concomitant SIADH.

❐❐   **What are the symptoms of SIADH?**

When the serum Na+ is between 110 and 120 mEq/L one may see nausea, vomiting, irritability, confusion and mental status changes. Once the Na+ goes below 110 mEq/L, seizures and coma may occur.

❐❐   **How is SIADH treated?**

Most important is treating the underlying condition. Fluid restriction and democlocycline have been proven to increase serum Na+. In emergent situations furosemide in conjunction with 300 ml/M2 of 1.5% NaCl may be used.

❐❐   **What is the emergent treatment for a hyponatremic child suffering from SIADH?**

3 ml/kg of 3% saline Q10-20 minutes until the symptoms resolve. A single dose of 1 mg/kg of furosemide may be used. 5 - 10 mg/kg of phenytoin IV can be used to inhibit ADH secretion as well as help to prophylax against possible seizures. Treating the underlying condition however is still the most important consideration.

❐❐   **What is the danger of correcting the Na+ to vigorously?**

Central pontine mylenolysis.

❐❐   **What is central diabetes insipidus?**

A lack of ADH secretion which results in an inability to concentrate the urine despite functioning kidneys.

❐❐   **What specific disease process should be considered in a child who presents with dehydration, hypernatremia, decreased urine osmolarity and a high level of circulating ADH?**

Nephrogenic diabetes insipidus

❐❐   **How is the diagnosis of diabetes insipidus made in a child?**

By finding hypernatremia, increased serum osmolarity and decreased urine osmolarity.

❐❐   **Are central causes of diabetes insipidus generally acquired or congenital?**

Acquired.

❐❐   **If a child presents with hypernatremia and dehydration, how is the free water deficiency calculated?**

Free water = [Na+measured - 145 mEq/L] x 4 ml/kg x (wt in kg before dehydration).

❐❐   **What additional adjuncts can be used in addition to volume replacement in a patient with diabetes insipidus?**

Intranasal administration of DDAVP at 0.4 g/kg.

❐❐   **What should the physician consider if the patient with diabetes insipidus continues to diurese despite repeated doses of DDAVP?**

The patient most probably has nephrogenic diabetes insipidus which is due to unresponsive kidney receptors for ADH regardless of whether the ADH is endogenous or exogenous.

❐❐   **If nephrogenic diabetes insipidus is assumed, what further pharmacological treatment may be helpful?**

Thiazide diuretics have a paradoxical effect in patients with diabetes insipidus and may work in decreasing fluid losses.

❏❏   **How frequently should the physician monitor the serum Na+ and urine osmolarity when correcting a hypernatremic state in a child with diabetes insipidus?**

At least every two hours.

❏❏   **What is acromegaly?**

A condition resulting from overproduction of growth hormone in children with closed epiphyses.

❏❏   **How does acromegaly differ from gigantism?**

Acromegaly occurs in children with closed epiphyses while gigantism is found in children whose epiphyses are still open.

❏❏   **What are the clinical manifestations of acromegaly?**

Coarse facial features, enlarged tongue, enlargement of the distal extremities and hypogonadism.

❏❏   **What medical modality can be used to suppress exogenous growth hormone production?**

Octreotide, an analogue of somatostatin.

❏❏   **What pituitary tumor is most common among adolescents?**

Prolactinomas.

❏❏   **What is the primary hormone responsible for the initiation of puberty in children?**

Gonadotropin-releasing hormone (GnRH).

❏❏   **What is the first sign of puberty in females? In males?**

In females, it is the appearance of breast buds; in males, it is enlargement of the testes.

❏❏   **What is the definition of precocious puberty?**

The onset of secondary sexual characteristics before age eight in a female and nine in a male.

❏❏   **What is Cushing's disease?**

Pituitary adenomas leading to increased ACTH secretion with resultant bilateral adrenal hyperplasia and elevated cortisol levels.

❏❏   **Is Cushing's disease different than Cushing's syndrome?**

Cushing's disease results from pituitary adenomas while Cushing's syndrome is elevated cortisol levels from various causes including; paraneoplastic syndromes, primary adrenal tumors, and exogenous use of cortisol.

❏❏   **How is Cushing's syndrome diagnosed?**

Using the dexamethasone suppression test. Patients with ACTH dependent Cushing's demonstrate suppression with the larger doses of dexamethasone while those with ectopic tumors cannot be suppressed at any level.

❏❏   **What is the most common cause of excess cortisol production in infants?**

A functioning adrenocortical tumor.

❏❏   **What are the clinical manifestations of primary aldosteronism?**

Hyperplasia of the zona glomerulosa leading to hypertension, sodium and water retention, hypokalemia and decreased serum renin levels.

❏❏   **What are the clinical manifestations of primary hypogonadism?**

Failure of development of the secondary sexual characteristics with abnormally small penis and testes.

❏❏   **What is hypogonadotropic hypogonadism?**

A delayed onset of puberty due to decreased levels of FSH and LH with functioning ovaries or testes.

❏❏   **How is the diagnosis of primary hypogonadism made?**

The levels of FSH and LH are abnormally elevated for the corresponding age. Testosterone levels remain low and show little response to the administration of hCG.

❏❏   **What is the deficient hormone in secondary hypogonadism?**

FSH or LH. The defect is in the pituitary rather than in the testes or ovaries.

❏❏   **What is Kallmann's syndrome?**

Hypogonadotropic hypogonadism with anosmia.

❏❏   **Is the pituitary gland responsible for parathyroid regulation?**

No. Unlike the thyroid gland, the parathyroids are not regulated by the pituitary gland but rather by circulating calcium levels.

❏❏   **What is the most common cause of childhood hyperparathyroidism?**

A single parathyroid adenoma.

❏❏   **What are the clinical manifestations of hyperparathyroidism regardless of cause?**

Anorexia, nausea, vomiting, constipation, polydipsia, polyuria, fever, weight loss, kidney stones and muscular weakness.

❏❏   **Explain the difference between primary and secondary hyperparathyroidism?**

In primary hyperparathyroidism the defect is in the parathyroid gland i.e., an adenoma or hyperplasia while in secondary hyperparathyroidism the elevated PTH is a physiologic response to a low calcium level usually as a result of renal disease.

❏❏   **What are the diagnostic laboratory findings seen in hyperparathyroidism?**

Elevated serum calcium and PTH with concomitant decreased phosphorous levels.

❏❏   **What is Von Recklinghausen's disease?**

Hyperparathyroidism leading to cystic changes in bone due to osteoclastic resorption with fibrous replacement forming non-neoplastic "brown tumors".

❏❏   **What is pseudohypoparathyroidism?**

It is an autosomal recessive disorder characterized by kidney unresponsiveness to PTH, shortened fourth and fifth metacarpals and metatarsals, and short stature all occuring without evidence or parathyroid dysfunction.

❏❏   **What is the glucose concentration in most standard oral rehydration solutions?**

According to the World Health Organization (WHO) 2% is optimal.

❏❏   **How much water should a newborn baby receive in addition to infant formula or breast feeding?**

In normal situations newborns need no additional free water. In fact excess free water is the major cause for water intoxication in infancy and the development of subsequent hyponatremic seizures.

❏❏   **What are the 3 most common side effects of Depo-Provera?**

Menstrual irregularities, amenorrhea, and weight gain.

❏❏   **A child with adrenal insufficiency also has hyperpigmentation of the skin. Is his adrenal insufficiency most likely to be primary or secondary?**

Primary. This would be due to the increased output of POMC (pro-opiomelanocorticotropin).

❏❏   **Are girls or boys more likely to be diagnosed early with congenital adrenal hyperplasia (CAH)?**

Girls, due to the presence of ambiguous genitalia.

❏❏   **A child with a past history of frequent viral infections is currently displaying the signs and symptoms associated with hypoparathyroidism. What is your presumptive diagnosis?**

DiGeorge syndrome. This is a congenital T-cell deficiency secondary to aberrant embryonic development of the third and fourth brachial arches.

❏❏   **A child comes into the emergency room after being struck on the head with a baseball yesterday. He is vomiting, and has a decreasing level of consciousness. Your STAT CT scan is normal. However, his electrolytes show a sodium level of 131. What is the diagnosis?**

SIADH (syndrome of inappropriate ADH).

❏❏   **The water deprivation test can be used to diagnose what syndrome?**

Diabetes insipidus

❏❏   **A 3 year old girl has a cafe-au-lait spot with a "coast of Maine" appearance, polyostotic fibrous dysplasia and precocious puberty. What is your diagnosis?**

McCune-Albright syndrome. This is a disease characterized by autonomous hyperfunction of multiple glands in association with the above mentioned abnormalities.

❏❏   **What is the insulin requirements of post-pubertal individuals?**

0.5-1.0 units/kg/day, obviously with individual adjustment depending on level of activity and caloric intake.

❏❏   **What is the Somogyi phenomenon?**

Rebound hyperglycemia after an incidence of hypoglycemia. It is believed to be due to an increased response of counter-regulatory hormones as a response to insulin-induced hypoglycemia. Tighter glucose control raises the risk of this occurring.

❏❏   **What is the dawn phenomenon?**

Hyperglycemia in the dawn hours (5-9 a.m.) without a preceding hypoglycemic episode. This is thought to be due partly from the early morning rise in growth hormone and cortisol, which you'll recall antagonize the effects of insulin.

❏❏   **How long after the diagnosis of diabetes are microscopic changes detectable in the glomerular basement membrane?**

2 years.

❏❏   **How long after the onset of proteinuria do most diabetics require dialysis?**

About 5 years. The mortality is about 12 years after the onset of proteinuria.

❏❏   **The HbA1C level can be used as an indicator of overall glucose level over what time period?**

The life of a red blood cell - 120 days.

❏❏   **What is the cause of hypoglycemic unawareness?**

The capacity to release catecholamines in response to hypoglycemia can become diminished in patients with diabetes. As the signs and symptoms of hypoglycemia are mostly catecholamine induced, this results in lack of awareness of the low levels of blood sugars by the patient.

❏❏   **A 45 kg child presents in ketoacidosis. How much fluid needs to be given in the first hour?**

900 cc's (20cc/kg) of isotonic saline.

❏❏   **What are the indications for bicarbonate therapy for children with DKA?**

Symptomatic hyperkalemia, cardiac instability, and inadequate ventilatory compensation.

❏❏   **Is a constitutional delay in reaching puberty or menarche familial?**

Yes.

❏❏   **How can radiographs assist in differentiating between genetic disease and familial short stature?**

They can be used to compare chronological age versus bone age, which will be comparable in familial short stature. There are standards of normal skeletal maturation by radiograph. The rate of bony maturation can be determined by a single bone age determination (i.e. left hand and wrist).

❏❏   **A newborn with ambiguous genitalia and midline abnormalities (i.e. cleft palate), most likely has a dysfunction of which gland(s)?**

Hypothalamus and pituitary.

❏❏   **Development of pubic hair before what age is considered 'precocious puberty'?**

8 years old in females and 9 years old in males.

❏❏   **Are girls or boys more likely to have precocious puberty?**

Girls (80%)

❏❏   **What is the most common cause of acquired hypothyroidism in the U.S.?**

Chronic Lymphocytic Thyroiditis (Hashimoto's)

❏❏   **How do most patients with Hashimoto's thyroiditis present?**

Asymptomatic goiter.

❏❏   **What is the prognosis of euthyroid Hashimoto's thyroiditis?**

About half of these patients will have complete resolution, the other half will eventually need thyroxine replacement therapy.

❏❏   **What is the most common cause of hyperthyroidism?**

Grave's disease.

❏❏   **What are the three types of therapy available for children with Grave's disease?**

I^{131} therapy, anti-thyroid medication (Methimazole, carbimazole or Propylthiouracil) or sub-total thyroidectomy.

❏❏   **How concerned should you be over an incidental finding of a solitary thyroid nodule in a 12 year old?**

Fairly. Though these "incidentalomas" are usually benign in adults, they tend to be cancerous in a much larger percentage of children.

❑❑   **What should be the first test you order for this child with a single thyroid nodule?**

Fine needle aspiration. Only if this is suspicious or inconclusive do you order a thyroid uptake scan.

❑❑   **In a child with suspected hyperthyroidism, what would you expect to see from the following tests: Total T4, T3 Resin Uptake, and Free Thyroxine Index?**

All would be increased.

❑❑   **What is the "DKA Triad"?**

Uncontrollable hyperglycemia, ketosis and acidemia.

❑❑   **What are the diagnostic criteria for DKA?**

Blood glucose >250 mg/dL, an arterial pH <7.3, and a bicarbonate level <15 mEq/L.

❑❑   **A newborn infant is brought to your office with a history of poor feeding, vomiting and convulsions. What five causes need to be considered?**

Hypoglycemia, hypocalcemia, infection, pyloric stenosis, and metabolic disorder.

❑❑   **The child in the above question was unresponsive to intravenous glucose and calcium, and septic workup is underway. If you are considering a metabolic disorder, what would be the next appropriate step?**

Obtain plasma ammonia, pH and CO_2 levels. If acidotic, consider organic acidemias. If all are normal, consider galactosemia or aminoacidopathies. A high ammonia and normal pH and CO_2 should make you consider urea cycle defects.

❑❑   **What is the most common form of inheritance of metabolic disorders?**

Autosomal recessive

❑❑   **What clinical manifestations are suggestive of inborn errors of metabolism?**

Unexplained mental retardation, convulsions, developmental delay, unusual odors, episodes of vomiting, hepatomegaly and renal stones.

❑❑   **What are the clinical findings in a child with classic PKU?**

Blond hair and blue eyes are common. A mousy/musty odor on body and in urine. An eczematoid rash, microcephaly, and hyperactive DTR's are also commonly seen.

❑❑   **What is the criteria for diagnosis of classic PKU?**

Plasma phenylalanine level above 20; a normal plasma tyrosine level; normal tetrahydrobiopterin (BH4); increased urinary levels of phenylpyruvic and o-hydroxyphenylacetic acids (metabolites of phenylalanine).

❑❑   **T/F: Patients with hyperphenylalaninemia can be treated with only a diet low in phenylalanine.**

False. Some patients with hyperphenylalaninemia have deficiency in the cofactor BH4 (tetrahydrobiopterin) also need BH4 supplementation as well as neurotransmitter precursors to avoid neurological damage.

❑❑   **What is the cause of death of most children with tyrosinemia?**

Hepatic failure. In children with hepatitis and/or evidence of hepatic failure, tyrosinemia needs to be considered, along with galactosemia, hereditary fructose intolerance and giant cell hepatitis.

❑❑   **What are the two major forms of generalized albinism (oculocutaneous)?**

Tyrosine positive (type II), which is most common, and tyrosine negative (Type I), which is most severe. They are classified according to whether or not a hair bulb can produce melanin when incubated in a medium with tyrosine.

❑❑   **What are the two main clinical manifestations seen in alcaptonuria?**

Arthritis and ochronosis.

❑❑   **What is ochronosis?**

A darkening of tissue. Seen as dark spots on the sclera, cornea and ear cartilage.

❑❑   **High levels of what compound in the urine confirms the diagnosis of alcaptonuria?**

Homogentisic acid.

❑❑   **What two disease entities commonly present with tall, thin body habitus, arachnodactyly, scoliosis, ectopia lentis, and pectus carinatum or excavatum?**

Marfan's syndrome and Homocystinuria Type I.

❑❑   **What clinical and laboratory findings are commonly seen with early-onset severe galactosemia?**

Jaundice, hypoglycemia, liver enzyme elevation (AST and ALT) and *E. coli* sepsis.

❑❑   **What is the most common disorder of tryptophan metabolism?**

Hartnup disorder, a usually benign and often asymptomatic disease.

❑❑   **A mother of a four month old infant has noticed that the diaper is blue when the child has a bowel movement. What causes this?**

This condition is most likely from indicanuria, a condition where tryptophan is poorly absorbed, most commonly from bowel stasis, and oxidized by bacteria and enzymatic action to indican.

❑❑   **What is the most remarkable routine laboratory finding in patients with Maple Syrup Urine Disease (MSUD)?**

Severe metabolic acidosis.

❑❑   **The absence or presence of what three features are used to distinguish the cause of organic acidemias?**

Ketosis, skin manifestations, and characteristic odor.

❑❑   **What is the treatment for a child in a state of acute hyperammonemia?**

Clear the ammonia with benzoate, phenylacetate, arginine, and, if ineffective, then dialysis. Also, keep child from going into catabolic state by supplying all nutrients, electrolytes, fluid and calories.

❑❑   **Routine labs on a premature, SGA (small for gestational age) baby reveals ammonia level of 45uM. What should you do?**

Nothing. A majority of these children have a mild, transient increase. They have no neurological sequelae.

❑❑   **A child is born with a epicanthal folds, a high forehead with shallow supraorbital ridges, low/broad nasal ridge, micrognathia, weakness, seizures and corneal clouding. What two syndromes should you suspect?**

Down's syndrome and Zellweger syndrome

❏❏   **What is the life expectancy of a newborn with Zellweger syndrome?**

A few months.

❏❏   **What causes Zellweger cerebrohepatorenal syndrome?**

Absence of, or reduction in, peroxisomes with peroxisome enzyme abnormalities.

❏❏   **What drug can be given to relieve the painful muscle spasms associated with adrenoleukodystrophy?**

Baclofen (*Lioresal*), 5 mg BID up to 25 mg QID.

❏❏   **What therapeutic measures are suggested for children with ALD?**

"Lorenzo's Oil" (4:1 glycerol triolate and glyceryl trierucate) and bone marrow transplantation (in certain circumstances).

❏❏   **When should you consider bone marrow transplantation in children with ALD?**

When there are early neurological changes and the MRI shows brain abnormalities consistent with ALD.

❏❏   **Of Niemann-Pick Disease, Gaucher disease, and Tay-Sachs, which does not have CNS involvement?**

Gaucher. These diseases differ in, among other things, where the sphingolipid is stored. In Gaucher disease, it is only in the periphery, in Tay-Sachs only in CNS, and in Neimann-Pick disease it is stored in both.

❏❏   **In a physical exam of an infant you notice a cherry-red spot on the macula, but no hepatomegaly. What disease is this most probably due to?**

Tay-Sachs. Although many sphingolipidoses manifest themselves with the cherry red spot on the macula, Tay Sachs is the only one that is limited to the CNS.

❏❏   **Tay-Sachs disease occurs most commonly among people of what descent?**

Ashkenazi Jews

❏❏   **What are the first signs of Tay-Sachs disease?**

Hyperacusis, decreased eye-contact, hypotonia, and a cherry-red spot of the macula.

❏❏   **What enzyme is deficient in Tay-Sachs disease?**

Hexosaminidase A

❏❏   **What is the defect in Niemann-Pick Disease (Type A)?**

Sphingomyelinase

❏❏   **What are the initial manifestations of Niemann-Pick Disease (Type A)?**

Failure to thrive and difficulty feeding. These usually appear between three and four months.

❏❏   **What is the expected life span of a child diagnosed with Niemann-Pick Disease (Type B)?**

The child is expected to have a normal life span. This form of sphingomyelinase deficiency is benign as there is no CNS involvement.

❏❏   **What is the defect in Gaucher disease?**

Beta-glucosidase is deficient. This leads to accumulation of glucocerebroside in the reticuloendothelial system.

❏❏   **What is the first sign of Gaucher disease?**

Splenomegaly. Lab findings include anemia, leukocytosis, and thrombocytosis.

❏❏   **Gaucher disease occurs most commonly among people of what descent?**

Ashkenazi Jews (1 in 500, making it 7-8 times more common in this population than Tay-Sachs).

❏❏   **What is the current treatment for Gaucher disease?**

Enzyme replacement therapy. *Ceredase* or *Cerezyme* at 8-30 units/Kg/2 wks IV.

❏❏   **What is the mode of inheritance of Fabry disease?**

X-linked recessive

❏❏   **What is the enzyme deficiency in Fabry disease?**

Alpha-galactosidase

❏❏   **T/F: Mental retardation is not seen in Fabry disease.**

True.

❏❏   **What organ systems are affected by Fabry disease?**

Musculoskeletal (pain in extremities), cardiac (mitral insufficiency), renal (kidney failure), and integumentary (angiokeratomas).

❏❏   **An 18 month old child is brought in for examination of nodules and painful swelling over many joints. There are not, however, any findings of rheumatoid arthritis. What do you do next?**

Order an assay of WBC's for ceramidase activity to rule out Farber disease.

❏❏   **The increase in plasma cholesterol seen in early adulthood is due mostly to which form of cholesterol?**

LDL cholesterol. Additionally, the HDL levels in females remains constant, whereas it starts to decline in men in the second decade.

❏❏   **Children should be considered hypercholesterolemic if their plasma cholesterol is above what percentile?**

75th. Above this they are at risk for heart disease as adults.

❏❏   **What children should be screened for hypercholesterolemia?**

Those with family history of a total cholesterol level >240 mg/dL, and those with other risk factors that make them more susceptible for coronary heart disease.

❏❏   **What is the equation for calculating the LDL cholesterol levels?**

LDL cholesterol=total cholesterol - [HDL cholesterol+(total triglycerides/5)]. Levels greater than 130 are considered elevated (for this equation to be accurate, the triglyceride level must be below 400 mg/dL).

❏❏   **Why is it not advisable to institute fat-limiting diets in children under 2 years old?**

Their rate of growth demands more calories, including fats. Additionally, their CNS systems are developing and they need the fats for their myelin, among other things.

❏❏   **What is the mainstay of therapy for children with familial hypercholesterolemia (FH)?**

Appropriate diet along with cholestyramine or colestipol resin.

❏❏   **This xanthoma striate palmaris is seen in what condition?**

These xanthoma are seen on the palm of the hand and occur in familial dysbetalipoproteinemia.

❑❑   **Why are patients with Tangier disease at increased risk for coronary heart disease?**

The defects in this disease are abnormal and reduced HDL particles. Thus, these patients do not benefit from the protective effects of HDL.

❑❑   **What is the most common familial disorder of lipoprotein metabolism?**

Familial Combined Hyperlipidemia (FCHL) is now more commonly detected than Familial Hypercholesterolemia. Both are dominantly inherited.

❑❑   **A newborn infant presents with failure to thrive, jaundice, cataracts, ascites, and hepatosplenomegaly. What are these infants at risk for?**

The diagnosis in this child is most likely galactosemia. These infants are at high risk for *E. coli* sepsis, which is often the initial presentation.

❑❑   **What triad is commonly found in patients with galactosemia secondary to a deficiency of galactokinase?**

Cataracts, galactosemia and galactouria.

❑❑   **T/F: Hereditary fructose intolerance can be diagnosed easily by doing a fructose tolerance test.**

False. Such a test may lead to hypoglycemia, shock and death. This is bad. Detection of urinary reducing substances by tests such as Clinitest, followed by chromatography will reveal the elevated fructose.

❑❑   **A 12 year old child complains of easy fatigue and severe muscle cramps well above that of his peers, after strenuous exercise. What enzyme deficiencies might produce these symptoms?**

Deficiencies of either muscle *phosphoglycerate mutase* or muscle type *lactate dehydrogenase* (LDH).

❑❑   **What clinical symptoms characterize Leigh subacute necrotizing encephalopathy (SNE)?**

Optic atrophy, seizures, vomiting, lactic acidosis, psychomotor retardation, and hypotonia.

❑❑   **Generally speaking, what should you suspect in a newborn with ketonuria and acidosis?**

An inborn error of metabolism.

❑❑   **A child with urine that smells like cabbage should be investigated for what inborn error of metabolism?**

Tyrosinemia type I

❑❑   **Patients with disorders of which biochemical pathways are more likely to present with hepatomegaly in the acute stages?**

Disorders of fatty acid or carbohydrate metabolism.

❑❑   **What cholesterol level is considered high for children and adolescents?**

>200

❑❑   **In children, what is the most common form of hyperlipidemia?**

Type IIa (familial hypercholesterolemia with increased cholesterol and LDL)

❑❑   **What type of hyperlipidemia is most likely to present in childhood?**

Type I (hyperlipoproteinemia)

☐☐ **What is the defect in Type IIa hyperlipidemia?**

Lack of functioning LDL receptors.

☐☐ **How does Type I hyperlipidemia usually present?**

Hepatosplenomegaly with recurrent abdominal pain.

☐☐ **What is the most common lipid storage disease?**

Gaucher disease.

☐☐ **In expectant mothers with PKU who are not maintaining a phenylalanine free diet, what is the risk of fetal injury?**

100%

☐☐ **What is the most common cause of a positive PKU blood screen test in a premature infant?**

Hyperphenylalaninemia from transient tyrosinemia of the newborn.

☐☐ **In premature infants with a positive PKU test, how does administration of vitamin C help?**

It increases metabolism of tyrosine and phenylalanine.

☐☐ **The child with dark urine in the diaper, ochronosis, and degenerative arthritis likely has what metabolic disorder?**

Alkaptonuria

☐☐ **How do you clinically distinguish between Marfan's syndrome and homocystinuria?**

By examining the joints, which are normal to contracted in homocystinuria, and hyperextended in Marfan's syndrome.

☐☐ **What causes the "blue diaper" syndrome?**

Tryptophan malabsorbtion.

☐☐ **Most females with classic galactocemia treated with galactose-free diets still suffer what complication?**

Ovarian insufficiency.

☐☐ **What metabolic derangement is commonly seen in hereditary fructose intolerance?**

Hypophosphatemia.

☐☐ **A patient who develops severe cramps after exercise and increasing fatigue is noted to have normal lactate levels and low post-exertional lactate levels. What 2 metabolic diseases should you suspect?**

McArdle disease and Tarui disease.

☐☐ **What tests are used to diagnose the different organic acidemias?**

Gas chromatography and mass spectrometry.

☐☐ **Before the commonly described self-destructive behavior seen in Lesch-Nyhan syndrome is seen, what features have already manifested themselves in the first year of life?**

Hypotonia, frequent vomiting, dystonia, and chorea.

☐☐ **The mother of a child with "the flu" wants to give him Pepto-Bismol to relieve his upset stomach. Should you let her?**

No, because of the theoretical risk of "Reyes syndrome" from the bismuth subsalicylates.

☐☐   **What is that funky name for the ocular abnormalities seen in Wilson's disease?**

Kayser-Fleischer rings.

☐☐   **What is the drug of choice for patients with Wilson's disease?**

D-penicillamine.

☐☐   **Why do females with porphyria encounter greater problems than their male counterparts?**

Estrogen is an inducer of ALA-synthase, the rate-limiting step in heme biosynthesis.

☐☐   **Zellweger syndrome is a disorder of what organelle?**

The peroxisone (you were already told this so you only get 1/2 credit)

☐☐   **What is "Lorenzo's oil" used to treat?**

Adrenoleukodystrophy (a.k.a. Lou Gehrig's disease).

☐☐   **What is Mela's syndrome?**

Mitochondrial Encephalopathy with Lactic Acidosis and strokes.

☐☐   **What is the most common procedure to diagnose inborn errors of metabolism prenatally?**

Enzyme analysis of cultured fibroblasts

☐☐   **What is the definition of malnutrition?**

A nutritional deficit associated with increase risk of adverse clinical events, and decreased risk of such events when corrected.

☐☐   **What is the primary goal of nutritional support in critically ill patients?**

To provide usable substrates to meet energy needs, conserve lean body mass, and restore physiologic homeostasis.

☐☐   **What proportion of critically ill and injured patients are catabolic or hypermetabolic?**

Nearly all.

☐☐   **Are immunocompetence and vital organ function dependent upon nutritional support?**

Absolutely. Both are secondary goals of nutritional support.

☐☐   **What is the predominant energy source used during starvation by a healthy subject?**

Lipids.

☐☐   **How long does the body's reserve of carbohydrates last during starvation?**

Glycogen stores are consumed within 24 hours.

☐☐   **Does the metabolic rate increase or decrease during starvation in a healthy subject?**

Decrease.

☐☐   **Are adaptation mechanisms seen with starvation similar to those seen in critically ill patients?**

No. There is impaired protein conservation and a persistent hypermetabolic response in the critically ill patient.

❏❏ **With the onset of critical illness, what factors are thought to raise resting energy expenditure and protein turnover?**

Catecholamines and cortisol.

❏❏ **How does the insulin resistance associated with critical illness affect substrate use?**

Insulin resistance decreases the peripheral use of glucose and increases proteolysis.

❏❏ **Is there any rationale for overfeeding or underfeeding critically ill patients?**

No. Both have been shown to be detrimental. The goal is to meet the metabolic needs of the patient.

❏❏ **What is the utility of anthropometric (e.g., weight change), biochemical (e.g., serum albumin level), or immunologic (e.g., absolute lymphocyte count) indices as a measures of nutritional status in the critical care setting?**

Low. Too many other factors such as fluid retention, changes in protein synthesis priorities, and underlying infections make these indices less reliable than in otherwise healthy patients.

❏❏ **What are the serum half-lives of albumin and prealbumin?**

18 days and 2 to 3 days, respectfully.

❏❏ **What two methods are frequently used to assess nutritional status in critically ill patients?**

Indirect calorimetry and nitrogen balance.

❏❏ **As a patient's FIO_2 requirements increases, is indirect calorimetry more or less accurate in measuring energy expenditure?**

Less.

❏❏ **What other factors are sources of errors with indirect calorimetry?**

Air leak from endotracheal tubes and the need for extrapolation of measurements to 24 hours.

❏❏ **Can lipid emulsions be useful in patients needing volume restriction or demonstrating carbohydrate intolerance?**

Yes. Lipids are calorie dense compared to dextrose solutions.

❏❏ **What clinical symptoms are seen with hypophosphatemia brought on by refeeding a malnourished patient?**

Weakness and congestive heart failure.

❏❏ **Besides an energy source, what role does glutamine play in the gut?**

It is thought to be important in maintaining intestinal structure and function.

❏❏ **Is glutamine an essential amino acid?**

No. However, during times of metabolic stress, intracellular glutamine stores are markedly depleted indicating supplementation may be beneficial.

❏❏ **When should nutritional support be started?**

As soon as a hypermetabolic state (e.g., trauma or sepsis), underlying malnutrition, or an expected delay in resuming an oral diet of > 5-10 days is recognized.

❏❏ **Has early initiation of enteral feedings been shown to decrease septic complications in trauma patients compared to early parenteral nutrition?**

Yes. It appears those most severely injured gain the greatest benefit.

❑❑   **What complications are associated with enteral nutrition?**

Complications involving routes of access to the GI tract (e.g., feeding tube displacement or obstruction), the GI tract itself (e.g., nausea, vomiting, diarrhea), or metabolic (e.g., hyperglycemia, hypophosphatemia).

❑❑   **T/F: Bowel sounds are a good index of small bowel motility.**

False.

❑❑   **Has preoperative nutritional support for malnourished patients been shown to reduce postoperative morbidity?**

Yes, for those with severe malnutrition.

❑❑   **In which patients is parenteral nutritional support indicated?**

When enteral access is unobtainable, enteral feeding contraindicated, or when level of enteral nutrition fails to meet requirements.

❑❑   **In which patients is intravenous nutritional support unlikely to be of benefit?**

Those expected to start oral intake in 5 to 7 days or with mild injuries.

❑❑   **Can lipids be given through a peripheral vein?**

Yes. They are isosmotic, unlike the concentrated dextrose solutions that should be infused centrally.

❑❑   **What are some of the complications of parenteral nutrition?**

Those associated with catheter insertion (e.g., pneumothorax), with the indwelling line (e.g., line sepsis, thrombosis), with lipid emulsions (e.g., pancreatitis, reticuloendothelial dysfunction), and GI tract complications (e.g., cholestasis, acalculous cholecystitis).

❑❑   **T/F: It is not recommended to place patients simultaneously on enteral and parenteral feedings.**

False. On the contrary, a small amount of nutrition delivered enterally may be all that is required to gain the positive effects of this route while the parenteral route supplies the balance of caloric and protein needs.

❑❑   **What is the most common cause of hyponatremia in infants?**

"Water Intoxication" caused by improper mixing of infant formula.

❑❑   **What is the major complication of hyponatremia in infants?**

Hyponatremic seizures.

❑❑   **What are the major complications of hypernatremic dehydration?**

Cerebral edema and hemorrhage.

❑❑   **Significant elevations of serum potassium levels result in what cardiac rhythm disturbance?**

Ventricular fibrillation.

❑❑   **What are the major clinical manifestations of severe hypokalemia?**

Paralysis and respiratory failure.

❑❑   **Which type of renal tubular acidosis is associated with Fanconi syndrome?**

Type II - proximal RTA.

❑❑   **What is Fanconi syndrome?**

A syndrome associated with genetically transmitted inborn errors of metabolism (galactosemia, Wilson's disease, tyrosinemia, etc.) or it can be acquired secondary to environmental toxins (lead, mercury, etc.).

Fanconi Syndrome causes rickets associated with multiple defects of the proximal renal tubule (Type II RTA). Most commonly associated with glucosuria, phosphaturia, aminoaciduria, and carnitinuria.

❑❑　　**What type of RTA usually presents as an isolated condition?**

Type I - distal RTA.

❑❑　　**What are the characteristic acid-base/electrolyte abnormalities associated with type I and type II RTA?**

Hypokalemic, hyperchloremic metabolic acidosis.

❑❑　　**What are the characteristic acid-base/electrolyte abnormalities associated with type IV RTA?**

Hyperkalemic, hyperchloremic metabolic acidosis.

❑❑　　**What is the underlying cause of type IV RTA?**

Decreased sodium reabsorption secondary to lack of aldosterone effect.

❑❑　　**What diseases are associated with type IV RTA?**

Diseases of the adrenal gland; most commonly Addison's disease and Congenital Adrenal Hyperplasia.

❑❑　　**What is the preferred method of rehydration in infants and children?**

The preferred method is oral rehydration with standardized electrolyte solutions assuming the patient is not in shock, vomiting, or unable to take oral fluids adequately. In those situations I.V. rehydration is the preferred method.

❑❑　　**21 Hydroxylase deficiency accounts for 95% of all cases of congenital adrenal hyperplasia. 75% of these cases are the salt losing variety and the other 25% are the classic virilizing form. What are the electrolyte abnormalities associated with the salt losing variety?**

Hyponatremia and hyperkalemia.

❑❑　　**What are the sodium concentrations of the most common commercially available IV fluids?**

0.9 normal saline = 154 meq/l
0.45 normal saline = 77 meq/l
0.3 normal saline = 54 meq/l
0.2 normal saline = 33 meq/l

❑❑　　**What are the most common conditions in pediatrics associated with metabolic alkalosis?**

Chronic vomiting- pyloric stenosis and anorexia/bullemia.
Nasogastric suctioning - post-op usually.
Chronic diuretic treatment - infants with Bronchopulmonary Dysplasia (BPD).

FETUS, NEONATE AND INFANT

"Variability is the law of life, and as no two faces are the same, so no two bodies are alike, and no two individuals react alike and behave alike under the abnormal conditions which we know as disease."
- William Osler (1849-1919)

❑❑   **What are the Wessel criteria for the diagnosis of infantile colic?**

33333! Crying or irritability lasting longer than 3 hours a day, 3 days a week, or 3 weeks total, all in an infant under 3 months old. Colic usually subsides after the age of 3 months.

❑❑   **What percentage of infants have colic?**

25%. The etiology is unknown.

❑❑   **When does physiological jaundice of the newborn occur?**

2–4 days after birth. Bilirubin levels may rise up to 5–6 mg/dl.

❑❑   **A neonate presents with a history of poor feeding, vomiting, respiratory distress, has abdominal distention, and is found to have hyperbilirubinemia. What is the likely cause of this complex?**

This neonate is septic.

❑❑   **Name some causes of jaundice occurring in the first day of life.**

Sepsis, congenital infections, ABO/Rh incompatibility.

❑❑   **Outline the Apgar scoring system.**

Index	0 points	1 point	2 points
Pulse	Ø	< 100	> 100
Resp. effort	Ø	Weak cry	Strong cry
Color	Cyanotic	Extremities cyanotic	Pink
Tone	Flaccid	Weak tone	Strong
Response	Ø	Motion	Cry

❑❑   **Sudden Infant Death Syndrome (SIDS) is the <u>most</u> <u>common</u> cause of death for infants in the first year of life. It occurs at a rate of 2/1000, or 10,000/year. What are 6 risk factors associated with SIDS?**

1) Prematurity with low birth weight.
2) Previous episode of apnea or apparent life-threatening event (ALTE).
3) Mother is a substance abuser.

4) Family history of SIDS.
5) Male gender.
6) Low socioeconomic status.

☐☐ **What is the normal pulse rate of a newborn?**

120–160 bpm.

☐☐ **External chest compressions should be initiated for a newborn with assisted ventilation when the heart rate is less than how many beats per minute?**

50 bpm.

☐☐ **SIDS has a bimodal distribution. At what ages do the peaks occur?**

2.5 and 4 months.

☐☐ **Define failure to thrive (FTT).**

FTT is defined as infants who are below the third percentile in height or weight or whose weight is less than 80% of the ideal weight for their age. Almost all patients with FTT are under 5 years old, while the majority of children are 6–12 months old.

☐☐ **What is the most common cause of FTT?**

Poor intake is responsible for 70% of FTT cases. One third of these cases are educational problems, ranging from inaccurate knowledge of what to feed a child to over-diluting formula to "make it stretch further."

☐☐ **What is the prognosis for patients with FTT?**

Only 1/3 of patients with FTT due to environmental factors have a normal life. The remainder grow up small for their size, and the majority also have developmental, psychological, and educational deficiencies.

☐☐ **Do term babies have functioning sweat glands?**

Yes, but they are hyporesponsive compared with that of adults.

☐☐ **How do infants generate heat?**

Metabolism of brown fat and muscular activity.

☐☐ **What induces the lipolysis of brown fat stores?**

Norepinephrine and thyroid hormones.

☐☐ **What abnormalities should be considered if the umbilical cord has not fallen off after 30 days?**

Neutropenia or a functioning abnormality of the neutrophils.

☐☐ **What is a good rule of thumb in estimating the necessary size of an umbilical catheter?**

The measured distance from the umbilicus to the shoulder.

☐☐ **How common is discordant growth in twin pregnancies?**

Very, as it is seen in almost one-third of twin pregnancies.

☐☐ **Is the first or second born twin at greater risk of developing respiratory distress syndrome (RDS)?**

The second born.

☐☐ **What is funisitis?**

The sense of urgency a child feels in an amusement park. Alternately, it also means inflammation of the umbilical cord vessels.

☐☐   **Preterm infants of what age should be evaluated for retinopathy of prematurity (ROP)?**

<30 weeks.

☐☐   **What specimen from the newborn is most apt to confirm the suspicion of maternal drug abuse?**

Meconium

☐☐   **What is the most common type of clavicular fracture during delivery?**

Greenstick fracture.

☐☐   **What are the two most common causes of fetal death?**

Congenital malformations and chromosomal abnormalities.

ADOLESCENCE

"He who cures a disase may be the skillfullest, but he that prevents it is the safest physician."
- Thomas Fuller (1564-1661)

❏❏ **A female with breast budding and a small amount of pubic hair near the labia is in what Tanner stage of development?**

Stage II (ages 8–15).

❏❏ **At what Tanner stage of development do males have facial hair development?**

Stage IV (ages 12–17).

❏❏ **How much does the average teenager grow during adolescence?**

Teenagers generally double their weight and increase their height by 15–20%.

❏❏ **What are the <u>most</u> <u>common</u> causes of delayed puberty?**

Constitutional growth delay, familial short stature, and chronic illness.

❏❏ **What percentage of teenage girls have eating disorders?**

20%.

❏❏ **When is the female growth spurt in respect to menarche?**

Females have menarche just after their peak growth spurt. This is just the opposite in males, who are well on their way through puberty before they hit their peak growth spurt.

❏❏ **What is the first sign of puberty in the male?**

Their amazingly mature personality (just teasing, of course). Puberty in the male begins with the growth of the testes followed by thinning and pigmentation of the scrotum, growth of the penis, and lastly the development of pubic hair.

❏❏ **By what age will a child reach half his/her adult height?**

2 years; however, by 2 years, children are only 20% of their adult weight.

❏❏ **How can you distinguish between short stature in a child due to heredity and short stature due to a constitutional delay in growth?**

Bone age determination. In children with familial short stature, bone ages will be normal. In children with constitutional growth delay, the bone ages will also be delayed, as will sexual maturation.

❏❏ **A 15 year old adolescent male has developed small breasts. The parents want this situation surgically corrected. What do you recommend?**

Surgery is a consideration if the physical abnormality is causing severe psychological pain or if the breasts have persisted for a long time. Otherwise, surgery is not a commonly recommended treatment as gynecomastia in adolescence generally lasts only 1–2 years. It has been reported that gynecomastia occurs in 36–64% of pubertal males.

❏❏ **What drugs can cause gynecomastia?**

Marijuana, hormones, digitalis, spironolactone, cimetidine, ketoconazole, antihypertensives, antidepressants, and amphetamines.

❑❑   **According to Erikson, what is the main psychosocial task of adolescence?**

Establishing a sense of identity.

❑❑   **What is the difference between adolescence and puberty?**

Adolescence is a time of psychosocial transition from being a child to being an adult. Puberty is the spectrum of physical changes that happen in the body. The two commonly occur at nearly the same time.

❑❑   **How common is smoking among adolescents?**

10-15% with females more common than males.

❑❑   **What percentage of deaths in the 15-19 year old range is due to injury?**

75-85%.

❑❑   **What percentage of all adolescent deaths are due to alcohol related automobile accidents?**

25%.

❑❑   **What percentage of fatalities in African American teenagers are due to firearms?**

About 50%.

❑❑   **Who are more likely to develop chronic fatigue syndrome, females or males?**

Females.

❑❑   **A 13 year old girl just started menarche. Is she capable of having children at this time?**

Generally not. Most girls do not ovulate for 1-2 years after menarche.

❑❑   **What is the most common breast tumor in adolescence?**

Fibroadenoma (>90%).

❑❑   **How useful is mammography in identifying lesions in adolescents?**

Not very as the breast tissue is too dense.

❑❑   **What endocrine abnormalities can lead to galactorrhea in a teenage girl?**

Hypothyroidism and an increase prolactin (i.e. from a pituitary adenoma).

❑❑   **Which is most common, primary or secondary dysmenorrhea?**

Primary. This is due to increased levels of PGF and PGE produced from the arachidonic acid released from sloughing endometrium.

❑❑   **In an adolescent female without a history of PID, what is the most common cause of chronic pelvic discomfort?**

Endometriosis.

❑❑   **When is the pain of endometriosis most severe?**

Right before menses.

What are the most common etiologies of secondary amenorrhea?

Structural abnormalities, foreign bodies (i.e. IUD), endometriosis and endometritis.

☐☐ **What are the four components, according to the DMS-IV criteria, that are necessary for the diagnosis of anorexia nervosa?**

1. Fear of becoming obese (not diminished by weight loss)
2. Dysmorphia-disturbance in way body is perceived
3. Refusal to keep weight over age/height minimum,
4. Absence of 3 or more menstrual cycles in post-menarchal females.

☐☐ **What are the 2 subclassifications of anorexia nervosa?**

Restricts - limit intake and Bulimia - binge eating followed by countermeasures.

☐☐ **How do you diagnose bulimia nervosa?**

A history of overeating followed by forced purging is all that is needed. Erosion of the tooth enamel and back of second and third fingers in the dominant hand should lead you to suspect the diagnosis.

☐☐ **What electrolyte abnormalities are commonly seen in bulimia nervosa?**

Hypokalemia, hypochloremia and metabolic alkalosis.

☐☐ **What are the main causes of death in patients with anorexia nervosa?**

About 10% of these patients end up dying from complications (i.e. electrolyte imbalances, arrhythmias, or congestive heart failure).

☐☐ **What is the Female Athlete Triad?**

Amenorrhea, disordered eating and osteoporosis.

☐☐ **What is the treatment for the Female Athlete Triad?**

Calcium supplements and oral contraceptives.

☐☐ **What is the most common structural anomaly that causes primary amenorrhea?**

Imperforate hymen.

☐☐ **How do you diagnose primary amenorrhea?**

By one of three criteria: 1) No menses by the age of 16; 2) No menses within one year of breast or pubic hair development having reached Tanner stage V; or 3) No menses within 3 years of the development of secondary sex characteristics.

☐☐ **Assuming your patient with primary amenorrhea is not pregnant, what are the next tests of choice?**

Karyotype analysis to rule out the presence of a Y chromosome (Testicular Feminization), TSH, TFT's and prolactin levels, as indicated after a thorough history and physical.

☐☐ **What is secondary amenorrhea?**

A history of no periods for 6 months in a previously menstruating female or a history oligomenorrhea followed by no periods in 12 months.

☐☐ **A 17 year old female comes to your office complaining that she has had no period for over a year. What should be the next step in defining the cause of her amenorrhea?**

Serum Prolactin and TSH, to rule out hyperprolactinemia and hypothyroidism, respectively. If these are both normal, proceed with a progesterone challenge to rule out anovulation.

☐☐ **What is the most common cause of chronic anovulation?**

Polycystic Ovary Syndrome (PCO)

□□   **How common is a varicocele?**

Dilation of the veins of the spermatic cords occurs in about 15% of adolescents (usually on the left side).

□□   **What is the most common solid tumor in adolescent males?**

Testicular seminoma.

□□   **What is the cure rate of testicular seminoma if the tumor is confined to the testicle?**

95% with orchiectomy and radiation.

□□   **Of epididymitis and testicular torsion, which will present with a positive Prehn sign?**

Testicular torsion (pain persists with elevation of the testes).

□□   **How long after the onset of testicular torsion do irreversible changes develop?**

About 4.5-5 hours.

□□   **During a routine examination of a 12 year old male, you encounter in the upper scrotum, a boggy enlargement. Should you (and he) be concerned?**

No. This is most likely a varicocele, which is very common. About 15-17% of adolescent males have an asymptomatic varicocele.

□□   **How soon after conception is the average home pregnancy kit able to detect the HCG and register as positive?**

Depending on sensitivity, anywhere from 1 to 3 weeks.

□□   **In a normal uterine pregnancy, what is the doubling time of the HCG levels?**

48 hours. This can be used as one of several screening measures to rule out a hydatiform mole.

□□   **How effective are condoms in pregnancy prevention as used by adolescents?**

Not very, with up to a 15% failure rate.

□□   **How effective are birth controls pills (BCPs) in pregnancy prevention as used by adolescents?**

Very, with a pregnancy rate of about 0.8% per year.

□□   **A vaginal smear of an adolescent with primary amenorrhea shows a positive estrogen effect. What can you give to induce menses?**

Medroxyprogesterone 10 mg po QD for 5 days every 6-12 weeks.

□□   **A 17 year old females comes to the ED complaining of excessive uterine bleeding. What hormonal adjunct can you give to stop the flow?**

Norethyrodrel (25 mg) usually stops blood flow within 24 hrs.

□□   **At what Tanner development stage do girls achieve menarche?**

SMR stage 3 (30%) or stage 4 (90%).

□□   **At what point in the menstrual cycle is a gonorrhea infection most likely to present?**

In the first 7 days of menses (80-90%)

□□   **A 17 year old female complains of vaginal irritation. She has a whitish discharge with a "fishy" odor on exam. Smear reveals clue cells. What is your diagnosis and treatment?**

Gardnerella vaginitis. Treatment is with metronidazole cream or tablets.

❑❑ **How do you treat the first episode of genital herpes?**

Oral acyclovir (200 mg 5 times/day for 10 days)

❑❑ **What is the most common STD in sexually active teenage males?**

Non-gonococcal urethritis due to *Chlamydia trachomatis*.

❑❑ **How long after intake can marijuana still be detected in the urine?**

From 3 days after one episode to 28 days in a frequent user.

❑❑ **How much more likely to become an alcoholic is the son of the town alcoholic as compared to the son of the town priest?**

Four times.

❑❑ **A fifteen year old teenager has his first cigarette at a party. What is the risk that he will become a regular smoker by the age of 18?**

About 65-75%

❑❑ **How soon after the last cigarette can nicotine withdrawal effects begin?**

Within two hours, with a peak around 24 hrs.

GROWTH AND DEVELOPMENT

"Let us spend one day as deliberately as Nature, and not be thrown off the track by every nutshell and mosquito's wing that falls on the rails."
- Henry David Thoreau

❏❏   **Child development: At what age are infants able to perform the following motor skills?**

1) Sit up by themselves.
2) Walk.
3) Crawl.
4) Walk up stairs.
5) Smile.
6) Hold their head up.
7) Roll over.

Answers: (1) 5–7 months, (2) 11–16 months, (3) 9–10 months, (4) 14–22 months, (5) 2 months, (6) 2–4 months, and 7) 2–6 months.

❏❏   **At what age are infants capable of the following language skills?**

1) "Mama/Dada" sounds.
2) One word.
3) Naming body parts.
4) Combine words.
5) Understandable speech.

Answers: (1) 6–10 months, (2) 9–15 months, (3) 19–25 months, 4) 17–25 months, and (5) 2 years–4 years.

❏❏   **At what age will a child be able to uncover a toy that is hidden by a scarf?**

9–10 months. This is called object permanence—the understanding that "out of sight" is not "out of existence."

❏❏   **Joe Montana (the greatest quarterback of all time) comes to you with his 3 year old son distressed that he can't catch a ball to save his life. You reassure Joe that children are not expected to perform that motor skill until they are what age?**

5–6 years old.

❏❏   **How many times a day should a healthy infant feed in the first 3 months of life?**

Infants should average 6–8 feedings a day. The schedule should be dictated by the infant (i.e., when he/she is hungry). By 8 months, feedings are generally only 3–4 times a day.

❏❏   **What, if any, nutritional value does cow's milk have over breast milk?**

Cow's milk has a higher protein content than breast milk. Both have the same caloric content (20 kcal/oz). Breast milk has a higher carbohydrate concentration, a greater amount of polyunsaturated fat, and is easier for the infant to digest. For the obvious immunological advantage, "breast is best."

❏❏   **A mother of a 2 month old breast fed infant comes to you complaining of breast pain, swelling, fever, and a red coloration just above her left nipple. She is a strong believer in the axiom**

"Breast is Best" and wants to know if she can continue to breast feed her infant. What do you tell her?

She most likely has bacterial mastitis, which is most common in the first 2 months of breast feeding. This is most frequently caused by *Staphylococcus aureus*. The mother should apply antibiotics and may continue breast feeding if she chooses.

❏❏ **At what age should solid foods be introduced?**

4–6 months. One food should be introduced at a time with 1–2 week intervals between the introduction of a new food. This way potential allergies can be defined.

❏❏ **How much weight should an infant gain per day in the first 2 months of life?**

20–30 gm/day. Newborns commonly lose 10% of their body weight during the first week of life due to a loss of extracellular water and a decrease in caloric intake. Healthy infants soon double their birth weight in 5 months and triple their weight in a year.

❏❏ **When do infants begin teething?**

By 6 months. They may become irritable with a decreased appetite and excessive drooling. Acetaminophen can be used to control the pain.

❏❏ **When should toilet training be started?**

Not until at least 18 months.

❏❏ **Short stature with normal weight should make you think of what general categories for investigation?**

Familial height history (constitutional delay, familial short stature), chondrodysplasias, endocrinopathies (hypothyroidism, GH deficiency, cortisol excess).

❏❏ **The mother of an 8 year old boy is worried that her child has attention deficit hyperactivity disorder. She states that for the last 4 months he has been fidgety, unable to stay seated, and talks incessantly and out of turn in school. At home, however, he seems relatively calm. What do you tell her?**

Although the symptoms are suspicious for ADHD, it is too early to make this diagnosis. In order to meet the DSM-IV criteria, the symptoms have to last at least 6 months and occur in more than one setting.

❏❏ **What neurological condition may mimic some of the symptoms of ADHD?**

Petit mal epilepsy can present as concentration and attention problems.

❏❏ **What is the treatment for ADHD?**

Behavioral and psychosocial therapy along with stimulant medications.

❏❏ **What is the most commonly used stimulant in the treatment of ADHD and how effective is it?**

Methylphenidate (Ritalin), given at 0.3-1.0 mg/kg, is efficacious in 75-80% of children.

❏❏ **What is the "parachute reflex" and when does it usually develop?**

At about 8 months of age, the infant will extend the arms and legs as a protective gesture when lowered head first in a prone position.

❏❏ **When do the Moro, rooting, and palmar grasp reflexes usually disappear?**

At about 5-6 months of age.

❏❏ **What age group is the Wechsler Intelligence Scale (WISC) used for?**

It measures the IQ's of 5-15 year olds.

❑❑   **At what age do most children stop sucking their thumbs?**

4 years old

❑❑   **At what age do most children achieve bladder control?**

About half of all American children achieve bladder control at 2.5 years of age. Girls showing toilet-training earlier than boys.

❑❑   **When does the anterior fontanelle usually close?**

Between 9-14 months of age.

❑❑   **What should you be concerned about in a child with early closure of the fontanelles?**

Premature cranial synostosis.

❑❑   **A 20 month old child still has a palpable anterior fontanelle. What conditions could cause this?**

Rickets, hypothyroidism, hydrocephalus, hypophosphatemia, or Trisomy 18.

❑❑   **How do you calculate the size of a fontanelle?**

Take the length (which is the anterior-posterior dimension) plus the width (which is the transverse dimension) and divide by 2.

❑❑   **What is craniosynostosis?**

Early fusion of cranial suture lines. This can lead to asymmetric growth, bridging of the sutures and deforming of the skull.

❑❑   **What four conditions can give you craniotabes?**

Rickets (in infancy), hypervitaminosis A, syphilis, and hydrocephalus.

❑❑   **Which are the first teeth to erupt? When does that happen?**

At 5-9 months the central incisors appear, after which there is about 1 new tooth per month. At 6-7 years, the first permanent teeth erupt (also central incisors).

❑❑   **You push a sitting infant sideways, and it reflexively holds its hand out to protect its fall. What is this called?**

Lateral propping reflex.

❑❑   **What are the first four of Ericson's life-cycle crises?**

Trust vs. mistrust (infancy), autonomy vs. shame and doubt (early childhood), initiative vs. guilt (early childhood), and industry vs. inferiority (school age).

❑❑   **In regards to acquisition of verbal skills, who develop faster-twins, or single birth infants?**

Single birth infants

❑❑   **A 10 month old infant is showing preference for his right hand. Should this be a cause of concern?**

Yes, children usually develop hand dominance by 18-24 months. Anytime hand dominance develops prior to this, you should be alert for possible cerebral palsy.

❑❑   **At what age can a child follow a simple, two-step command?**

24 months

❏❏   **What are the 2 most common causes of death in 1-6 month olds?**

SIDS and abuse.

❏❏   **T/F: Full-term infants and preterm infants have comparable risk of child abuse.**

False, preterm is much higher (3 times as much).

❏❏   **A 4 year old child present with increased hearing impairment and asymptomatic hematuria. What is your diagnosis?**

Alport syndrome (aka hereditary nephritis). This is an autosomal dominant disease that more commonly afflicts males.

❏❏   **At what age should a child with stuttering have your concern?**

5-6 years, as most children have outgrown stuttering by this age.

❏❏   **T/F: Most children with autism are mentally retarded.**

True. About 75% have an IQ less than 70.

❏❏   **At what age do most autistic children exhibit signs and symptoms of their disease?**

Usually before 3 years of age.

❏❏   **What are common predisposing factors for pica?**

Mental retardation and lack of parental nurturing.

❏❏   **When should you be concerned over a 1 year old child who constantly ingests non-nutritional items?**

As pica usually starts at 1-2 years of age, this should be high in your differential. However, mouthing objects is extremely common at this age, so a look at the family structure and signs of other disorders (i.e. schizophrenia, autism) can be investigated, and arrange for follow-up visits.

❏❏   **How successful is positive reinforcement alone in eliminating enuresis?**

80-90%.

❏❏   **If positive reinforcement is insufficient in eliminating enuresis in a child, what else can be done?**

Imipramine (needs about 5 mo. of treatment to be effective), or Desmopressin nasal spray (DDAVP).

❏❏   **What is range of IQ is considered average?**

90-109

❏❏   **What range of IQ is considered mild mental retardation?**

50-69

❏❏   **What is the most common preventable cause of mental retardation worldwide?**

Iodine deficiency. This leads to maternal and fetal hypothyroxinemia.

❏❏   **What are the 2 most common childhood psychiatric disorders?**

Attention Deficit Hyperactivity Disorder (ADHD), and Oppositional Disorder.

❏❏   **Are children of parents with an affective disorders more likely to have psychiatric problems?**

25% will have a major affective disorder and 45% will have a psychiatric disorder themselves.

❑❑   **How is skeletal age determined?**

By comparing the presence or absence of certain ossification centers to known standards. This is useful in the evaluation of short stature.

❑❑   **The parents of a 3 year old boy is concerned about an episode where he held his breath until he lost consciousness and actually had a small seizure. What do you tell them?**

This is fairly common and there is no risk of the child developing a seizure disorder. Advise them to ignore the child when he holds his breath and leave the room. Without any reinforcement the child will soon discontinue the behavior.

❑❑   **Which children have more nightmares?**

Girls > boys, usually starting at < 10 years old. More common in children with anxiety and affective disorders.

❑❑   **How do you treat Obsessive-Compulsive Disorder in children?**

SSRI's (such as Fluoxetine, Sertraline, and Paroxetine) and counseling.

❑❑   **Children with what psychological disorder are at relatively high risk of developing antisocial personality disorder as adults?**

Conduct disorder.

❑❑   **With regards to hallucinations, can you distinguish organic psychosis from psychiatrically based psychosis?**

Yes. Psychiatrically based psychosis is more likely to induce auditory hallucinations, whereas organic psychosis induces more visual, tactile, or olfactory hallucinations.

❑❑   **What is the average time that an American child watches TV per day?**

3-4 hours.

❑❑   **Who are more likely to have learning disabilities, boys or girls?**

Boys are two times more commonly diagnosed with learning disabilities in comparison with their female counterparts.

❑❑   **What percentage of school-age children are diagnosed with a learning disability?**

5%

❑❑   **A mother comes to you complaining that her child is failing in school. What tests would you perform initially?**

Hearing and vision tests should be done routinely. Evaluation for learning disabilities and IQ deficits should be performed as well.

❑❑   **Which infants tend to sleep for shorter periods and awaken more frequently at night - breast-fed or non breast fed?**

Breast fed infants

❑❑   **What sleeping position is best for infants?**

The supine position has been found to drastically decrease the incidence of SIDS.

❑❑   **The mother of a 6 week old infant complains that her child cries almost 3 hours a day. Does she have cause for concern?**

No. This is normal in that age group. This should decline to about 1 hour a day at 12 weeks.

□□   **What is the definition of infantile colic?**

Fits of crying for over 3 hours a day more than 3 days a week in an otherwise healthy infant.

□□   **When do infants sleep through the night?**

70% will sleep through the night without waking at 3 months of age. This increases to about 90% by 6 months of age.

□□   **By what age do infants generally no longer need night feedings?**

About 6 months old.

□□   **The mother of an eight year old child is worried about her child's occasional episodes of sleep walking. What do you tell her?**

This is fairly common in this age group, and it usually disappears by age 15. Imipramine or diazepam can be used for severe cases.

□□   **How long does an episode of pavus nocturnus usually last?**

Night terrors last between 30 seconds to 5 minutes. The child does not remember the episode in the morning.

□□   **What percentage of newborns have pseudostrabismus?**

30%

□□   **How do you easily differentiate pseudostrabismus from strabismus?**

In pseudostrabismus, one can observe full range of extraocular motion, corneal reflections of a light source 12 inches or more away that are symmetric, and a normal red reflex by direct ophthalmoscopy.

□□   **What is amblyopia?**

Visual deficits that can not be corrected in the developing eye. Seen in 2% of American children.

□□   **What is the treatment for nasal lacrimal duct obstruction?**

Nothing. About 95% resolve spontaneously by six months. After this time period, referral to an ophthalmologist is recommended.

□□   **How are regular color blindness and blue color blindness inherited?**

X-linked and autosomal dominant, respectively.

□□   **By what age are 90% of children walking?**

15 months.

□□   **What percent of children still wet the bed at night by school entry age?**

10% (Up to 30% of boys still wet the bed 1-6 times per year and up to 15% of girls at school entry; however more frequent bedwetting or never been dry for > 3 months involves about 10% of children, boys more than girls).

□□   **A child is sitting well, is saying, "dadada," and has a neat pincer grasp. How old is he?**

9 months.

□□   **Premature thelarchy commonly occurs before what age?**

2 years.

❑❑   **Describe premature thelarchy.**

Breast buds without other signs of pubertal development, and later onset with normal cadence and timing of pubertal development.

❑❑   **What is precocious puberty?**

When the onset of puberty (adrenarchy, thelarchy, menarche) occurs at two or more standards before its expected onset.

❑❑   **What is the average age of the onset of puberty in patients of both genders?**

Females: 10 years.
Males: 12 years.

❑❑   **What is the earliest age and typical presentation of puberty in boys?**

Age: 9.5 years.
Presentation: Testicular enlargement.

❑❑   **What is the earliest age and typical presentation for normal onset of puberty in females?**

Age: 8 years
Presentation: Breast bud development and growth spurts.

❑❑   **What is the typical length of time from onset of puberty to menarche?**

2.5 years.

❑❑   **In what Tanner stage do girls begin to menstruate?**

Stage II: 10%
Stage III: 20%
Stage IV: 60%
Stage V: 10%

❑❑   **Colic (a.k.a. paroxysmal fussing) usually begins and ends between what ages?**

2 weeks to 3-4 months.

❑❑   **What is the most common time of the day for colic to occur?**

Late afternoon and evening.

❑❑   **What helps colic?**

Holding, correct positioning, and gentle rocking.

❑❑   **What is the normal range of infant crying in the first 3 months of life?**

Two Weeks: 2 hours per day
One Month: 3 hours per day
Three Months: 1 hour per day

❑❑   **How many stools does the average breast fed infant have per day during their first 1 week to 2 months of life?**

4 - 10. Hey, parents will quiz you on this.

❑❑   **Open vowel sounds (ows and ahs) are usually made by what age?**

3-4 months.

□□ **By what age should an infant begin to swipe (bat) intentionally at objects?**

4 months.

□□ **By what age does the automatic/involuntary grasp response disappear?**

5 months.

□□ **At what age is a mature pincer grasp usually attained?**

9-11 months.

□□ **A 9 month old child begins to scream and cry whenever anyone besides his mother approaches. What is your diagnosis, and is this something to be concerned about?**

Stranger anxiety. This is a normal developmental stage that generally occurs in the second half of an infant's first year. The child's temperament, along with his developmental age, will determine the severity this reaction. The parent(s) should be reassured that the child is developing normally. This stage may last weeks to months. In very shy children, this may last longer.

□□ **Separation anxiety also develops late in the first year of life. What is it and how should parents be advised?**

The realization that a parent is not present occurs because the infant has developed object permanence. The child can remember the parents, even in their absence. Short leaves, with open statements of return, should be offered to reassure the infant (even if he/she understands little of the discussion).

□□ **By what age does a child generally begin to demand that he feed himself?**

12 months. By this time, a child has a well developed pincer grasp, is beginning to use a spoon, and has decreased energy needs; the child is quite determined to feed him/her self.

□□ **Dropping food over the side of a highchair and looking for it on the floor is typical activity for a child of what age?**

9 months. However, he may continue this activity for months.

□□ **Object permanence is well developed by what age?**

9-10 months.

□□ **When do children begin to climb stairs?**

Between 8-18 months.

□□ **A child is beginning to read competently, understands simple addition and subtraction, and can count easily to 100+. He cannot ride a bike. What is his developmental age?**

Likely 6-7 cognitively, however he may have motor delays or no exposure.

□□ **How many children use a transitional object? What is its purpose?**

About 2/3 of toddlers have an inanimate object for comfort. This security object is most often used for falling asleep or in times of stress. Use continues through the 4th birthday and even later by some.

□□ **How do you counsel a parent who is interested in potty training a 2 year old?**

Toilet training is an exciting and key developmental stage for child. Parents should realize that the child wants to imitate and please parents, that this is a time when the child will take control of his environment and achieve a sense of mastery. Child must be able to complete a series of motor tasks, but must also be able to respond to a bodily feeling. Children may be ready when they can walk well, undress/take pants off easily, get to the bathroom, sit on the potty chair. Children who identify and dislike wet/dirty diapers may be nearing but not necessarily ready for training. The child must be able to understand feeling of fullness in bladder or bowel and anticipate voiding, he must have voluntary control of sphincters.

☐☐   **What is the peak age for tantrums?**

2-4 years, however the peak in anger outbursts is at 18 months in both girls and boys.

☐☐   **Do children who are exposed to 2 languages (e.g., live in bilingual households) have delayed onset of language skills?**

No, there is no evidence that being exposed to a bilingual household delays language, although it may appear that children have temporary delays in expressive abilities. Delayed language may be a manifestation of a broad variety of social/familial conflicts or developmental delays.

☐☐   **Fears are common throughout childhood. List typical fears at ages 1, 3, 6, 8, 10, and 13-17 years of age.**

1 year olds: Separation, strangers, crowds, sudden movements;
3 year olds: Masks, old people, distortions and deformities, dark, animals;
6 year olds: Supernatural, hidden people (robbers in room), bodily injury, being left alone;
8 year olds: School and personal failure, mockery by friends/peers;
10 year olds: Wild animals, criminals, older children, loss of possessions, world catastrophes;
Teens: Body changes, sexuality and other sexual fears, loss of face, world events.

☐☐   **A lack of understanding of cause and effect, despite rather mature language skills is typical in what age child?**

4-5 year old has thought patterns exemplified by juxtapositions (does not understand cause and effect, just closeness in time - I took a bath because I was clean), egocentrism (things evolve around the child - why does it snow? so I can go sledding), animism (belief that inanimate objects are alive; why is the sun shining? because he is awake), and artificialism (thinking that things/events are caused by humans - what made you sick? because I was bad).

☐☐   **At what ages should children copy a circle, cross, square, triangle, diamond?**

3, 3-4, 4-5, 5-6, 6-7 (easy to remember 3,4,5,6,7)

☐☐   **What are the 3 broad areas of difficulty in patients with Attention Deficit Disorders?**

Impulse control, inattentiveness, hyperactivity.

☐☐   **How long must difficulty with impulse control, inattentiveness or hyperactivity be present to consider ADHD?**

It generally begins before age 7, and lasts at least 6 months.

☐☐   **What else do you need to consider when a teacher tells you a child has ADHD?**

Depression, learning disabilities, other psychiatric problems, other significant social or emotional problems (i.e., anxiety), global cognitive delays (mental retardation), and chronic illness.

☐☐   **What are some typical psychological changes experienced by an adolescent?**

Prefers friends/peers to parents/family, interest in sex and sexuality, nocturnal emissions (wet dreams), and masturbation.

☐☐   **At what age would you be concerned about the lack of pubertal development in a girl?**

14, with no secondary signs of puberty; 16, with no menarche.

☐☐   **At what age would you consider referral of a boy who has not begun puberty?**

16 years.

☐☐ **What does the ELMS test?**

Early Language Milestones is a test of receptive, expressive, and visual language for 0-36 month olds.

☐☐ **At what age do the first teeth erupt?**

5-7 months (range 0-13 months).

NEUROLOGY

"It is impossible for anyone to find the correct function of any part unless he is perfectly acquainted with the action of the whole instrument."
- Galen

☐☐   **A 14 year old female with hearing loss over the last 6 months presents at 2 a.m. with vertigo that has progressively become worse over the last 2 months. On exam, she is mildly ataxic. What is the diagnosis?**

Eighth nerve lesion, possibly an acoustic schwannoma or meningioma.

☐☐   **What is a vestibular schwannoma?**

An acoustic neuroma or a tumor of the eighth cranial nerve. In addition to hearing loss and vertigo, patients also present with tinnitus. Surgical removal is the treatment of choice because this tumor may spread to the cerebellum and the brainstem.

☐☐   **Where are congenital berry aneurysms located?**

In the circle of Willis.

☐☐   **What three bacterial illnesses present with peripheral neurologic findings?**

Botulism, tetanus, and diphtheria.

☐☐   **Which type of bacteria is most commonly cultured from brain abscesses: aerobic or anaerobic?**

Anaerobic.

☐☐   **A child complains of blurry vision. On exam she has an abnormal pupil reflex and a white reflex on funduscopic examination. What is the treatment?**

Surgical removal of the eye. This is a retinoblastoma that can metastasize to other sites in the brain or body. This is an inherited condition, and she should be counseled on the dangers when she is ready for children.

☐☐   **A patient presents with facial droop on the left and weakness of the right leg. Where is the most likely site of the lesion?**

Brainstem, specifically the left pons.

☐☐   **What area of the brain is dysfunctional when a patient has Cheyne-Stokes respirations?**

The cortex. The nervous system is relying on diencephalic control.

☐☐   **What causes cerebral palsy?**

70% of the cases are idiopathic. Other causes are in utero infections, chromosomal abnormalities, or strokes. Cerebral palsy is a defect in the central nervous system that occurs prenatally, perinatally, or before the age of 3.

☐☐   **What is the <u>most</u> <u>common</u> cause of floppy baby syndrome?**

Cerebral palsy.

❐❐   **A 16 year old presents with progressively severe intermittent vertigo for 6 months and progressive unilateral hearing loss for 3 months. What is the diagnosis?**

Cerebellopontine angle tumor. Confirm diagnosis with a MRI scan.

❐❐   **A 15 year old presents with a history of being knocked unconscious for 10 seconds while playing touch football one week ago. Since then, he has had intermittent vertigo, nausea, vomiting, blurred vision, a headache, and malaise. His neuro exam and CT are normal. What is the diagnosis?**

Post concussive syndrome. Most individuals recover fully over a 2 to 6 week time span. However, a few of these cases have persistent deficits.

❐❐   **Differentiate between decerebrate and decorticate posturing.**

Decerebrate posturing is when the elbows and legs are extended which is indicative of a lesion below the red nucleus, usually in the midbrain.
Decorticate posturing is when the elbows are flexed and the legs are extended. This suggests a lesion above the red nucleus, usually in the midbrain. Remember: DeCORticate = hands by the heart (cor).

❐❐   **When is the onset of epilepsy most common?**

Before the age of 20. In acquired epilepsy, onset usually occurs in patients younger than 20 or older than 60.

❐❐   **How long must a generalized tonic-clonic seizure last without a period of consciousness to be considered status epilepticus?**

30 minutes. Status epilepticus may result from a variety of causes most commonly anticonvulsant therapy withdrawal (missed doses).

❐❐   **A patient opens his eyes to voice, makes incomprehensible sounds, and withdraws to painful stimulus. What is his GCS?**

9.
Glascow coma scale:

Eye opening	Best verbal response	Best motor response
4 spontaneously	5 oriented x 3	6 obeys commands
3 on request	4 confused conversation	5 localizes to pain
2 to pain	3 words spoken	4 withdraws from pain
1 no opening	2 groans to pain	3 flexes either arm
	1 no response	2 extends arm to pain
		1 no response

N.B. This scale is for children >5, there are variations under that age. For example, infants under 1 can achieve a motor score of 5 only, as they cannot obey commmands, and best verbal would be a smile, coo, or appropriate cry.

❏❏ **Differentiate between partial seizures and generalized seizures.**

Partial seizures arise from a single focus and may spread out, whereas generalized seizures involve the whole cerebral cortex. Absence and grand mal seizures are examples of generalized seizures. Generalized and complex partial seizures involve a loss of consciousness. Simple partial seizures do not result in a loss of consciousness.

❏❏ **Recurrent seizures in patients with a history of febrile seizures generally occur in what time frame?**

About 85% occur within the first 2 years. The younger the child, the more likely recurrence will happen. If a patient has a febrile seizure in the first year of life the recurrence rate is 50%. If it occurs in the second year, the recurrence is only 25%.

❏❏ **What will happen if you shine a light in the eyes of a patient who is in a diabetic coma?**

The pupils will constrict.

❏❏ **Distinguish between the gait of a patient with a cerebellar lesion and the gait of a patient with an extrapyramidal lesion.**

The patient with a cerebellar lesion will have truncal ataxia, which is an unsteady, irregular gait with broad steps. A patient with extrapyramidal lesion will have a festinating gait. In the latter case, the patient takes several small, shuffling steps without swinging his/her arms.

❏❏ **The Weber's test is performed on a patient complaining of hearing loss. This patient hears the sound more loudly in his right ear. Which type of hearing loss does this patient have?**

Conductive hearing loss on the right or sensory hearing loss on the left.

❏❏ **What are the expected results when the Rinne's test is conducted on this patient?**

The Rinne's test is performed by placing the tip of the tuning fork on the mastoid process until the patient can no longer hear the tone. The fork is then relocated to just in front of the pinna until the patient can no longer hear the tone. In normal patients, the ratio is 1:2. This patient may not hear the tone any longer when the fork is placed adjacent to the pinna.

❏❏ **What is the _most_ _common_ cause of a subarachnoid hemorrhage?**

Saccular aneurysm.

❏❏ **What are other common causes of a subarachnoid hemorrhage?**

Rupture of cerebral artery aneurysm and arteriovenous malformation. These patients present with an abrupt onset of the worst headache of their lives which can then progress to syncope, nausea, vomiting, nuchal rigidity, and non-focal neurological changes.

❏❏ **Damage to the middle meningeal arteries results in what kind of hematoma?**

An epidural hematoma.

❏❏ **A 16 year old male presents after having his head pounded into the concrete. The patient had a brief episode of LOC but was then ambulatory and alert. Now he appears drowsy and just threw up on you. What is the diagnosis?**

Epidural hematoma.

❏❏ **Which is more common, a subdural hemorrhage or an epidural hemorrhage?**

A subdural. Subdurals can result from the tearing of the bridging veins. Bleeding occurs less rapidly because the veins, not arteries, are damaged.

❏❏ **A patient with back pain who cannot walk on his/her toes has a lesion at what level?**

S1.

❏❏ **A patient with back pain who cannot walk on his/her heels has a lesion at what level?**

L5.

❏❏ **What is wrong with a patient who has back pain when his hip and knee are flexed and the sciatic nerve is "plucked" or "strummed" in the popliteal fossa?**

A disc herniation with nerve root impingement produces this "strum sign."

❏❏ **A 16 year old woman complains of a throbbing, dull, unilateral headache that lasts for hours then goes away with sleep. She also has been nauseous and has vomited twice. She reports small areas of visual loss plus strange zig-zag lines in her vision. What is the diagnosis?**

A classic migraine headache. This title is a misnomer because the classic migraine is in fact rare, accounting for only 1% of migraines. It can be differentiated from the common migraine, the most frequently occurring migraine, because visual disturbances of scotomata and fortification spectra arise in addition to all the other migraine symptoms.

❏❏ **What factors may precipitate migraine headaches?**

Bright lights, cheese, hot-dogs and other foods containing tyramine or nitrates, menstruation, monosodium glutamate, and stress.

❏❏ **Describe the key signs and symptoms of a classic, a common, an ophthalmoplegic, and a hemiplegic migraine headache.**

1) Common: This headache is indeed the most common. It is a slow evolving headache that lasts for hours to days. A positive family history as well as two of the following are prevalent: Nausea or vomiting, throbbing quality, photophobia, unilateral pain, and increase with menses. Distinguishing feature from "Classic" migraine is the lack of visual symptoms.

2) Classic: Prodrome lasts up to 60 minutes. Most common symptom is visual disturbance, such as homonymous hemianopsia, scintillating scotoma, fortification spectra, and photophobia. Lip, face, and hand tingling, as well as aphasia and extremity weakness may occur. Nausea and vomiting may also result.

3) Ophthalmoplegic: Most frequently manifests in young adults. Patient has an outwardly deviated, dilated eye, with ptosis. The third, sixth, and fourth nerves are typically involved. s.

4) Hemiplegic: Unilateral motor and sensory symptoms, mild hemiparesis to hemiplegia are exhibited with this type of headache.

❏❏ **How can you tell if a headache is really caused by of an intracranial tumor?**

By obtaining a CT or MRI. However, everyone who walks into the office complaining of a headache cannot be subjected to these procedures. If the patient complains of the "worst headache of their life," he/she has written a ticket for a scan and LP. Other signs that may suggest a serious underlying disease are headaches that (1) wake patients from their sleep, although cluster headaches may do this, (2) are worse in the morning, (3) increase in severity with postural changes or Valsalva maneuvers, (4) are associated with nausea and vomiting even though migraines have similar symptoms, (5) are associated with focal defects or mental status changes, and (6) occur with a new onset of seizures.

❏❏ **A baby girl was born to a man who developed Huntington's chorea at the age of 44. What are her chances of developing the same disease?**

50%. Huntington's chorea is an autosomal dominant disorder that first manifests itself between the ages of 30-50. Unfortunately, this little girl can expect to become demented, amnesiac, delusional, emotionally unstable, depressed, paranoid, antisocial, and irritable if she inherits the disease. She will also develop chorea, bradykinesia, hypertonia, hyperkinesia, clonus, schizophrenia, intellectual impairment, and bowel incontinence. She will eventually die a premature death 15 years after the onset of her symptoms.

❑❑   **Which chromosome carries the genetic defect in patients with Huntington's chorea?**

The short arm of chromosome #4.

❑❑   **A 17 year old woman with a history of flu like symptoms (URI) one week ago now presents with vertigo, nausea, and vomiting. No auditory impairment or focal deficits are noted. What is the most likely cause of her problem?**

Labyrinthitis or vestibular neuronitis.

❑❑   **At what age is bacterial meningitis <u>most</u> <u>common</u>?**

Infants under 1.

❑❑   **Which bacteria is the <u>most</u> <u>common</u> cause of meningitis in infants under 1?**

Group B *Streptococci* and *E. coli.*

❑❑   **Which organism is frequently responsible for bacterial meningitis in adults?**

Neisseria meningitides.

❑❑   **How does bacterial meningitis differ from viral meningitis in terms of the corresponding CSF lab values?**

Bacterial meningitis will indicate low glucose and high protein levels, while viral meningitis will have normal glucose and a normal protein.

❑❑   **On LP, opening pressure is markedly elevated. What should be done?**

Close the 3-way stopcock, remove only a small amount of fluid from the manometer, abort the LP, and initiate measures to decrease the intracranial pressure.

❑❑   **A patient presents with acute meningitis. When should antibiotics be initiated?**

Immediately. Do not wait. Patients should receive a CT prior to LP only if papilledema or focal deficit is present.

❑❑   **What is the most worrisome diagnosis of a purpuric, petechial rash in an infant?**

Meningococcemia. Other causes include *Hemophilus influenzae, Streptococcus pneumoniae,* and *Staphylococcus aureus.*

❑❑   **Mononeuropathies are <u>most</u> <u>commonly</u> due to what?**

Trauma that results in compression or entrapment of the involved nerve.

❑❑   **A 16 year old female complains of weakness and tingling in her right arm and leg for 2 days. She reports an episode of right eye pain and blurred vision that resolved over one month, but the onset of that pain started 2 years ago. She also recalls a two week episode of intermittent blurred vision the previous year. What is the diagnosis?**

Presumptive multiple sclerosis. Confirm with MRI and CSF (look for oligoclonal bands).

❑❑   **What is the <u>most</u> <u>common</u> presenting symptom of MS?**

Optic neuritis (about 25%).

❑❑   **A patient with MS presents with a fever. The nurse asks, "Should I give the patient Tylenol?" What is your response?**

Yes! Lowering the temperature is important for MS patients because small increases in temperature can worsen existing signs and symptoms.

☐☐ **Which is the <u>most</u> <u>common</u> type of muscular dystrophy?**

Duchenne's muscular dystrophy

☐☐ **Which forms of muscular dystrophy are autosomal dominant and which forms are X-linked?**

Myotonic dystrophy and Fascioscapulohumeral dystrophy are autosomal dominant. Duchenne's muscular dystrophy and Becker muscular dystrophy are X-linked.

☐☐ **Pseudohypertrophy of the calves is characteristic of which type of muscular dystrophy?**

Duchenne's muscular dystrophy. Hypertrophy is due to fatty infiltration of the muscles.

☐☐ **What neoplastic process is <u>most</u> <u>commonly</u> associated with myasthenia gravis?**

Thymoma.

☐☐ **Which is the <u>most</u> <u>common</u> medication associated with Neuroleptic Malignant Syndrome?**

Haloperidol. Other drugs, especially antipsychotic medications, are also causative.

☐☐ **What is the hallmark motor finding in Neuroleptic Malignant Syndrome?**

"Lead pipe" rigidity.

☐☐ **What is Shy-Drager syndrome?**

A rare, gradually progressive degeneration of the autonomic nervous system characterized by very low blood pressure, lack of coordination, muscle wasting, stiffness, and lack of bladder and/or bowel control. This syndrome occurs more often in young people.

☐☐ **What is the <u>most</u> <u>common</u> cause of syncope?**

Vasovagal or simple fainting (50%).

☐☐ **In order for a patient to faint from cardiac causes, to what level must the cardiac output fall?**

50% the normal capacity. Cardiac syncope can occur because of mechanical causes, such as aortic or pulmonic obstruction and arrhythmias, or because of ischemic causes, such as MI or aortic dissection.

☐☐ **A child that you have been following since birth is brought to you at age 9 months because he is having frequent convulsions and cannot control his muscles enough to even hold his head up anymore. You noted a developmental road block at the age of 6 months, and now it seems the child is regressing in both motor and cognitive skills. On exam, the patient has a cherry-red macula. What is the patient's prognosis?**

This patient probably has Tay-Sachs disease and will go blind and become demented and paralyzed. He will die before the age of 4.

☐☐ **What is the probable ethnic background of the patient described in the above case?**

Eastern European Jewish or French Canadian.

☐☐ **For the following clinical presentations, identify if each is associated with peripheral vertigo or with central vertigo.**

1) Intense spinning, nausea, hearing loss, diaphoresis.
2) Swaying or impulsion, worse with movement, tinnitus, acute onset.
3) Unidirectional nystagmus inhibited by ocular fixation, fatigable.

4) Mild vertigo, diplopia, and ataxia.

5) Multi-directional nystagmus not inhibited by ocular fixation, non-fatigable.

Answers: peripheral vertigo: (1), (2), and (3); central vertigo: (4) and (5).

☐☐   **What maneuver can be performed to determine whether vertigo is peripheral or central?**

The Nylen-Barany maneuver. It is performed as follows: The patient is rapidly brought from the sitting to the supine position, and the head is then turned 45°. If unidirectional nystagmus is seen, the cause is most likely peripheral. If the nystagmus generated is non-fatiguing and multidirectional, search for a more central cause.

☐☐   **A patient has an irritative lesion in the left hemisphere. Which way do his eyes deviate?**

To the right, away from the lesion.

☐☐   **What is the significance of bilateral nystagmus with cold caloric testing?**

It signifies that an intact cortex, midbrain, and brainstem are present.

☐☐   **What are the main stages in brain development, when do they occur, and what are the clinical abnormalities seen?**

Neurulation occurs between 3-7 weeks gestational age and results in the formation of the primitive neural tube. Failure of neurulation results in neural tube defects ranging from anacephaly to spina bifida. Neural proliferation occurs between 2-4 months gestational age and defects can result in both macrocephaly and microcephaly. Neuronal migration occurs between 3-5 months gestational age and abnormalities lead to lissencephaly, pachy-and polymicro-gyria, and neuronal heterotopias. Organization occurs from 5 months gestational age to years post-natal and defects are likely causes of mental retardation. Finally, myelination takes place from birth to years post-natal and these syndromes have not been well described.

☐☐   **What is the brain structure which is most likely to be involved in intraventricular hemorrhage in a premature infant?**

The germinal matrix.

☐☐   **What is the most common motor deficit seen in premature infants after a periventricular hemorrhage?**

Spastic diplegia. Since the axons that carry information from the motor neurons controlling the legs run the closest to the ventricles, these are the most often affected, resulting in a spastic diplegia. Upper extremities can also be involved but usually to a lesser degree.

☐☐   **What symptoms form the classic tetrad seen in kernicterus?**

Choreoathetosis, supernuclear ophthalmoplegia, sensorineural hearing loss, and enamel hypoplasia.

☐☐   **What are the two classic forms of brachial plexopathy seen after birth trauma?**

Erbs palsy results from damage to the upper plexus (C5 and C6 roots) due to stretching from traction on the shoulder. This is the most common and results in the 'waiter's tip' positioning of the arm. Klumpke's palsy results from traction on the abducted forearm causing injury to the lower plexus and an absent or weak grasp.

☐☐   **What are the four types of Arnold-Chiari malformations?**

Type I consists of downward displacement of the cerebellar tonsils, may be associated with syringomyelia and presents mainly in adolescents with symptoms related to either hydrocephalus or syringomyelia. However, type I is typically asymptomatic. Type II is more severe and associated with a myelomenigocele. It presents in newborns with hydrocephalus and myelomenigocele. Type III is associated with encephalocele and is analogous to type I and II. Type IV includes cerebellar hypoplasia but is not associated with any spinal malformations. While it is included in Chiari's original description, it is not considered to be caused by the same mechanism.

☐☐   **What are the two main forms of neurofibromatosis?**

Type 1 (NF1), von Recklinghausen disease or peripheral neurofibromatosis, consists of cafe-au-lait spots, neurofibromas, plexiform neuromas, iris hamartomas (Lisch nodules), optic gliomas, and osseous lesions. It is caused by a mutation in the gene on chromosome 17, and accounts for 85% of all neurofibromatosis. Type 2 (NF2), central neurofibromatosis, involves tumors of cranial nerve VIII and the gene is linked to chromosome 18.

☐☐   **What are the main intracranial lesions of tuberous sclerosis (TS)?**

Tubers, subependymal nodules and subependymal giant cell astrocytomas.

☐☐   **What cardiac abnormality is associated with TS?**

Rhabdomyomas appear in infancy and can be large enough to cause heart failure and death in as many as one quarter of the patients. They often resolve spontaneously.

☐☐   **What are the renal lesions associated with TS?**

These include angiomyolipomas and renal cysts.

☐☐   **What is the immunological abnormalities associated with ataxia-telangiectasia?**

These include increased susceptibility to sinopulmonary infections and increased risk of malignancy, such as lymphoma. Often absent or low levels of IgA, normal or low levels of IgG and increased or normal levels of IgM can be utilized to help make the diagnosis.

☐☐   **How is Prader-Willi syndrome and Angelman syndrome related?**

Both syndromes are caused by deletions of chromosome 15q11q13. If the deletion is on the paternal chromosome, the Prader-Willi syndrome consisting of hypotonia, hyperphagia, hypogenitalism and mild to moderate retardation is seen. If the deletion is on the maternal chromosome then the 'happy puppet' syndrome of Angelman is seen. This consists of severe mental retardation, ataxia with jerking of the limbs and trunk and a happy demeanor.

☐☐   **What is the most common cranial suture involved in craniosynastosis and what is the shape of the head that results?**

The sagittal suture. The head is long and narrow (scaphocephaly).

☐☐   **Intrauterine seizures can be seen with which vitamin deficiency?**

Pyridoxine (vitamin B6).

☐☐   **What are the two disorders involving copper metabolism?**

Wilson's disease (hepatolenticular degeneration) with diminished ceruloplasmin and copper accumulation and Menkes disease (Kinky hair disease) with maldistribution of copper leading to decreased synthesis of copper-containing enzymes.

☐☐   **What is the enzyme defect in Lesch-Nyhan disease?**

Hypoxanthine-guanine phosphoribosyltransferase (HGPRT).

☐☐   **What is the pathology associated with Rett syndrome?**

Rett syndrome is a neurodevelopmental disorder only seen in females. It presents with acquired microcephaly, psychomotor retardation, spasticity, seizures and characteristic hand-wringing movements. The brains at autopsy are found to be small and the neurons have decreased numbers of dendrites.

❏❏   **What is done to try to prevent the sensorineural hearing loss in children with bacterial meningitis?**

Sensorineural hearing loss occurs in 10% of children with bacterial meningitis, with it being bilateral in 4%. This is usually a severe to profound loss and more common with *H. influenzae* infections. Starting the patient on steroids just prior to giving antibiotics has been shown to reduce the frequency of hearing loss. Due to the rapid decline of H. flu meningitis, secondary to vaccination, this is not done routinely.

❏❏   **Ampicillin is used in the treatment of meningitis in newborns to cover which organism?**

Listeria monocytogenes.

❏❏   **Which are the two most common organisms to cause meningitis in patients with a ventriculo-peritoneal (VP) shunt?**

Staphylococcus epidermidis and *Staphylococcus aureus.*

❏❏   **Which vitamin should be given routinely during the treatment of tuberculous meningitis?**

Isoniazid can induce a peripheral neuropathy which can be prevented by the co-administration of vitamin B6.

❏❏   **What are the three most common predisposing factors in the formation of a brain abscess?**

Cyanotic heart disease, otitis and sinusitis.

❏❏   **What is the most common cranial neuropathy seen in Borreliosis (Lyme disease)?**

Unilateral or bilateral facial palsy. Less frequently, the VIII nerve can also be affected.

❏❏   **What is the characteristic EEG abnormalities seen with subacute sclerosing panencephalitis (SSPE)?**

SSPE is a chronic encephalitis caused by an atypical infection by measles virus. It presents with marked personality changes and a dementia that is characterized by aphasia, apraxia, and agnosia. Myoclonic jerks are common and eye findings such as chorioretinitis are seen. The EEG consists of pseudo-periodic EEG complexes.

❏❏   **Which virus is thought to be associated with Mollaret recurrent meningitis?**

Mollaret meningitis is a multirecurrent meningitis characterized by the presence of Mollaret cells, large mononuclear cells, in the CSF. It is thought to be caused by an atypical herpes simplex infection.

❏❏   **What is the most common paraneoplastic syndrome seen in children?**

Opsoclonus-myoclonus ('dancing eyes-dancing feet') is seen with neuroblastoma. Unlike most paraneoplastic syndromes seen in adulthood, it is responsive to immunosuppressive therapy.

❏❏   **What are growing skull fractures?**

These are seen as a complication of skull fracture in children under three years of age. They are caused by the presence of leptomeningeal cyst that is formed by an unrecognized dural laceration. It prevents the two sides of the bone from aligning together during recovery.

❏❏   **When should steroids be used in the treatment of increased intracranial pressure (ICP)?**

Steroids are beneficial in the treatment of vasogenic edema, so should be used to treat increased ICP associated with tumors, abscesses and brain trauma.

❏❏   **What cutaneous manifestation is seen in patients with Sturge-Weber disease?**

A Port-wine stain, or angiomatous naevus, is seen in the distribution of cranial nerve V. This may be associated with pial angiomas. Seizures are the main clinical manifestation but hemiparesis can also be seen.

❏❏ **What are the typical EEG findings of absence seizures?**

Typically, absence seizures are preceded by a run of 3 Hz spike and wave. This can be brought out by hyperventilation during the EEG.

❏❏ **What is the West syndrome?**

Infantile spasms, hysparrhythmia on EEG, and developmental delay.

❏❏ **What is the drug of choice in juvenile myoclonic epilepsy?**

Valproate.

❏❏ **What is the main difference in the history obtained between seizures and breath-holding spells?**

Breath-holding spells are always provoked. Cyanotic breath-holding spells are provoked by crying precipitated by fright, anger, pain, or frustration. Pallid breath-holding spells are provoked by pain, especially a minor bump to the head.

❏❏ **Why is a family history of deafness important in evaluating a patient with episodes of sudden loss of consciousness?**

Jervell-Lange-Nielson syndrome is associated with prolonged Q-T and neurosensory hearing loss. Prolonged Q-T syndromes must be identified because they can lead to sudden death.

❏❏ **What is Sandifer syndrome?**

Opisthotonic posturing which occurs because of GE reflux due to hiatal hernias may be mistaken for seizures, spasticity or other movement disorders.

❏❏ **What percent of migraine patients have their onset of headaches prior to age 5 years of age?**

20%.

❏❏ **Ophthalmoplegic migraine most commonly affects which cranial nerve?**

Cranial nerve III.

❏❏ **In which stage(s) of sleep does night terrors (parvor nocturnus) occur?**

They occur during stage III and IV of sleep, distinguishing them from nightmares which occur during REM sleep.

❏❏ **What are the clinical findings of Klein-Levin syndrome?**

This syndrome occurs in adolescent males and presents with episodes of hypersomnia, hyperphagia and frontal lobe-type personality changes.

❏❏ **Which metabolic peripheral neuropathy can be clinically misdiagnosed as Friedreich's ataxia?**

Vitamin E deficiency.

❏❏ **Which toxic neuropathy can be clinically misdiagnosed in infants as Guillian-Barre syndrome?**

Botulism. Unlike in older patients that ingest the toxin, infants are usually colonized by the bacteria. A risk factor seems to be feeding the infant honey.

❑❑   **What is the difference between neonatal myasthenia and congenital myasthenia?**

Neonatal myasthenia is transiently seen in newborns of mothers with myasthenia gravis. The symptoms begin a few hours after birth, can last for up to three days, and are due to circulating maternal antibodies. Congenital myasthenia presents at birth with ophthalmoplegia and is caused by the lack of various proteins important to the transduction of the signal across the synaptic cleft.

❑❑   **What components of the history are the most important in evaluating a child with neurological problems?**

Developmental, perinatal, birth and family.

❑❑   **What is the significance of a mildly depressed and pulsatile fontanelle in an infant?**

Nothing. This is normal.

❑❑   **What does the clasp-knife phenomenon indicate?**

That the child has some spasticity, indicating upper motor neuron (CNS) dysfunction. This is elicited by sensing resistance to passive movement followed by sudden release of resistance.

❑❑   **What would you expect to find in a child with rigidity?**

Cogwheeling, or constant resistance to passive movement.

❑❑   **What are the inheritance patterns for Duchennes muscular dystrophy and Becker muscular dystrophy?**

Both are inherited in an X-linked fashion.

❑❑   **What is Gower's sign?**

A specific way to rise to standing from the supine position that is seen in certain forms of muscular dystrophy, indicative of maximal muscular weakness. The child first rolls over onto hands and knees. Then the child stands up by "walking" his/her hands up the leg.

❑❑   **Two days after surgery, an adolescent complains of left lower leg weakness. CSF analysis shows elevated protein but normal WBC count. What idiopathic disease might be at work here?**

Guillain-Barré syndrome.

❑❑   **What is the most useful test to diagnose multiple sclerosis in children?**

MRI showing multiple white matter plaques in the periventricular regions.

❑❑   **In a child in a coma you elicit positive doll's eyes reflex. Does this mean the eyes move with the head, or away from the head?**

Away from the movement of the head. This sign determines viability of the brainstem. A positive sign means the brainstem function is intact.

❑❑   **Which way do the eyes move in normal caloric testing?**

Remember the mnemonic COWS- Cold Opposite, Warm Same. Absence of the nystagmus occurs with eighth nerve damage.

❑❑   **What is the most common cause of acute onset, painless monocular blindness in patients between 15-45?**

Optic neuritis. 60% of these patients eventually develop multiple sclerosis.

❑❑   **Patients diagnosed with pseudotumor cerebri should be periodically tested for what development?**

Loss of visual fields.

☐☐   **What is the most effective way to reduce the incidence of post lumbar puncture headaches?**

Use the smallest gauge possible (in the original studies that describe this phenomenon, 16 gauge needles were used and up to 12 cc of fluid was removed!).

☐☐   **A Babinski sign is indicative of an abnormality of what tract?**

Corticospinal. It is indicative of an upper motor neuron lesion.

☐☐   **In an extremely ticklish patient that will not let you perform the Babinski maneuver, or makes it difficult to interpret, what other maneuver could be used?**

The Chaddock maneuver. In this maneuver, the outer part of the dorsum of the foot is stroked. Extension of the toe is indicative of an upper motor neuron lesion.

☐☐   **What is the incidence of a child with a history of febrile seizures developing a convulsive disorder compared with a child who has never had a febrile seizure?**

It is the same.

☐☐   **What is the drug of choice for febrile seizures?**

Trick question, no treatment is usually given. However, if treatment is used, the drug of choice is Phenobarbital.

☐☐   **What type of movement disorder is associated with rheumatic fever?**

Sydenham chorea.

☐☐   **A child is brought in with a new onset "tic". What is your treatment?**

None at this time. Simple clonic motor tics usually resolve spontaneously in less than a year.

☐☐   **How do you diagnose Tourette's syndrome?**

Clinically. The patient must have complex tics for > 6 months, with vocal components (such as coprolalia), in the absence of any other medical etiology.

☐☐   **What other problems are commonly seen in patients with Gilles de la Tourette's syndrome?**

ADHD, learning difficulties, emotional problems, or social problems.

☐☐   **What is the drug of choice in the treatment of Tourette's syndrome?**

Haloperidol or pimozide.

☐☐   **What can you give to ameliorate the dystonic reactions sometimes seen in a patient taking haloperidol?**

Benztropine (Cogentin).

☐☐   **What metabolic abnormalities can cause neonatal seizures?**

Hypoxemia, hypoglycemia, hypocalcemia, hypomagnesemia and hyponatremia.

☐☐   **Why should you look in the eyes of a patient with neurofibromatosis (Von Recklinghausen's disease)?**

To look for Lisch nodules and optic glioma.

☐☐   **What are these Lisch nodules you are looking for?**

Pigmented iris hamartomas.

❏❏   **On a routine newborn examination of a full term black infant you notice a large cafe-au-lait spot on the thigh. What is the most likely diagnosis?**

Normal examination.

❏❏   **A 5 year old is brought to the ED for a new onset seizure. On examination you notice a rash on the face and a large, rough lesion in the lumbosacral area. What is the most likely diagnosis?**

Tuberous sclerosis. The skin lesion on the back is a Shagreen patch.

❏❏   **What disease classically presents with a port wine stain on the face?**

Sturge-Weber syndrome.

❏❏   **What is the treatment for infant botulism?**

Trivalent immune serum as well as respiratory support.

❏❏   **What is the definition of ataxia?**

Ataxia is an impairment in the coordination of movement without the loss of muscle strength.

❏❏   **What is the most common posterior fossa tumor?**

Astrocytoma.

❏❏   **What clinical features are found in patients with ataxia-telangiectasia?**

Clinical features include: 1) neurologic dysfunction, which primarily manifests as ataxia, choreoathetosis, involuntary myoclonus and abnormalities of oculomotor function; 2) telangiectasias of the bulbar conjunctiva, which appear between the ages of 2-5; 3) endocrine dysfunction, such as abnormal glucose tolerance; 4) agenesis of the ovaries; 5) predisposition to cancers, such as Non-Hodgkin lymphoma. Some patients may have immunodeficiency as well.

❏❏   **Can ataxia be a manifestation of Guillain Barre syndrome?**

Yes- if there is a significant sensory neuropathy present, there may be an impairment of afferent sensory input to the cerebellum, causing a "sensory ataxia", in addition to the muscle weakness and areflexia seen in these patients.

❏❏   **What is the definition of "status epilepticus"?**

Status epilepticus is defined as either continuos or repetitive seizures that last longer than 30 minutes; the patient does not regain consciousness during this time.

❏❏   **What clinical features define a simple febrile seizure?**

1) Brief duration, usually less than 15 minutes
2) Generalized seizure
3) Occur within the first 24 hours of a febrile illness
4) Occur in children between 1-4 years of age, who have
5) Normal neurologic development
6) Normal neurologic examination after the seizure

❏❏   **Will a child with simple febrile seizures have a normal electroencephalogram (EEG)?**

Yes-an interictal EEG will be normal except for possible post-ictal generalized background slowing.

❏❏   **What is the likelihood of a second febrile seizure in a child with a normal neurologic exam and normal psychomotor development?**

The recurrence rate after the first simple febrile seizure is approximately 30%.

❐❐ **What clinical features characterize children with benign paroxysmal vertigo?**

Clinical features include : 1) age less than 4 years; 2) sudden onset of vertigo, which manifests as sudden imbalance, where the child will cry out, appear frightened and try to hold onto a stabilizing object; 3) autonomic symptoms, such as nausea, vomiting and sweating; 4) nystagmus, which will be present during the episode and often helps diagnose this condition. There is no loss of consciousness during these episodes.

❐❐ **Why is lorazepam preferable to diazepam as a first line medication to stop seizure activity?**

Lorazepam has the same efficacy as diazepam to stop seizure activity; it also shares with diazepam similar side effects, such as sedation, respiratory and cardiovascular depression. However, lorazepam has a longer effective half-life (up to 3 hours), which may preclude adding a second anticonvulsant.

❐❐ **What side effects of valproic acid limit its usefulness in young children with generalized seizures?**

Though valproic acid is very effective in treating generalized seizures, it has been shown to cause irreversible hepatic dysfunction and bone marrow failure, leading to death, in children less than 2 years of age.

❐❐ **What side effects limit the long term use of phenytoin to treat generalized seizures in young children?**

Though gingival hyperplasia can be managed with good dental hygiene, phenytoin can cause problematic cosmetic effects, such as hirsutism and coarsening of the facial features, which limit its usefulness in treating young children with generalized epilepsy.

❐❐ **What type(s) of seizures are well controlled with carbamazepime?**

Generalized tonic-clonic, partial and complex partial seizures.

❐❐ **What type(s) of seizures are well controlled with ethosuximide?**

Absence (petit mal) seizures.

❐❐ **Clonazepam is a useful adjunct therapy to treat what type(s) of seizures?**

Akinetic and generalized motor seizures.

❐❐ **What clinical features are seen in children with cluster headaches?**

Cluster headaches are unilateral and are associated with autonomic nervous system symptoms as tearing and rhinorrhea. Episodes occur close together, or in "clusters".

❐❐ **What criteria must be met before the diagnosis of migraine headache can be made?**

In addition to repeated episodes of headache, at least three of the following symptoms must be present: 1) family history of migraine headache; 2) visual, sensory, motor or vertiginous aura prior to the onset of the headache; 3) nausea/vomiting or recurrent abdominal pain accompanying the headache; 4) unilateral head pain that is throbbing or pounding; 5) relief of pain by a brief period of sleep.

❐❐ **What symptoms and signs distinguish transverse myelitis from Guillain-Barre syndrome?**

Both transverse myelitis and acute polyneuritis share the acute onset of lower extremity weakness and paresthesias as presenting symptoms and signs. Patients with transverse myelitis will initially complain of back pain (in the absence of trauma) and urinary retention. Patients with Guillain-Barre syndrome will have bowel and bladder dysfunction later in the course. On physical examination of patients with transverse myelitis, a distinct "sensory level" will also be elicited; impairment of touch, pain and temperature sensation will be seen, but proprioception will remain intact.

☐☐   **What is the pathophysiology of Guillain-Barre syndrome?**

The pathologic hallmark of acute polyneuritis is demyelination of motor and sensory nerves, thought to be due to an autoimmune process, causing the classic ascending paralysis, areflexia and paresthesias seen in these patients.

☐☐   **What is the "Fisher variant" of Guillain-Barre syndrome?**

Patients with the Fisher variant of acute polyneuritis will have areflexia, oculomotor palsies and ataxia as the predominant physical findings.

☐☐   **What is the pathophysiology of myasthenia gravis?**

Antibodies against the acetylcholine receptor of the post-synaptic neuromuscular junction-this results in failure of neuromuscular transmission, with consequent fluctuating muscle weakness.

☐☐   **What are the presenting signs and symptoms of juvenile myasthenia gravis?**

The juvenile form of myasthenia gravis accounts for 25% of all cases and is the predominant form seen in the pediatric population, usually in school-age children. Most patients will have ptosis, oculomotor palsies and truncal or limb weakness that becomes progressively worse with continued muscle activity.

☐☐   **What is the "Tensilon test"?**

The Tensilon test secures the diagnosis of myasthenia gravis. Edrophonium (Tensilon), which is an anticholinesterase drug, is given slowly by the intravenous route. Patients with myasthenia gravis will have a brief, but dramatic, resolution of their muscle weakness.

☐☐   **A 4 year old presents with the acute onset of unsteadiness of gait. He has otherwise been well, except for a recent upper respiratory infection. Examination reveals ataxia, tremor and bilateral dysmetria. What is the most likely diagnosis?**

Acute cerebellar ataxia, which is characterized by the acute onset of ataxia in an otherwise healthy child, usually between the ages of 1 and 4 years. Antecedent viral infections precede the onset of symptoms in over half of patients. Resolution of symptoms usually occurs within 2 weeks of the onset of symptoms.

☐☐   **What must be excluded in the above patient before the diagnosis of acute cerebellar ataxia?**

A posterior fossa mass or tumor.

☐☐   **What other organ systems are involved in patients with Duchenne muscular dystrophy?**

Cardiomyopathy, to varying degrees, is found in nearly every patient, as well as intellectual impairment, most often in the form of learning disabilities.

☐☐   **Is Lyme disease a common cause of seventh nerve palsy?**

Yes. There is a subset of patients with Lyme disease who present solely with an isolated seventh nerve palsy. This is especially true in patients with bilateral seventh nerve palsies.

☐☐   **What is the likelihood that a patient with Bell's Palsy will completely recover?**

Complete recovery is seen in up to 80% of patients, usually within three weeks of the onset of symptoms.

☐☐   **What are some clinical findings that may be present in patients with myelomeningoceles?**

Deficits in lower extremity motor function; disturbances in bowel and bladder function; hydrocephalus, which is seen in up to 75% of cases; and arthrogryposis, which are contractures of the lower extremities due to lack of lower extremity movement in utero.

☐☐   **What CNS malformation may be seen in patients who have myelomeningocele and hydrocephalus?**

Arnold-Chiari malformations.

❑❑   **What is the defect responsible for spina bifida occulta?**

Spina bifida occulta occurs because of a vertebral defect, usually in the lumbosacral region, that does not lead to a herniation of the contents of the spinal canal.

❑❑   **What are the cutaneous manifestations that may be seen in patients with spina bifida occulta?**

Some patients may have a hairy tuft or a "birth mark" at the base of the spine. Occasionally, there may be a sinus tract that leads to an intraspinal cyst. Most patients, however, are asymptomatic.

❑❑   **What is the definition of " non-communicating" hydrocephalus?**

If the obstruction to the flow of cerebrospinal fluid occurs within the ventricular system, then non-communicating hydrocephalus results.

❑❑   **What is the definition of "communicating" hydrocephalus?**

If the obstruction to the flow of cerebrospinal fluid occurs outside the ventricular system at the level of any of the exit foramina or if there is an excessive production of cerebrospinal fluid, then communicating hydrocephalus results.

❑❑   **What clinical features make up the Dandy-Walker syndrome?**

The clinical features making up the Dandy-Walker syndrome include: 1) failed formation of the cerebellar vermis; 2) cyst in the floor of the fourth ventricle; 3) anterior compression of the aqueduct of Sylvius; 4) obstruction of the exit foramen of the fourth ventricle.

❑❑   **How do neonatal seizures differ from seizures in older children?**

In contrast to older children, in whom idiopathic epilepsy is common, seizures in neonates are usually secondary phenomena of underlying disease.

❑❑   **What are some of the underlying disease states that may lead to neonatal seizures?**

- Metabolic disturbances, such as hypoglycemia, hypocalcemia, hypomagnesemia, hyponatremia;
- Hypoxic ischemic encephalopathy;
- Intracranial hemorrhage;
- CNS infections, both bacterial and viral;
- Pyridoxine dependent seizures;
- Maternal drug abuse in the third trimester, such as methadone addiction or passive exposure ex-utero, such as that from crack cocaine;
- Local anesthetic intoxication;
- Familial neonatal convulsions.

❑❑   **What is the most common cause of neonatal seizures?**

Hypoxic-ischemic encephalopathy, which accounts for nearly 60% of cases.

❑❑   **What is the treatment for infantile botulism?**

Therapy is supportive, such as nasogastric feeding and support of respiration. Antibiotics do not halt the progression of the disease.

❑❑   **What is the definition of macrocephaly?**

Macrocephaly is defined as a head circumference two standard deviations above the mean.

❑❑   **What is the definition of microcephaly?**

Microcephaly is defined as a head circumference two standard deviations below the mean.

❑❑   **What agents are useful to decrease the production of cerebrospinal fluid (CSF) in patients with hydrocephalus?**

Acetozolamide, furosemide and glycerol have all been used to decrease CSF production.

❑❑   **What is "benign intracranial hypertension" (pseudotumor cerebri)?**

Benign intracranial hypertension is a syndrome in which patients have symptoms and signs (headache, papilledema) of increased intracranial pressure; however, physical examination shows no focal neurologic deficits or encephalopathy and there is no evidence of an intracranial mass or obstruction to the flow of CSF. CSF analysis will be normal except for increased opening pressure.

❑❑   **What drugs are thought to be associated with the development of benign intracranial hypertension (pseudotumor cerebri)?**

Antibiotics, such as tetracycline, minocycline, penicillin, gentamycin; oral contraceptives; steroids; NSAIDS such as indomethacin; thyroid; hormone; lithium carbonate.

❑❑   **Deficiency of what vitamin may cause benign intracranial hypertension (pseudotumor cerebri)?**

Vitamin A.

❑❑   **What is the most common cause of intracranial bleeding in children?**

Congenital malformations of cerebral blood vessels, such as arteriovenous malformations (AVM's).

❑❑   **What are the two most common presentations of arteriovenous malformations (AVM's) in children?**

50-75% of patients with AVM's will present with intracranial hemorrhage (usually subarachnoid hemorrhage), while 25-40% will present with seizures.

❑❑   **What is the most common complication from a linear skull fracture?**

A subgaleal hematoma is the most common complication. These hematomas can become very large, especially if they liquefy and dissect through the subgaleal space.

❑❑   **A 5 month old child presents with coma. There is no history of reported trauma or viral prodrome. On examination the child is afebrile, comatose, with decerebrate posturing and fixed, dilated pupils and a bulging fontanel. What other physical examination finding would help to confirm the diagnosis?**

Fundoscopic examination-if retinal hemorrhages are present, then this is most likely a case of a shaking-impact injury. A CT scan may show subdural or intracranial hemorrhage.

❑❑   **Can significant head trauma, causing intracranial bleeding, lead to hypovolemic shock in a child?**

As a general rule, closed head trauma, no matter how significant, rarely causes hypovolemic shock in children. However, children less than 12 months of age who have large epidural hematomas with overlying skull fractures may decompress the hematoma into the scalp to a degree that significant blood loss can occur. This is the one rare exception to the rule.

❑❑   **A child with a significant closed head injury develops generalized seizures. Which (intravenous) anticonvulsant should be administered?**

Phenytoin, as it will not cloud the sensorium or cause sedation, so that subsequent neurologic examinations can be done easily.

❑❑   **What is the first cranial nerve abnormality seen in the early stages of transtentorial herniation?**

Because of its course along the parahippocampal gyrus of the temporal lobe, which is that portion of the brain that herniates through the tentorium, the third cranial nerve is compressed, leading to a unilateral fixed, dilated pupil.

⬜⬜   **A child presents with severe somnolence and a two week history of gradually worsening headache. On examination he is somnolent and responsive only to pain. He also has bilateral sixth nerve palsies. What is the cause of his symptoms?**

A diffuse increase in intracranial pressure, probably the result of an intracranial mass.

⬜⬜   **What clinical signs are present in patients with cerebellar tonsillar herniation (through the foramen magnum)?**

These patients often have a "head tilt", usually to the side of the tonsillar herniation. If bilateral tonsillar herniation is present, patients will have neck pain that is alleviated by extension of the neck.

⬜⬜   **An otherwise healthy child presents with high fever, headache, stiff neck and somnolence. On examination he has a left hemiparesis. What is the cause of these signs and symptoms?**

This child most likely has a subdural empyema, which can occur alone or with meningitis.

⬜⬜   **What is the mechanism for the development of a subdural empyema?**

Subdural empyemas occur most often as a sequelae of chronic sinusitis; there may be direct extension of bacterial pathogens from sinus cavities that are contiguous with the CNS or from septic venous thromboses. Subdural empyemas may also occur on first presentation, or after several days of therapy, in patients with bacterial meningitis

⬜⬜   **Which procedure is more sensitive to detect subarachnoid hemorrhage- a lumbar puncture or CT scan of the head?**

A lumbar puncture is a more sensitive procedure than CT to detect subarachnoid hemorrhage, as it can detect small amounts of blood in the subarachnoid space. An atraumatic lumbar puncture that is bloody, but does not "clear" (the number of RBC's in the first tube is not greater than that in the last tube) is suggestive of a subarachnoid hemorrhage. CT scan is 97.5% sensitive by itself, according to recent literature, but LP is still considered standard of care after CT.

⬜⬜   **What are the four major groups of signs and symptoms seen in children with brain tumors?**

1) Severe, recurrent headaches, with/without vomiting; 2) Cerebellar ataxia; 3) Acute deterioration in level of consciousness; 4) Acute onset of cranial nerve palsies.

⬜⬜   **What signs and symptoms are suggestive of a mass lesion/tumor in the infratentorial region?**

Patients with infratentorial mass lesions will more often present with cerebellar dysmetria, gait ataxia, vomiting and cranial nerve palsies.

⬜⬜   **What signs and symptoms are suggestive of a mass lesion/tumor in the supratentorial region?**

Patients with supratentorial mass lesions will more often present with intellectual disturbances, speech difficulties, visual field cuts, seizures and hemiparesis.

⬜⬜   **What is "lissencephaly"?**

Lissencephaly is an unusual disorder that is characterized by the absence of cerebral gyri and poorly formed sylvian fissures, leading to a smooth appearance of the surface of the brain. This defect is caused by faulty migration of neuroblasts during embryogenesis.

❑❑   **What clinical features are found in infants with lissencephaly?**

These infants present with failure to thrive, microcephaly, marked developmental delay, hypoplasia of the optic nerve, microopthalmia and severe seizures.

❑❑   **What infectious agents may cause myositis?**

Infectious causes of myositis are usually viral in origin and include Influenza A and Coxsackie virus, types A and B. Multiple abscesses of muscle from *Staphylococcus aureus* and trichinosis are unusual causes of myositis.

❑❑   **What type of breathing pattern is seen in patients with "Cheyne-Stokes" respirations?**

Patients with Cheyne-Stokes respirations will have periods of hyperpnea followed by shorter periods of apnea.

❑❑   **Where is the dysfunction in the CNS in patients who have Cheyne-Stokes respirations?**

Patients with Cheyne-Stokes respirations have bilateral cerebral hemisphere dysfunction with normal brainstem function.

❑❑   **Can otitis media be a cause of vertigo in children?**

Yes; children with acute otitis media may often complain of decreased hearing and impaired balance, but occasionally purulent otitis media may lead to a serous labyrinthitis, resulting in vertiginous symptoms and temporary hearing loss.

❑❑   **What is the most common cause of labyrinthitis in children?**

Labyrinthitis in children is most often due to viral causes, such as influenza, measles and mumps.

❑❑   **Which symptoms help to distinguish vestibular neuronitis from labyrinthitis in children?**

Both labyrinthitis and vestibular neuronitis are causes of vertigo in children and often are associated with coexisting viral infection. However, children with labyrinthitis will have hearing loss, while those with vestibular neuronitis will not.

❑❑   **What clinical features characterize children with cyclic vomiting?**

Cyclic vomiting is a migraine variant that may present in young children. These patients will have cyclic, or even monthly, episodes of vomiting with abdominal pain that are alleviated by periods of deep sleep. Later in life, these children often develop migraine headaches.

❑❑   **What clinical features characterize children with acute confusional states?**

Acute confusional states are migraine variants that have unusual presentations, such as the onset of headache that is followed by a period of vomiting, lethargy and confusion, disorientation and unresponsiveness. These episodes of "acute confusion" may last for several hours, after which the patient may have no memory of the event. There will be a family history of migraine headache.

❑❑   **How does one make the diagnosis of acute confusional state?**

The diagnosis is often made by a history of headache followed by a period of confusion or unresponsiveness that is not due to any other organic cause and a family history or migraine headache. An EEG may reveal localized areas of slowing during and shortly after the attack, after which the EEG will be normal.

❑❑   **What skin manifestation is seen in nearly every patient with neurofibromatosis?**

Cafe-au-lait spots > than 5 that are 5 mm in diameter in prepubertal patients, > than 6 that are 15 mm in diameter in postpubertal patients.

❑❑   **What two skin manifestations may be present in patients with neurofibromatosis?**

Axillary or inguinal freckling; and cutaneous neurofibromas, which appear during adolescence or pregnancy and are small, rubbery purplish masses.

❑❑ **What other clinical features are seen in patients with neurofibromatosis, type 1?**

In addition to cafe-au-lait spots, axillary freckling and neurofibromas, patients may have Lisch nodules, which are hamartomas of the iris; osseous lesions, such as dysplasia of the sphenoid wing and bowing of the tibia and fibula; and optic gliomas. Patients may also have CNS abnormalities, such as seizures, learning disabilities, and difficulty paying attention.

❑❑ **What clinical feature distinguishes patients with neurofibromatosis, type 2?**

Bilateral acoustic neuromas, which are a cause of hearing loss, problems with balance and facial weakness, are most characteristic of patients with neurofibromatosis, type 2.

❑❑ **What neurocutaneous syndrome may be seen in patients with infantile spasms?**

Tuberous sclerosus.

❑❑ **What characteristic skin lesions are present in the majority of patients with tuberous sclerosus?**

Hypopigmented patches, occasionally resembling an "ash leaf", are seen in nearly 90% of patients with tuberous sclerosus.

❑❑ **What instrument may aid in the identification of the hypopigmented patches in patients suspected of having tuberous sclerosus?**

A Wood's lamp, which provides an ultraviolet light source, will aid in the identification of patients with tuberous sclerosus.

❑❑ **What two skin manifestations may be seen in patients with tuberous sclerosus?**

1. "Shagreen patches", which are raised lesions with an "orange peel" consistency, often found in the lumbosacral region;
2. Sebaceous adenomas, which are red nodules of the nose and cheeks that are seen in children over 4 years of age.

❑❑ **What cardiac lesions are seen in some patients with tuberous sclerosus?**

Cardiac rhabdomyomas, which can be present in up to 50% of patients with tuberous sclerosus, are often found in the left ventricle .

❑❑ **Are patients with tuberous sclerosus at an increased risk of malignancy?**

Yes-tubers of the CNS can occasionally progress to malignant astrocytomas.

❑❑ **Which clinical features characterize patients with Sturge-Weber syndrome?**

- Facial nevus, or port wine stain;
- Seizures;
- Mental retardation;
- Intracerebral calcifications;
- Hemiparesis.

❑❑ **Do all infants with facial port wine stains need an evaluation for Sturge-Weber syndrome?**

No. Only those patients with port wine stains that involve the distribution of the trigeminal nerve require evaluation.

❑❑ **What opthalmologic complications may be found in patients with Sturge-Weber syndrome?**

The following complications involving the eye ipsilateral to the facial nevus may occur: enlargement of the eye , bupopthalmos, and glaucoma.

☐☐   **What type of seizures are seen in patients with Sturge-Weber syndrome?**

Most often, focal tonic-clonic seizures that involve the side of the body contralateral to the facial nevus.

☐☐   **What is the most common movement disorder in childhood?**

Transient tic disorder, which presents most often in boys. The movements consist of eye-blinking, throat clearing or other repetitive facial movements. These "tics" usually regress after one year and do not require drug treatment. Family history is often positive for "tics".

☐☐   **How does one distinguish patients with transient tic disorder from those with *Gilles de la Tourette* syndrome?**

In contrast to patients with transient tic disorder, patients with Gilles de la Tourette syndrome will sometimes have coprolalia (repetitive use of obscene words), echolalia (repetition of words addressed to the patient), palilalia (repetition of one's own already spoken words) and echokinesis (imitation of others' movement). These tics are lifelong.

☐☐   **What other neurologic conditions may be associated with *Gilles de la Tourette* syndrome?**

Attention deficit-hyperactivity disorder may be seen in up to 50% of patients with *Gilles de la Tourette* syndrome.

☐☐   **What drug therapy is most often successful in treating patients with *Gilles de la Tourette* syndrome?**

Haloperidol.

☐☐   **The patient in the question above also has clear fluid leaking from his nares. How do you distinguish between excessive nasal secretions and a CSF leak?**

By checking the fluid for the presence of glucose. Glucose will be present in CSF but not nasal secretions.

☐☐   **A 7 year old presents with a generalized seizure. His mother also mentions that she has noted a deteriorating performance in school, as well as difficulty controlling his temper and clumsy gait. On physical examination his skin seems darkly pigmented, even in the perineal region. He also has hyperreflexia and clonus. What test would help with your diagnosis?**

This is a common presentation of adrenoleukodystrophy. A CT scan or MRI of the brain may demonstrate periventricular demyelination.

☐☐   **How do you explain his darkly pigmented skin?**

Up to 50% of patients with adrenoleukodystrophy will have primary adrenal insufficiency.

☐☐   **What is the prognosis for this patient?**

Most patients with adrenoleukodystrophy will die within 10 years of the onset of symptoms.

☐☐   **A 6 year old child falls 5 feet, hitting his head on concrete and then has a generalized seizure lasting less than 1 minute. His neurological exam is completely normal. What is the most likely diagnosis?**

Post-traumatic seizure.

☐☐   **His parents want to know the likelihood of another seizure. What do you tell them?**

Approximately 25% of children with post-traumatic seizure will have additional seizures beyond one week after the injury.

□□   A 3 year old child presents with coma. He had intractable, non-bilious vomiting for hours prior to the onset of coma. There is no history of trauma. SGOT and SGPT are elevate but the serum bilirubin is normal. What is the most likely diagnosis?

Reye's syndrome.

INFECTIOUS DISEASES

"Medicine is a science of uncertainty and an art of probability."
- William Osler

☐☐   **What are the 3 stages of measles and what are the associated signs and symptoms?**

Incubation stage (10-12 days), which has no signs or symptoms; prodromal (or catarrhal) stage, which is characterized by Koplik spots, low grade fever, coryza, and cough; and the final stage, with the classic rash and high fever.

☐☐   **What is the classic rash of measles?**

Maculopapular, and sometimes confluent, rash on face, neck, upper arms, and upper chest initially. The rash spreads downwards and fades in the same direction.

☐☐   **What laboratory test is used for diagnosis of measles?**

None, as you probably knew, as this is a clinical diagnosis.

☐☐   **How does Rubeola differ clinically from measles?**

Sorry for the trick question. Measles is Rubeola.

☐☐   **What are some complications of measles?**

Photosensitivity, pharyngitis, encephalitis, subacute sclerosing panencephalitis (SSP), and DIC.

☐☐   **When should children be immunized against rotavirus?**

At 2,4, and 6 months.

☐☐   **Describe the pathophysiologic features of HIV.**

HIV attacks the T4 helper cells. The genetic material of HIV consists of singlestranded RNA. HIV has been found in semen, vaginal secretions, blood and blood products, saliva, urine, cerebrospinal fluid, tears, alveolar fluid, synovial fluid, breast milk, transplanted tissue, and amniotic fluid. There has not been documentation of infection from casual contact.

☐☐   **How quickly do patients infected with HIV become symptomatic?**

Five to ten percent develop symptoms within three years of seroconversion. Predictive characteristics include a low T4 count and a hematocrit less than 40. The mean incubation time is about 8.23 years for adults and 1.97 years for children less than 5 years old. When AIDS develops, the survival duration is about 9 months. However, new treatments may prolong this time period.

☐☐   **What is the second <u>most</u> <u>common</u> complication of AIDS?**

Kaposi's sarcoma. PCP is the most common.

☐☐   **What is the <u>most</u> <u>common</u> cause of focal encephalitis in AIDS patients?**

Toxoplasmosis. Symptoms include focal neurologic deficits, headache, fever, altered mental status, and seizures. Ring enhancinglesions are evident on CT.

☐☐   **The differential diagnosis of ring enhancing lesions in AIDS patients is what?**

Lymphoma, cerebral tuberculosis, fungal infection, CMV, Kaposi's sarcoma, toxoplasmosis, and hemorrhage.

□□   **An AIDS patient complains of decreased visual acuity, photophobia, redness, and eye pain. What is the diagnosis?**

Retinitis or malignant invasion of the periorbital tissue or eye.

□□   **What is the most common cause of retinitis in AIDS patients?**

Cytomegalovirus. Findings include photophobia, redness, scotoma, pain, or a change in visual acuity. On exam, fluffy white retinal lesions may be evident.

□□   **What is the most common opportunistic infection in AIDS patients?**

PCP. Symptoms may include a nonproductive cough and dyspnea. A chest x-ray may reveal diffuse interstitial infiltrates or it may be negative. Although, Gallium scanning is more sensitive, false positives occur. Initial treatment includes TMPSMX. Pentamidine is an alternative.

□□   **What is the most characteristic sign of Rubella?**

Adenopathy. This is most notable in the retroauricular, posterior occipital, and posterior cervical chains. The adenopathy usually disappears before the rash.

□□   **Aside from the rash, what are some findings in German Measles?**

Rubella can present concomitantly with polyarthritis, splenomegaly, and low grade fever. Myalgias, malaise, and photophobia are NOT seen.

□□   **When is the child with Rubella infectious?**

One week before and one week after the rash is a good rule of thumb.

□□   **What are some common complications of mumps?**

Orchitis/epididymitis, meningoencephalitomyelitis (that's a $20 diagnosis), mild pancreatitis, and unilateral nerve deafness.

□□   **When is the child with mumps considered infectious?**

Again, a good rule of thumb is a week before the parotid gland swelling and just over a week after its disappearance.

□□   **A patient is infected with *Treponema pallidum*; what is the treatment?**

The type of treatment depends upon the stage (1°, 2°, 3°) of the infection. Stages 1° and 2° syphilis are treated with benzathine penicillin G (2.4 million units IM X 1 dose) or doxycycline (100 mg bid po for 14 day). Stage 3° syphilis is treated with benzathine penicillin G, 2.4 million units IM X 3 doses 3 weeks apart.

□□   **Describe the lesions associated with lymphogranuloma venereum.**

LV caused by *Chlamydia* presents as painless skin lesions with lymphadenopathy. Lesions may be papular, nodular, or herpetiform vesicles. Sinus formation, involving the vagina and rectum, are common in females.

□□   **What is the cause of chancroid?**

Hemophilus ducreyi. Patients with this condition present with one or more painful necrotic lesions. Suppurating inguinal lymphadenopathy may also be present.

□□   **What is the cause of granuloma inguinale?**

Calymmatobacterium granulomatis. Typically the onset occurs with small papular, nodular, or vesicular lesions that develop slowly into ulcerative or granulomatous lesions. Lesions are painless and are located on mucous membranes of the genital, inguinal, and anal areas.

❑❑   **Which is the <u>most</u> <u>common</u> tapeworm in the U.S.?**

Hymenolepsis nana. Infections occur in institutionalized patients.

❑❑   **List 3 common protozoa that can cause diarrhea.**

1) *Entamoeba histolytica.* Occurs worldwide. Although half of the infected patients are asymptomatic, the usual symptoms consist of N/V/D/F, anorexia, abdominal pain, and leukocytosis. Determine the presence of this organism by ordering stool tests and performing an ELISA for extraintestinal infections. Treatment is with metronidazole or tinidazole followed by chloroquine phosphate.

2) *Giardia lamblia.* Occurs worldwide. This organism is one of the most common intestinal parasites in the U. S.. Symptoms include explosive watery diarrhea, flatus, abdominal distention, fatigue, and fever. The diagnosis is confirmed via a stool examination. Treatment is with metronidazole.

3) *Cryptosporidium parvum.* Occurs worldwide. Symptoms are profuse watery diarrhea, cramps, N/V/F, and weight loss. Treatment is supportive care. Medications may be needed for immunocompromised patients.

❑❑   **Explain the pathophysiology of rabies.**

Infection occurs within the myocytes for the first 48 to 96 hours. It then spreads across the motor endplate and ascends and replicates along the peripheral nervous system, axoplasm, and into the dorsal root ganglia, spinal cord, and CNS. From the gray matter, the virus spreads by peripheral nerves to tissues and organ systems.

❑❑   **What are the signs and symptoms of rabies?**

Incubation period of 12 to 700 days with an average of 20 to 90 days. The initial signs and symptoms begin with fever, headache, malaise, anorexia, sore throat, nausea, cough, and pain or paresthesias at the bite site.

During the CNS stage, agitation, restlessness, altered mental status, painful bulbar and peripheral muscular spasms, bulbar or focal motor paresis, and opisthotonos are exhibited. As in the Landry-GuillainBarré syndrome, 20% develop ascending, symmetric flaccid and areflexic paralysis. In addition, hypersensitivity to water and sensory stimuli to light, touch, and noise may occur.

The progressive stage includes lucid and confused intervals with hyperpyrexia, lacrimation, salivation, and mydriasis along with brainstem dysfunction, hyperreflexia, and extensor planter response.

In the final stages, coma, convulsions, and apnea occur followed by death between the fourth and seventh day for the untreated patient.

❑❑   **What is the diagnostic procedure of choice in rabies?**

Fluorescent antibody testing (FAT).

❑❑   **How is rabies treated?**

Prevention is the most effective treatment. Wound care of a suspected rabies bite should include debridement and irrigation. The wound must not be sutured; it should remain open. This will decrease the rabies infection by 90%. RIG 20 IU/kg, half at wound site and half in the deltoid muscle, should be administered along with HDCV, 1mL doses IM on days 0, 3, 7, 14, and 28, also in the deltoid muscle.

❑❑   **What is the second <u>most</u> <u>common</u> tick borne disease?**

Rocky Mountain spotted fever (RMSF). The causative agent is *Rickettsia rickettsii* and the vectors are the female Ixodi ticks, *Dermacentor andersoni* (wood tick) and *D. variabilis* (American dog tick). Lyme disease is the most common tick borne disease.

❏❏ **A patient presents with fever up to 40 °C followed by a rash which is erythematous, macular, and blanching. The rash becomes deep red, dusky, papular, and petechial. The patient also complains of a headache, vomiting, myalgias, and cough. Where did the rash begin?**

RMSF rash typically begins on the flexor surfaces of the ankles and wrists and spreads centripetally and centrifugally.

❏❏ **Which test should be performed to confirm RMSF?**

Immunofluorescent antibody staining of a skin biopsy or a serologic fluorescent antibody titer. The WeilFelix reaction and complement fixation tests are no longer recommended.

❏❏ **Which antibiotics are prescribed for the treatment of RMSF?**

Tetracycline or chloramphenicol. Antibiotic therapy should not be withheld pending serologic confirmation.

❏❏ **Which type of parasitic infection commonly occurs with a papular pruritic rash?**

Schistosoma.

❏❏ **Which type of parasite infections do not typically result in eosinophilia?**

Protozoa infections, such as amebas, Giardia, Trypanosoma, and Babesia.

❏❏ **Which is the most common intestinal parasite in the U.S.?**

Giardia. Cysts are obtained from contaminated water or passed by handtomouth transmission. Symptoms include explosive foul-smelling diarrhea, abdominal distention, fever, fatigue, and weight loss. Cysts reside in the duodenum and upper jejunum.

❏❏ **What is the most frequently transmitted tickborne disease?**

Lyme disease. The causative agent is spirochete, *Borrelia burgdorferi;* the vectors are *Ixodes dammini, I. pacificus, Amblyomma americanum*, and *Dermacentor variabilis.*

❏❏ **When are patients most likely to acquire Lyme disease?**

Late spring to late summer with the highest incidence in July.

❏❏ **How is Lyme disease diagnosed?**

Immunofluorescent and immunoabsorbent assays identify the antibodies to the spirochete. Treatment includes doxycycline or tetracycline, amoxicillin, IV penicillin, or erythromycin.

❏❏ **What is the most common cause of cellulitis?**

Streptococcus pyogenes. Staphylococcus aureus can also cause cellulitis though it is generally less severe and more often associated with an open wound.

❏❏ **What is the most common cause of cutaneous abscesses?**

Staphylococcus aureus is the most common aerobe in cutaneous abscesses; two-thirds are found in the upper torso, 97% are resistant to penicillin G. It is most commonly isolated in axilla abscesses.

❏❏ **What percentage of dog and cat bites become infected?**

About 10% of dog bites and 50% of cat bites become infected. *Pasteurella multocida* are the causative agents for 30% of dog bites and 50% of cat bites.

❏❏   A six year old child presents with headache, fever, malaise, and tender regional lymphadenopathy about a week after a cat bite. A tender papule develops at the site. What is the diagnosis?

Cat-scratch disease. This condition usually develops 3 days to 6 weeks following a cat bite or scratch. The papule typically blisters and heals with eschar formation. A transient macular or vesicular rash may also develop.

❏❏   What is the probable cause of an infection arising from an animal bite that develops in less than 24 hours? More than 48 hours?

Less than 24 hours is typically *P. multocida* or Streptococci. More than 48 hours is usually S*taphylococcus aureus*.

❏❏   What is the <u>most</u> <u>common</u> site of herpes simplex I virus infection?

The lower lip. First the lip itches and burns. Then the small vesicle with the red base appears. These lesions are painful and can frequently recur since the virus remains in the sensory ganglia. Recurrences are generally triggered by stress, sun, and illness.

❏❏   What are the most common causes of otitis media?

S. pneumoniae, H. influenza, and *M. catarrhalis.*

❏❏   An infant is brought to your office with fever and lethargy. On physical exam, you notice purulent rhinitis and an adherent membrane. The patient also has some shallow ulcers on the upper lip. What is your diagnosis?

Diptheria in nares. This is more common in infants.

❏❏   What should be your disposition for the above patient?

As this can spread to the pharynx and trachea, this child should be admitted and given antitoxin (after testing for hypersensitivity) and antibiotics (Penicillin or erythromycin).

❏❏   What are the 3 stages of pertussis? How long does each last?

Catarrhal, paroxysmal, and convalescent. Each stage lasts about 2 weeks.

❏❏   How do you calculate dosages for antibiotics in obese children?

Calculate their ideal weight from height and use that.

❏❏   What are the most common viral causes of pneumonia in the otherwise healthy child?

RSV, influenza, parainfluenza, and adenovirus.

❏❏   What viral cause of pneumonia can lead to acute fulminant pneumonia?

Some serotypes of adenovirus.

❏❏   In a child with the typical signs and symptoms of an upper respiratory tract infection, what antibiotic should you prescribe?

None. Viruses cause about 95% of URI's. The dangers of overuse and misuse of antibiotics are well known.

❏❏   In a child with the typical facial features of classic mumps, where else on the body should you look for suggestive signs?

Look for sternal edema (classic) and examine the testicles.

❏❏   **An 11 year old child stepped on a nail on his way home from school. The nail pierced through his sneaker and into his foot. His tetanus status is up to date. What is your main concern?**

Infection with Pseudomonas can lead to osteomyelitis. Pseudomonal infection is most commonly associated with hot, moist environments, such as sneakers.

❏❏   **Which is more fatal-Staphylococcal scalded skin syndrome or Group A Streptococcal toxic shock-like syndrome?**

Though both can be fatal, GASTSS is more common. (up to 50%).

❏❏   **What is the most common cause of infectious arthritis in patients with sickle cell disease? What joint is most commonly affected?**

Staph. aureus remains the most common cause, as in otherwise healthy children. However, *Salmonella* is more commonly seen in septic arthritis in children with hemoglobinopathies. The hip is most commonly affected.

❏❏   **What is the antibiotic regimen of choice after an appendectomy?**

Cefoxitin or clindamycin and gentamycin.

❏❏   **In the U.S. what is the recommended time of isolation for a dog or cat to rule out rabies?**

10 days.

❏❏   **What are the 2 causes of visceral larva migraines?**

Toxocara canis and Toxocara cati.

❏❏   **A 15 year old boy is brought to your office with a complaint of joint pains and general weakness. On physical exam, he has a slight fever and hepatosplenomegaly. The father states that the boy has been really depressed lately for no known reason- "why look how happy he was just 2 weeks ago when he shot his first elk!" The father shows a picture of the son holding onto his kill. What possible diagnosis is the picture a clue to?**

It should make you consider Brucellosis and Lyme disease.

❏❏   **Stool culture of a child reveals Cryptosporidium parvum. How should you treat it?**

Watchful waiting. The disease is usually self-limited and there is no effective antibiotic anyway.

❏❏   **What is the easiest way to distinguish residual formula in the mouth from thrush in an infant?**

Formula is easily scraped away with a tongue depressor, while the same maneuver in a child with thrush might lead to minute bleeding points.

❏❏   **Cerebral calcifications are most commonly associated with what 3 congenital infections?**

Toxoplasmosis, herpes simplex and cytomegalovirus.

❏❏   **Minimal to severe brain dysfunction can be a sequelae of what intrauterine infections?**

Toxoplasmosis, rubella, CMV, and herpes.

❏❏   **Which congenital infections are most common?**

CMV, though only about 5% will show any symptoms.

❏❏   **A newborn should be given varicella immune globulin (VZIG) if the mother develops varicella in what time period?**

5 days before to 2 days after delivery.

❑❑   **What are the most characteristic abnormalities of congenital rubella syndrome?**

Congenital heart lesions (esp. PDA), microphthmalia, corneal opacities, cataracts, glaucoma, and radiolucent bone lesions.

❑❑   **How is neonatal herpes usually contracted?**

Contact with genital secretions at delivery.

❑❑   **What is the characteristic triad of manifestations for late congenital syphilis?**

Hutchinson's triad consists of Hutchinson's teeth, interstitial keratitis, and eighth nerve deafness.

❑❑   **What is the most effective method of reducing fever in a child?**

Acetominaphen (and NSAIDS) can return the set-point to normal. Luke warm sponge baths can also help.

❑❑   **What organism is responsible for most cases of occult bacteremia in infants and toddlers?**

Streptococcus pneumoniae.

❑❑   **A child with a positive blood culture to what organism is most likely to develop meningitis?**

Meningiococcus.

❑❑   **How can the distribution of petechiae help one to evaluate the risk of a serious bacterial infection?**

Petechiae found only above the line of the nipples is rarely found in systemic disease.

❑❑   **What is necessary for the diagnosis of fever of unknown origin?**

1. History of fever over 1 week,
2. Documentation of fever by health provider,
3. Lack of a diagnosis after one week of investigation.

❑❑   **What specific substance in the body is the cause of fever?**

PGE.

❑❑   **Why should a child with suspected idiopathic thrombocytopenic purpura (ITP) be tested for HIV?**

Because thrombocytopenia may be the presenting sign for HIV infection.

❑❑   **How do viral meningitis and bacterial meningitis differ with regards to CSF pressure? CSF leukocytes? CSF glucose?**

The pressure in bacterial infection is increased, whereas it is normal or slightly increased in viral. The leukocytosis is greater than 1000 (up to 60K) in bacterial, and rarely over 1000 in viral meningitis. The glucose concentration is decreased in bacterial meningitis and is generally normal in viral.

❑❑   **What is the most common cause of bacterial meningitis in a child greater than 2 months old?**

H. influenza type b (decreasing since use of HIB vaccine), *Strep. pneumonia*, and *N. meningitidis.*

❑❑   **What antibiotic agent(s) should you start immediately in a toxic, febrile infant that is less than 3 months old?**

Ceftriaxone or cefotaxime and ampicillin.

❏❏ **What is the most common cause of death in children with HbSS?**

Infection.

❏❏ **How does the vaccination schedule of an HIV positive child differ from the standard schedule, if at all?**

OPV should be substituted with inactivated polio vaccine and, if symptomatic, they should also receive influenza and pneumococcal vaccine.

❏❏ **A premature infant is delivered at 32 weeks of age. How long after delivery should the infant be given his first vaccine?**

2 months after birth, same as a full-term baby.

❏❏ **Of measles, mumps, and rubella, which is the only vaccine component that is free of egg protein?**

Rubella.

❏❏ **In an immunocompetent individual, how long does the virus persist after receiving the OPV?**

Up to 2 months in the stool, but only 1-2 weeks in the blood.

❏❏ **What is the absolute contraindication to pertussis immunization?**

If the child had either an immediate anaphylactic reaction or an encephalopathy within one week of the previous vaccination.

❏❏ **An 8 year old child who has never received any vaccinations is brought to your office. Should this child be given pertussis vaccine?**

No. In children greater than 7 years old, it is not necessary.

❏❏ **A child with congenital HIV infection should receive a pneumococcal vaccine at what age?**

No earlier than 2 years.

❏❏ **Which children should receive a meningococcal vaccine?**

Children over 2 years of age with either asplenia or complement deficiency.

❏❏ **Why do so many patients with meningitis become hyponatremic?**

Because a majority of patients with this disease develop some degree of SIADH.

❏❏ **What is the *sine quo non* of botulism poisoning presentation?**

Bulbar palsy.

❏❏ **What disease may present with Magayama spots?**

These erythematous papules on the soft palate are commonly seen in patients with Roseola Infantum.

❏❏ **If the mother of a child with erythema infectiosum is infected, what would be her most likely presentation?**

Arthralgia and arthritis.

❏❏ **Which cephalosporins cover *Listeria monocytogenes*?**

None. That is why ampicillin is usually added to the antibiotic regimen when infection with this organism is a possibility.

❏❏   **Where does the rash of rocky mountain spotted fever usually start?**

On the wrists and ankles. It then spreads to the trunk and extremities within hours.

❏❏   **A worried mother calls you concerned that her daughter was exposed to chicken pox at the day care center. If she were exposed, how long would it take for the symptoms to appear?**

One and half to three weeks.

❏❏   **What is the most common cause of nosocomial bacteremia?**

S. epidermidis. This is usually successfully treated with methicillin.

❏❏   **What should you suspect in a child that presents with tender and swollen pectoral nodes?**

Cat-scratch disease.

❏❏   **What is the causative agent of cat-scratch disease?**

Bartonella henselae.

❏❏   **What is thought to be the mode of inoculation in cat-scratch disease?**

Rubbing the eye after contact with a cat.

❏❏   **A child is diagnosed with impetigo from group A streptococcus. What sequelae do you have to keep an eye out for?**

Acute post-streptococcal glomerulonephritis. It will not lead to rheumatic fever, however, for reasons that are not fully understood (possibly the strains for pharyngitis and impetigo are different).

❏❏   **What is the usual ideologic agent of a hordeolum (stye)?**

Staph. aureus.

❏❏   **For a hordeolum from a Staph infection, what is the therapy of choice?**

Hot soaks, and I & D, if necessary. Routine antibiotic use is not recommended.

❏❏   **What is considered to be the best therapy for patients with uncomplicated cat-scratch disease?**

Symptomatic relief. The use of antibiotic is controversial.

❏❏   **What are the major Jones criteria used to diagnose rheumatic fever?**

Carditis, chorea (Sydenham), erythema marginatum, migratory polyarthritis, and subcutaneous nodules. The diagnosis requires either 2 major or 1 major and 2 minor with evidence of previous strep infection.

❏❏   **What Jones criteria alone is sufficient for the diagnosis of rheumatic fever?**

Sydenham chorea. Deterioration in handwriting and increased clumsiness are commonly seen.

❏❏   **A 10 year old boy presents to your office with fever, tonsillopharyngitis, and lymphadenopathy. What laboratory tests will confirm your presumed diagnosis?**

CBC and Monospot should be all you need to confirm your suspicion of EBV (infectious mononucleosis).

❏❏   **What immunoglobulin characterizes acute infection with EBV?**

Anti-BCA IgM.

❏❏   **What would you expect to find on a peripheral blood smear of a patient with an acquired CMV infection?**

Absolute lymphocytosis and atypical lymphocytes.

❏❏ **What is the drug of choice for meningococcal disease?**

Aqueous penicillin G (250k-300k units/kg/day IV in 6 doses) is the ideal, though patients can be started effectively on empiric cefotaxime or ceftriaxone for suspected cases and in patients with penicillin allergy.

❏❏ **How often are fever and a bulging fontanelle present in an infant less than 2 months old with meningitis?**

Only about half have a fever, and only a third will have a bulging fontanelle.

❏❏ **How is CNS hemorrhage differentiated from a traumatic tap?**

A traumatic tap will have a decreasing RBC count in each successive tube and will not have crenated RBCs or xanthochromia of the supernatant.

❏❏ **Of bacterial, viral, fungal and tubercular meningitis, which typically presents with the greatest concentration of WBCs?**

Bacterial meningitis.

❏❏ **What is the formula to determine the true number of WBCs in the CNS of a traumatic tap?**

$$\text{True WBCs (CSF)} = \frac{[\text{WBC (CSF)} - \text{WBC (blood)}] \times \text{RBCs (CSF)}}{\text{RBCs (blood)}}$$

❏❏ **In an infant with suspected meningitis, you plan to take both CSF samples and blood samples. Does it matter which order you take them in?**

Yes. The stress of an LP can acutely elevate the glucose levels.

❏❏ **In patients with bacterial meningitis, is intracranial pressure usually elevated?**

Yes, almost always.

❏❏ **Does antibiotic therapy before an LP affect the outcome of the CSF culture?**

If the causative agent is Haemophilus then no. But it might sterilize the CSF in the cases with meningococcus and pneumococcus meningitis.

❏❏ **In children with meningitis, how soon after the initiation of antibiotics is the CSF considered sterile?**

Within 1 1/2 to 2 days.

❏❏ **In what circumstances would it be advisable to re-tap a child with meningitis?**

If there is no clinical response to antibiotic therapy within one to two days, or if cultures indicate that penicillin-resistant *Streptococcus pneumonia* is the causative agent.

❏❏ **Meningitis due to what organism most commonly presents with a sub-dural effusion?**

H. influenzae.

❏❏ **Should people who have had contact with patients with meningococcal meningitis be given prophylactic antibiotics?**

Yes. Rifampin or ceftriaxone are recommended.

❏❏ **What is, overall, the most common cause of aseptic meningitis?**

Enteroviruses.

❏❏ **Generally speaking, how do exudates of viral conjunctivitis differ from bacterial conjunctivitis?**

Viral is serous, and bacterial is mucopurulent or purulent.

❏❏ **What is the recommended initial treatment for cases of gonorrhea?**

Third generation cephalosporins (especially ceftriaxone) plus either doxycycline (100 mg BID for seven days) or azithromycin (1 gram PO x1) for presumptive coinfection with chlamydia.

❏❏ **What is the cause of epidemic keratoconjunctivitis?**

Adenovirus.

❏❏ **What is the initial therapy of gonococcal ophthalmia neonatorum?**

Ceftriaxone or cefotaxime and saline irrigation of the eye until resolution of the discharge.

❏❏ **Clinically, how can you distinguish orbital cellulitis from periorbital cellulitis?**

Extra-ocular muscle dysfunction, decreased pupillary reflexes, decreased visual acuity and changes in globe position are seen only in orbital cellulitis.

❏❏ **With a child you suspect has an otitis media from the history, but are unable to visualize the lumen secondary to cerumen obstruction, how should you proceed?**

Remove the cerumen and visualize the membrane.

❏❏ **What is the treatment for 'glue ear'?**

(Also known as serous otitis media) Myringotomy tubes after trial of appropriate antibiotic therapy.

❏❏ **What is the most common cause of hearing deficits in children?**

Secretory otitis media.

❏❏ **What is the drug of choice for streptococcal pharyngitis?**

Penicillin V.

❏❏ **After initiation of therapy for streptococcal pharyngitis, when should children be allowed back into school?**

At least 24 hours should elapse.

❏❏ **After finishing the prescribed dosage of penicillin for pharyngitis, your patients' repeat culture still shows streptococcus. What do you do?**

Nothing. Most people are asymptomatic carriers, and in most cases it is inconsequential.

❏❏ **What are the most common causes Herpangina?**

Coxsackievirus A and B, and Echovirus.

❏❏ **Does trismus more commonly occur with a peritonsillar abscess or peritonsillar cellulitis?**

Peritonsillar abscess.

❏❏ **Currently, what is the most common cause of epiglottitis?**

Group A Strep. The widespread use of the HiB vaccine has brought the number of Haemophilus induced epiglottitis cases down dramatically.

❏❏ **Are steroids effective in acute laryngotracheitis?**

Yes. The use of Dexamethasone (0.3-0.6 mg/kg) can lead to decreased need for intubation and more rapid improvement.

❏❏ **How often is sinus tenderness found in patients with sinusitis?**

Almost never.

☐☐   **What sinuses are most commonly involved in sinusitis?**

Ethmoid and maxillary sinuses.

☐☐   **What are the most common causes of acute sinusitis in children?**

Pneumococcus, H. influenzae, and *Moraxella catarrhalis* (same as otitis media).

☐☐   **Why does therapy for TB take several months, when other infections usually clear in a matter of days?**

Because the mycobacteria divide very slowly and have a long dormant phase, during which time they are not responsive to medications.

☐☐   **What is the most common side effect of rifampin?**

Orange discoloration of urine and tears.

☐☐   **What negative outcome can be avoided by supplementing pyridoxine in patients receiving isoniazid?**

Peripheral neuritis and convulsions.

☐☐   **Name at least three diseases that give false positive non-treponema (VDRL, RPR) tests for syphilis.**

Infectious mononucleosis, connective tissue diseases, tuberculosis, endocarditis, and intravenous drug abuse.

☐☐   **What are the organisms most commonly thought to be associated with Guillain-Barre Disease?**

CMV, EBV, coxsackie virus, Campylobacter jejuni, and Mycoplasma pneumoniae.

☐☐   **What is the age at which a single dose of HiB vaccine serves as the complete series?**

Fifteen months of age or older. Haemophilus influenza vaccine is no longer required at all after the patient reaches five years of age.

☐☐   **In what disease is cerebrospinal fluid albuminocytologic dissociation seen and what does it mean?**

Guillain-Barre Disease. An increase in cerebrospinal fluid protein without a corresponding increase in cerebrospinal fluid white cells is referred to as albuminocytologic dissociation.

☐☐   **Children with sickle cell disease most commonly are affected with what organisms?**

Streptococcus pneumoniae, Haemophilus influenzae B, and particularly severe Mycoplasma pneumoniae infections.

☐☐   **How does one go about making the diagnosis of allergic broncho pulmonary aspergillosis?**

Patients will have eosinophilia, Aspergillus fumigatus in the sputum and serum IgE to aspergillus.

☐☐   **What is the evaluation of foreign body in the lung?**

Chest x-ray and bronchoscopy.

☐☐   **What are some of the most convenient ways to make the diagnosis of Mycoplasma pneumoniae?**

Cold agglutinin levels of >=1:32 with consistent clinical findings will make a presumptive diagnosis. A complement fixation level to Mycoplasma pneumoniae may be seen of >= 1:256, or Mycoplasma pneumoniae specific IgA or IgM will be elevated.

□□   **What are the most common causes of non-infectious stomatitis?**

Behcet's syndrome, Stevens-Johnson syndrome, cancer chemotherapy, and Kawasaki syndrome.

□□   **Name at least five causes of parotitis in pediatric patients.**

An incomplete list of causes of parotitis include bacteria in general, viruses, especially mumps, echovirus, coxsackie A, lymphocytic choriomeningitis virus, parainfluenza 1 and 3, cytomegalovirus, Epstein-Barr virus, and HIV. Other causes include mycobacteria, histoplasmosis, post-typhoid fever, cat scratch disease, dehydration, collagen-vascular disease, cystic fibrosis, ectodermal dysplasia, familial dysautonomia, sarcoidosis, drugs, poisoning (including lead, copper and mercury), sialolithiasis, and tumors.

□□   **If a patient with underlying heart disease that has a tendency towards the development of endocarditis is undergoing a genito-urinary or gastro-intestinal procedure, what prophylactic antibiotic should be administered?**

Intravenous or intramuscular ampicillin and gentamicin thirty minutes prior to the procedure followed by the same, or amoxicillin eight hours after the procedure. Alternatively, intravenous vancomycin and gentamicin just prior to the procedure and repeated eight hours later is also acceptable. For a low risk procedure where the patient remains conscious, amoxicillin may be given one hour before and repeated six hours later.

□□   **When a child presents with more than one infected joint simultaneously, what organisms should be considered as the likely culprits?**

Staphylococcus aureus, salmonella or *gonorrhea*.

□□   **When a child has an underlying cardiac condition which predisposes him/her to endocarditis, what events and procedures do not require endocarditis prophylaxis?**

Dental procedures without gingival bleeding; injection of local intraoral anesthetic (except intraligamentary injections); shedding primary teeth; tympanostomy tube insertion; endotracheal intubation; flexible bronchoscopy, with and without biopsy; cardiac catheterization; gastrointestinal endoscopy, with and without biopsy; cesarean section; and, if there is no infection present, urethral catheterization; dilation and curettage; uncomplicated vaginal delivery, therapeutic abortion; sterilization procedures and insertion or removal of an intrauterine device.

□□   **Name at least five infectious agents associated with erythema nodosum.**

Erythema nodosum has been associated with many infectious and some non-infectious processes. Some of its better known associates are Group A streptococcus, meningococcus, syphilis, Mycobacterium tuberculosis, and Mycobacterium leprae, as well as histoplasmosis, coccidiomycosis, blastomycosis and herpes simplex virus. Some of the less common associates of erythema nodosum include Chlamydia trachomatis, Chlamydia psitacci, Corynebacterium diphtheriae, campylobacter, Haemophilus ducreyi, yersinia, Rochalimea henselae, trichophyton, filariasis, sarcoidosis, and various drugs.

□□   **Pediatric patients that have received transplantations have an increase in what infections?**

Staphylococcus, pseudomonas, klebsiella, candida, aspergillus, nocardia, Pneumocystis carinii, cytomegalovirus, and varicella zoster virus.

□□   **Name three common causes of pleural effusion without empyema in the pediatric age group.**

Staphylococcus aureus, Streptococcus pneumonia, HiB, Streptococcus pyogenes, and Mycoplasma pneumonia.

❑❑ **What is the most common complication of otitis media?**

Effusion and hearing loss.

❑❑ **What is the most common intracranial complication of otitis media?**

Meningitis. Other intracranial complications include epidural abscess, subdural abscess, brain abscess, encephalitis, lateral sinus thrombosis, communicating hydrocephalus, CSF otorrhea, and petrositis.

❑❑ **What is the most common extracranial complication of otitis media?**

Labyrinthitis, mastoiditis, facial nerve paralysis, subperiosteal abscess, labyrinthine fistulas, perilabyrinthitis, ossicular destruction, cholesteatoma and temporal osteomyelitis.

❑❑ **What are the indications for the prophylaxis of otitis media?**

Prophylaxis should be given after the third episode of otitis media under six months of age, or the fourth episode of otitis media before twelve months of age.

❑❑ **How does the perforation of the tympanic membrane associated with chronic supporative otitis media differ from the perforation associated with acute otitis media?**

Tympanic membrane perforation in chronic suppurative otitis media can be permanent

❑❑ **What malignancies in children are most likely to present as a fever of unknown origin?**

Leukemia, lymphoma, neuroblastoma, hepatoma, sarcoma, and atrial myxoma.

❑❑ **Name three diseases transmitted by tick bites.**

Lyme Disease, Rocky Mountain Spotted Fever, tularemia, relapsing fever secondary to borrelia, Colorado Tick Fever, ehrlichiosis and babesiosis.

❑❑ **Name two immunizations that are associated with post-vaccine aseptic meningitis.**

Measles, polio, rabies, and vaccinia.

❑❑ **If Creutzfeldt-Jakob disease (CJD) is a disease whose average age of presentation is 60 years, why has it suddenly become a concern of pediatricians?**

CJD was first described in the 1920's. It can be sporadic (no know cause), environmentally acquired (including pituitary hormones or dura mater grafts) or familial (due to mutations on chromosome 20). The recently diagnosed 21 patients in England were all under 50 years of age with an average age of 27 years. The "new variant" (nv) of CJD has in common with the classic CJD the features of progressive dementia, ataxia, and mild clonus. The unique characteristic of nvCJD are onset with psychiatric and/or sensory symptoms and an absence of characteristic electroencephalograph findings. The nvCJD seems to be associated with consumption of prion-contaminated beef.

❑❑ **What is the leading cause of meningitis in the United States?**

With the advent of conjugate vaccines against *Haemophilus influenza* type B, *Neisseria meningitidis* is now the leading cause of meningitis in children.

❑❑ **What four classes of contacts of a patient with meningococcal disease require prophylaxis?**

People who live in the same household, attendees of the same child care or nursery school in the previous seven days, those who have been directly exposed to the index case's secretions, such as by kissing or sharing of food, and health care providers whose mucous membranes were unprotected during resuscitation or intubation of the patient.

❑❑ **Why isn't the meningococcal vaccine in routine use in the United States?**

Serogroups B and C meningococci each cause approximately 50% of the meningococcal disease in the United States. The highest risk age group for meningococcal disease is in children under two years of age. The reason meningococcal vaccine is not routinely used in this country is because serogroup B polysaccharide is not represented in the vaccine and the serogroup C that is present is very poorly immunogenic in children under two years of age.

☐☐   **What infectious disease problem is both characteristic of and potentially devastating in patients with lupus, whether on steroids or not on steroids?**

Meningitis.

☐☐   **What rapid diagnostic test is now available to diagnose herpes simplex virus encephalitis in patients of all ages and how reliable is it considered to be?**

HSV polymerase chain reaction (PCR) on cerebrospinal fluid is considered to be highly sensitive and specific in the diagnosis of HSV encephalitis.

☐☐   **What percent of school age children with classic symptoms (dysuria, frequency, urgency) actually have a urinary tract infection?**

10%. The remainder have urethral irritation from such things as pinworms, masturbation, bubble baths or poor hygiene.

☐☐   **What is the only reliable result from a culture of urine collected by the bag method?**

No growth.

☐☐   **Any organisms that grow in the culture of a urine specimen obtained by suprapubic aspiration can be considered to represent true infection. In symptomatic children, how many colonies in a urine culture are required to make the diagnosis when the urine specimen is obtained by catheterization?**

At least 10,000 colonies per ml of a single organism.

☐☐   **What simple measures can be taken to prevent urinary tract infections in children?**

Taking showers instead of baths, avoiding bubble baths, treating pin worms, treating constipation and in sexually active females, post-coital voiding.

☐☐   **What children are candidates for influenza vaccine?**

Any child six months of age or older who is a resident of a chronic care facility; who has a chronic cardiovascular condition; or who has pulmonary, metabolic, hematologic, or an immunologic disorder (including asthma, diabetes, renal failure, sickle cell disease, immunosuppression and HIV infection). Also, children who are receiving aspirin therapy, or are the siblings of children who are in any of these high risk group, should have the influenza immunization as well.

☐☐   **What are the three questions that every victim of a dog bite should be asked?**

1. Was the attack provoked or unprovoked?
2. Was the dog known or unknown?
3. Has the dog had its rabies shots?

☐☐   **What are the most common organisms found in human bite wounds?**

Staphylococcus aureus, Streptococcus species, and *Eikenella corrodens*. Anaerobes are also commonly seen.

☐☐   **What is the risk of transmission of HIV from an HIV-infected person following a needle stick exposure?**

0.3%-0.5%.

PEDIATRIC MEDICAL STUDENT PEARLS OF WISDOM129

❑❑   **Children with sickle cell disease are started on prophylactic penicillin by two to three months of age. This should be continued until what age?**

Routine prophylaxis with penicillin has been shown to have no effect on reduction of the risk of invasive pneumococcal infections for children older than five years of age.

❑❑   **When should children with sickle disease be given the pneumococcal vaccine, and should they receive a booster dose of the vaccine?**

All children with sickle cell disease should receive the polyvalent pneumococcal vaccine at two years of age. A booster dose is often given at five years of age.

❑❑   **In a pediatric patient who is suspected of having meningitis, cranial computed tomography (CT) of the brain should be performed before lumbar puncture under what circumstances?**

When the patient is in a coma, has papilledema or focal neuroligic findings. When head CT is performed, patients should have blood cultures taken and then appropriate empiric antibiotic therapy started prior to the CT.

❑❑   **If a pediatric patient with an acute illness who is receiving a third generation cephalosporin becomes secondarily infected and bacteremic, what organism would be the usual offender?**

Enterococcus.

❑❑   **In the United States, which domestic animal is <u>most</u> <u>commonly</u> infected with rabies: the cat, or the dog?**

The cat. Among wild animals, rabies are most commonly found among raccoons, skunks, foxes and coyotes.

❑❑   **Would a child be likely to receive a rabies vaccine following a wild rat bite?**

No. Bites from rodents rarely pose a risk of rabies.

❑❑   **Since 1980, in the United States, what percentage of the 32 cases of human rabies has an associated history of animal bite?**

25%.

❑❑   **There are twenty indigenously derived cases of rabies in the United States between 1980 and 1996. How many series of post exposure rabies prophylaxis were given in the United States during that same time period?**

40,000 people received post exposure prophylaxis during that time period. Post exposure prophylaxis for rabies consists of 20 international units per kilogram of Human Rabies Immune Globulin (HRIG) and five doses of vaccine.

❑❑   **Which method is more reliable for the diagnosis of cytomegalovirus (CMV) infection in the newborn--the CMV lgM antibody, or the CMV culture of the urine or saliva?**

The presence of IGM antibody to CMV in the serum of a newborn is diagnostic of a congenital CMV infection. However, the sensitivity of most of these antibody methods is poor, with fewer than half of congenitally infected neonates being detected. The CMV culture has greater sensitivity.

❑❑   **Neonates with HSV infection may present with a localized skin, eye and mouth (SEM) infection, a disseminated infection or an encephalitis. What is the mortality rate of infants with disseminated HIV infection who are treated with acyclovir?**

Fifty percent.

❑❑   **What percentage of patients with localized skin, eye and mouth infection survive and what is the neurological outcome?**

All neonates with SEM treated with acyclovir survive and greater than 90% develop normally.

❑❑   **In the United States polio vaccine is no longer necessary to give after a person reaches which birthday?**

The 18th birthday.

❑❑   **Haemophilus influenzae B vaccine is not necessary after which birthday?**

The fifth birthday.

❑❑   **Pertussis vaccine is not recommended after which birthday?**

The seventh birthday.

❑❑   **Name three immunizations which are necessary at any age if they have not previously been given.**

The measles, mumps, and rubella (MMR), the tetanus-diphtheria vaccine, and, though not generally appreciated, the hepatitis B vaccine (HBV).

❑❑   **Is a pregnant mother in the household a contraindication to the immunization of a child in the house and, if so, to which vaccine?**

A pregnancy in the household is not a contraindication to vaccinating any household member other than the pregnant person herself. Pregnancy is a contraindication to live vaccines in general.

❑❑   **Would a time lapse of two years between the second and third dose of hepatitis B vaccine be an indication to restart the series?**

NO vaccine series ever has to be restarted, no matter what the time lapse between doses.

❑❑   **T/F: All vaccines may be given simultaneously.**

True. (The only exception to this rule is that cholera and yellow fever may not be given at the same time.)

❑❑   **What impact does breast feeding by the mother have on immunizations of the baby?**

All vaccines may be given to a baby who is breast feeding and all vaccines may be given to a mom who is breast feeding a baby.

❑❑   **May a child with contraindication or precaution against the use of DPT be given a DTaP?**

DTaP is contraindicated in anyone who may not use DPT. The patient may however by given the TD or Td.

❑❑   **If a child has received a course of chemotherapy, does the child need to be revaccinated?**

No.

❑❑   **If a child has had a bone marrow transplantation, will he or she need to be revaccinated?**

A child who has had a bone marrow transplant will receive some or all of the immunity of the donor. After recovery, consider giving the most important vaccines such as MMR and Td.

❑❑   **Following an immunoglobulin or blood product administration, how long should a patient wait before receiving a measles vaccination?**

It depends. If a child has received washed red blood cells, no wait whatsoever is required. If a child has received packed red blood cells, a five month interval is required. Children who have received tetanus immune globulin or immune serum globulin, either for Hepatitis A prophylaxis or international travel and patients who have received Hepatitis B immune globulin, are required to wait three months for the next measles vaccination. Various other immune globulins and blood products require longer waits. The longest waits are following the receipt of respiratory syncytial virus (RSV)--IGIV (a nine month wait) and intravenous immune globulin (IGIV) for Kawasaki Disease (eleven months).

☐☐   **T/F: A culture from a patient is reported as growing coagulase negative staphylococci. This should be interpreted to mean *staphylococcus epidermidis*.**

False. There are 15 different coagulase negative staphylococci that have been reported to cause diseases in or to colonize humans. An additional sixteen non-human coagulase negative staphylococci exist.

☐☐   **The laboratory report reads "*Streptococcus viridans*." What is wrong with that report?**

Clinically, we're splitting hairs here. Just for academic's sake, you should be aware that there is no such organism as *Streptococcus viridans*. The class of organisms being referred to is rightly called Viridans streptococci. Viridans streptococci are alpha hemolytic streptococci which are composed of at least eight separate species which cause diseases in man. Examples of Viridans streptococci include: S. milleri, S. constellatus, S. anginosus and S. mutans. While most laboratories will not normally speciate a Viridans streptococci for you because they may simply be contaminants, if they are seen in two or more blood cultures or grow in pure culture from a deep site, it is appropriate to ask for speciation. The species of the organism can point to the etiology of the disease. Certain Viridans streptococci are associated with endocarditis, while others are associated with such things as carcinoma and brain abscess.

☐☐   **A six year old child presents with a history of having had a PPD placed three weeks ago which was 4 mm in induration, measured by a reliable colleague. A repeat PPD was placed one week ago and the child's forearm demonstrated 14 mm of induration. This PPD was measured by the same physician. Which PPD should be accepted as reflecting the correct amount of induration?**

The second, or "boosted" response, is accepted as the reliable response. It is routine for many institutions to test their employees with two PPD's, separated by two weeks, in order to take advantage of this phenomenon.

☐☐   **A six year old child presents with a history classic for giardia and has a three year old brother who was documented to have the same symptoms. A complete stool work-up is performed and after the first day, the laboratory reports the identification of rotavirus. What is the most likely explanation?**

The six year old probably has both rotavirus and giardia, and probably caught them both from his three year old sibling. Like venereal diseases, more than one infectious agent is often transmitted at a time. Two pathogens or more are found in the stool of patients symptomatic with acute gastroenteritis at least 15% of the time.

☐☐   **An eighteen month old presents with an exudative pharyngitis, fever and mildly abnormal liver function test. You suspect mononucleosis. What study would you send?**

An EBVlgG and IGM (lgG and lgM antibody to viral capsid antigen or VCA). The chances that a mono spot will be positive in the presence of mononucleosis between 0 and 2 years of age is practically zero. The chances that a mono spot is positive between the second birthday and the fourth birthday is approximately 30%. Specific Epstein-Barr virus antibodies are much more useful for making the diagnosis in the first four years of life.

☐☐   **A ten month old presents with the signs and symptoms of pneumonia, which is confirmed by chest x-ray. What are the chances that this pneumonia is due to Mycoplasma pneumoniae?**

About 2%. Mycoplasma pneumoniae is hardly ever seen in the first year of life. It increases steadily as a cause of pneumonia in children into early adulthood. A convenient way to remember the chances of a child's pneumonia being due to mycoplasma is to assign a 2% chance per year of age into the twenties. By the mid-twenties, as many as 35-45% of all pneumonia is secondary to Mycoplasma pneumoniae.

❏❏   **Pasteurella multocida infection from an animal bite is best treated with which antibiotic?**

Penicillin is the drug of choice.

❏❏   **The intervention most likely to be successful in the treatment of onychomycosis of the toenail is: a) removal of the toenail or b) antifungal therapy for four to eighteen months?**

Drug therapy with Itraconazole (Sporanox) is the easiest and shortest term of the various antifungal drug regimens. Treatment can be given for one week each month for three to four months. Other medications that are useful include terbinafine, ketoconazole, and griseofulvin. Therapy with griseofulvin can take as long as eighteen months.

❏❏   **Polio most frequently affects which age group?**

Polio is now extremely rare in the US (i.e., 2 cases per year). When it does infect, it attacks the pediatric age group 3 months-16 years.

❏❏   **A mother brings her 5 year old son in because he was just bitten by the neighbor's dog. She is frantic because he will now develop rabies. What should you tell her to calm her fears?**

The incidence of rabies in the US is 0-3 cases a year. The likelihood that her son is infected is low. However, the dog should be quarantined for ≥ 10 days and observed if the dog has not been vaccinated or appears ill.

❏❏   **In the US, what animals are most likely to be infected with the rabies virus?**

Bats, skunks, and raccoons. Dogs are the usual carriers in developing countries.

❏❏   **Are rabies transmitted via a rat bite?**

No, rodents do not carry the virus.And, no, bats are NOT rodents with wings.

❏❏   **Name two common urinary pathogens that do not give a positive urine nitrate test.**

Enterococcus and *Staphylococcus saprophyticus.* Acinetobacter also fails to give a positive urine nitrate test.

❏❏   **Group B Streptococcus is known to have both an early and a late onset presentation in neonatal sepsis and meningitis. What other organism does the identical thing?**

Listeria monocytogenes.

❏❏   **What common minor surgical procedure is associated with a decreased incidence of pyelonephritis in males?**

Circumcision.

❏❏   **What percentage of the time do infants with documented pyelonephritis fail to demonstrate pyuria?**

Approximately 50% of the time.

❏❏   **What is the incidence of occult bacteremia in infants between six and twenty-four months of age with temperature higher than 40 degrees centigrade and a white blood count > 15,000/cu.mm?**

Approximately fifteen percent.

❏❏   **What could be concluded about the spinal fluid of a three day old infant with a CSF white count of 15 and a CSF protein of 90?**

That it is normal. At birth the CSF white count can be as high as 29. It may not fall to the expected "adult" normal of 6 or 7 until a month of age. The CSF protein can be up to 175 at birth and may take as long as three months to fall to the expected upper limit of normal of 45.

❑❑   **What is the risk and where is the risk of salmonella coming into a household in an ordinary package of a dozen eggs?**

In some studies, as many as 30% of commercial eggs are contaminated with salmonella. The organism can be found on the surface of the shell, may penetrate the egg itself, or may contaminate the egg yolk, having been transmitted from an ovarian infection.

❑❑   **What are the chances that salmonella will be introduced into a household on contaminated meats?**

Up to 50% of poultry samples, 15% of pork and 5% of beef have been demonstrated to be contaminated with salmonella.

❑❑   **What percent of dog and cat bites result in cellulitis?**

Approximately 30% of cat bites and 6% of dog bites.

❑❑   **Bartonella henselae is one of the causes of Parinaud's oculoglandular syndrome (a combination of conjunctivitis and ipsilateral preauricular adenitis) and is the most common cause of chronic lymphadenopathy in children. With what animal is this organism associated?**

The cat. It is the agent of cat scratch disease.

❑❑   **One day after sitting in a hot tub, a nine year old child and her mother develop papular and pustular skin lesions. What is the most likely explanation?**

Pseudomonas aeruginosa dermatitis has been reported to occur in healthy individuals following immersion in hot tubs. There may be a few scattered lesions or extensive involvement. Patients may also have malaise, fever, vomiting, sore throat, conjunctivitis, rhinitis, and swollen breasts.

❑❑   **What are the two most common organisms known to be transmitted by unpasteurized Mexican cheese?**

Brucella and listeria.

❑❑   **What is the most common infectious disease complication of both measles and influenza?**

Pneumococcal pneumonia.

❑❑   **Which rickettsial infection is most common in the United States?**

Rocky Mountain Spotted Fever caused by Rickettsia rickettsia.

❑❑   **In the treatment of a patient with cellulitis, what therapeutic maneuver is arguably as important as antibiotic therapy?**

Elevation of the affected part.

❑❑   **What prophylactic antibiotic should be given systemically to burn victims?**

None. Prophylactic agents with antibacterial activity should be given topically. Chief among these is Silvadene.

❑❑   **What is the most likely focus of infection in a patient who presents with gram negative enteric bacteremia?**

Urinary tract infection.

❑❑   **What is the most likely focus of infection in a patient who presents with periorbital cellulitis unassociated with skin trauma?**

Sinusitis.

❑❑   **A 3 month old infant presents with poor feeding, constipation, and hypotonia. There is a recent history of ingestion of honey. While you suspect infant botulism, you cannot rule out the possibility of sepsis. What class of antibiotics would you not give to this patient?**

Aminoglycosides. Gentamicin and related drugs can add to the blocked motor nerve terminals, and lead to respiratory failure in these patients.

❑❑   **A teenager presents with an irritating cough which is becoming gradually worse. The boy's father had a similar problem, which was treated with erythromycin and resolved after seven days. PPD's on both the father and the son have been negative. What are the three most likely etiologic agents for this problem?**

Mycoplasma pneumonia, Chlamydia pneumonia, and *Bordetella pertussis.*

❑❑   **What part of the body should you examine to confirm that a vesicular rash is related to chickenpox?**

The scalp. Vesicular and crusting lesions in the scalp are typical of chicken pox. It is extremely unlikely that other causes of vesicular lesions on the skin would be associated with scalp lesions.

❑❑   **It is well known that children with chickenpox may eventually have an episode or episodes of herpes zoster. Will herpes zoster follow an immunization with chickenpox vaccine?**

Yes. It occurs at approximately one-third to one-fifth the frequency that it does following the natural illness.

❑❑   **What's the earliest age at which a child may be immunized for influenza?**

At 6 months of age.

❑❑   **While older infants and children with respiratory syncytial virus infection (RSV) usually present with cough and wheezing, some infants may present with what other symptom?**

Apnea.

❑❑   **What is the name of the viral illness that presents predominantly with pharyngitis and conjunctivitis?**

Pharyngoconjunctival fever. Sometimes, your first guess is your best guess.

❑❑   **Since only a minority of children who present with fever and petechiae have meningococcemia, what etiologic agent accounts for the bulk of the remaining cases?**

The enteroviruses, including the Coxsackieviruses, and the ECHO viruses.

❑❑   **A ten month old infant presents with fever, diarrhea, and mild irritability. A spinal tap shows 68 white cells, no red cells, normal protein, normal glucose, and a CSF latex agglutination that is negative for all bacterial pathogens tested. What is the most likely diagnosis?**

Rotavirus. Aseptic meningitis is not uncommon in children with rotavirus gastroenteritis.

❑❑   **What parasitic agent should be included when mononucleosis and CMV are diagnosed?**

Toxoplasmosis.

❑❑   **When itchy lesions are seen on the palms and/or soles, what blood sucking ecoparasite should be high in the differential diagnosis?**

Sarcoptes scabiei, the etiologic agent of scabies.

❑❑   **Which intestinal parasites are known to cause anemia as their major manifestation?**

Hookworms.

❑❑   **What are the characteristic symptoms of bacterial meningitis?**

Headache, stiff neck, fever, and photophobia.

❑❑   **What are the usual CSF findings in bacterial meningitis?**

Neutrophilic pleocytosis, increased protein, hypoglycorrachia (CSF glucose <50% of serum glucose). Additionally, bacterial antigens may be positive.

❑❑   **What are the three most common causes of bacterial meningitis beyond the neonatal period?**

Pneumococcus, meningococcus and hemophilus influenza.

❑❑   **What are the common pathogens for meningitis in the neonates?**

Streptococcus group B, and *E. coli* (escherechia coli used to be the most common pathogen, but the incidence is now higher with streptococcus).

❑❑   **What is the most common sequela of pediatric bacterial meningitis?**

Hearing impairment.

❑❑   **What other deficits may develop following bacterial meningitis?**

Mental retardation, seizure, and spastic weakness.

❑❑   **What are the CSF findings in viral meningitis?**

Lymphocytic pleocytosis, normal to slightly elevated protein, and normal glucose.

❑❑   **What are the sequelae of viral meningitis?**

None.

❑❑   **What are the CSF characteristics of tuberculous meningitis?**

Lymphocytic pleocytosis, very high protein (several hundred to a thousand mg/dl), and very low glucose.

❑❑   **Where is the postulated site of the viral latency in HSV 1 that is responsible for HSV encephalitis?**

Gasserian ganglion of the Trigeminal nerve.

❑❑   **At which stage of Lyme disease does neurological involvement occur?**

The second and third stages.

❑❑   **What is the vector responsible for the transmission of Lyme disease?**

Deer tick (*Ixodus damnii*)

❑❑   **What important feature in a patient's history should be sought when neurological involvement from Lyme disease is being considered?**

History of Erythema Chronicum Migrans (ECM), which present in nearly 60-80% of patients early in this disease.

❑❑   **What is the currently recommended treatment for Lyme disease?**

For isolated VIIth cranial nerve palsy, oral amoxicillin, alternatively doxycycline. All other neuroborreliosis should be treated with intravenous Ceftriaxone.

☐☐ · **How is brucellosis spread?**

Through the ingestion of contaminated milk and milk products. It may also be spread by contact with an infected animal (usually cattle).

☐☐ **Which organism is responsible for brucellosis?**

Brucella Melitensis.

☐☐ **Which infectious disease characteristically causes dementia and a supranuclear palsy?**

Whipple's disease, which is caused by a gram positive argyrophillic bacillus.

☐☐ **What neurological findings are almost exclusively found in Whipple's disease?**

Oculo-facial-skeletal-myoarrythmia. In this condition, there is a convergence of the eyes or a pendular nystagmus that is synchronous with movements of the jaw or other parts of the body.

☐☐ **What is the neuropathological characteristic of Whipple's disease?**

A nodular ependymitis, mainly of the third and fourth ventricles and the cerebral aqueduct. There is also a microgranulomatous polioencephalitis that may involve the inferior frontal, temporal cortex and cerebellar nuclei. Spinal cord grey matter may be involved.

☐☐ **What is the diagnostic test for Whipple's disease?**

Examination of the jejunal mucosa, where PAS positive macrophages are seen in the lamina propria. These PAS positive structures are within the macrophages. They are the remnants of the bacilli, and are seen under the electron microscope.

☐☐ **What is the typical clinical presentation of progressive multifocal leucoencephalopathy (PML)?**

PML commonly presents with focal neurological signs such as hemisensory or motor signs, and visual field deficits.

☐☐ **PML is seen in which other immune disorders?**

Cell mediated immunedeficiencies. It is thus seen in HIV disease, chronic myeloid leukemia, Hodgekin's disease, chemotherapy patients and rarely sarcoidosis.

☐☐ **How is botulism contracted?**

Through the consumption of contaminated foods, by injury from non sterile objects (wound botulism), and (in infants) from intestinal colonisation by clostridium botulinum (lack of normal intestinal flora permit this colonization).

☐☐ **What are botulism's principle clinical features?**

A descending paralysis with complete ophthalmoplegia, bulbar and somatic palsy.

☐☐ **What is epidemic pleurodynia (Bornholm's disease)?**

An upper respiratory tract infection is followed by pleuritic chest pain and tender muscles.

☐☐ **Which is the organism responsible for causing Bornholm's disease?**

Coxsackie viruses are a group of enteroviruses that are responsible for the epidemic myalgia (Bornholm's disease) where pleurodynia is also a common feature. Specifically the disease is thought to occur due to a Coxsackie group B virus.

RHEUMATOLOGY, IMMUNOLOGY AND ALLERGY

"I don't want to achieve immortality through my work.
I want to achieve it through not dying."
- Woody Allen

□□ **Which class of immunoglobulins is responsible for urticaria (hives) and angioedema?**

Both are mediated by IgE.

□□ **Which class of immunoglobulins is responsible for food allergies?**

IgE.

□□ **What are the most common food allergies?**

Dairy products, eggs, and nuts.

□□ **When do the clinical manifestations of a new drug allergy usually become apparent?**

1-2 weeks after starting the drug.

□□ **Which class of drugs is commonly associated with angioedema?**

Severe and refractory angioedema of the face, lips, and tongue can occur from the use of angiotensin-converting-enzyme (ACE) inhibitors. A patient who has suffered angioedema from one ACE inhibitor should not be prescribed another ACE inhibitor. The complication can result from any member of this class of antihypertensive agents.

□□ **Which drug is the most common pharmaceutical cause of true allergic reactions?**

Penicillin accounts for approximately 90% of true allergic drug reactions and for more than 95% of fatal anaphylactic drug reactions. Parenterally administered penicillin is more than twice as likely to cause a fatal anaphylactic reaction than orally administered penicillin.

□□ **How long after exposure to an allergen does anaphylaxis occur?**

The symptoms of anaphylaxis may occur within seconds or may be delayed up to 1 hour.

□□ **Anaphylaxis-related deaths are primarily caused by penicillin. What is the second most common cause?**

Insect stings. Approximately 100 deaths in the U.S. occur annually because of anaphylaxis that is induced by insect stings.

□□ **Most children with mucocutaneous lymph node syndrome are below what age?**

MLNS, or Kawasaki disease, is predominantly found in children under 9 years of age.

□□ **Are the nodules of erythema nodosum most often symmetrically or asymmetrically distributed?**

Erythema nodosum produces distinctive bilateral tender nodules with underlying red or purple shiny patches of skin that develop in a symmetric distribution along the shins, arms, thighs, calves, and buttocks.

☐☐   **What therapy is effective for treating erythema nodosum?**

There is no therapy known to alter the course of the disease. The disease usually lasts several weeks but the pain associated with the tender lesions can be relieved with non-steroidal anti-inflammatory agents.

☐☐   **What percentage of patients with Kawasaki disease also develop acute carditis?**

Fifty percent will develop carditis, usually myocarditis with mild to moderate congestive heart failure. Pericarditis, conduction abnormalities, and valvular disturbances may occur but are less common.

☐☐   **A patient presents with fever, acute polyarthritis, or migratory arthritis a few weeks after a bout of Streptococcal pharyngitis. What disease should be suspected?**

Acute rheumatic fever. Although the early symptoms may be nonspecific, a physical exam eventually reveals signs of arthritis (60-75%), carditis (30%), choreiform movements (10%), erythema marginatum, or subcutaneous nodules.

☐☐   **What treatment should be started after the diagnosis of acute rheumatic fever has been made?**

Penicillin or erythromycin should be given even if cultures for Group A *Streptococcus* are negative. High-dose aspirin therapy is used at an initial dose of 75-100 mg/kg/day. Carditis or congestive heart failure is treated with prednisone, 1-2 mg/kg/day.

☐☐   **Cite an example of each of the 4 major types of allergic reactions: type I—immediate hypersensitivity; type II—cytotoxic, type III—Arthus reaction; and type IV—delayed hypersensitivity.**

Type I: Asthma, food allergies (IgE).
Type II: Transfusion reaction (IgG and IgM).
Type III: Serum sickness, post streptococcal glomerulonephritis (complex activates complement).
Type IV: Skin testing (activated T-lymphocytes).

☐☐   **Which of the four types of allergic reactions can be caused by a drug allergy?**

A drug allergy can produce all four types of allergic reactions.

☐☐   **Myocardial infarction can occur with which two rheumatic diseases?**

Kawasaki disease and polyarteritis nodosa (PAN).

☐☐   **What is the __most__ __common__ cause of anaphylactoid reactions?**

Radiographic contrast media.

☐☐   **A bacterial infection and an allergic phenomenon can both cause a generalized confluent exfoliation of skin. What are the two diseases, and what test should be performed to distinguish between the two?**

Ritter's disease, or dermatitis exfoliativa neonatorium, is caused by infection by *Staphylococcus* and thus is also known as Staphylococcal scalded skin syndrome (SSSS). This condition causes exfoliation at the superficial granular layer of the epidermis. Toxic epidermal necrolysis (TEN) appears very similar, but is an allergic phenomenon. A skin biopsy distinguishes the two conditions because the exfoliative cleavage plane is deeper at the dermal-epidermal junction or lower with TEN.

☐☐   **What is required to make a diagnosis of mucocutaneous lymph node syndrome, or Kawasaki disease, in a young patient with a prolonged fever?**

The diagnosis requires four of these five common clinical findings:

1) Conjunctival inflammation.
2) Rash.
3) Adenopathy.
4) Strawberry tongue and injection of the lips and pharynx.
5) Erythema and edema of extremities.

Desquamation of the fingers and the toes may be striking, but it is a late finding and is not one of the key clinical features of the disease.

❑❑ **How long should a patient with a generalized anaphylactic reaction be observed?**

Because recurrence of hemodynamic collapse and airway compromise is common within the first 24 hours, patients should be observed for at least that period of time. Treatment with antihistamines and steroids should be continued for 72 hours.

❑❑ **A patient who is on chronic steroids presents with weakness, depression, fatigue, and postural dizziness. What pathological process should be suspected? What is the treatment?**

Adrenal insufficiency. The treatment is to administer large "stress doses" of steroids.

❑❑ **If adrenal insufficiency is suspected, what test should be performed? Which drug should be prescribed?**

A serum cortisol level should be drawn before administering a large dose of steroids. Dexamethasone is the preferred agent because it does not interfere with subsequent tests that may be indicated.

❑❑ **What cardiac complication commonly occurs with SLE as well as with juvenile rheumatoid arthritis and rheumatoid arthritis?**

Pericarditis.

❑❑ **How should a potentially septic olecranon bursitis be treated?**

As much fluid as possible should be aspirated from the bursa via a large-bore needle, and antibiotics should be started immediately.

❑❑ **A 10 year old child presents limping and complaining of several weeks of groin, hip, and knee pain that worsens with activity. What diseases should be considered?**

Transient tenosynovitis of the hip, slipped capital femoral epiphysis, Legg-Calvé-Perthes, suppurative arthritis, rheumatic fever, juvenile rheumatoid arthritis, and tuberculosis of the hip.

❑❑ **What disease is suspected in an adolescent with a tender, purpuric dependent rash, colicky abdominal pain, migratory polyarthritis, and microscopic hematuria?**

Henoch-Schonlein purpura, a leukoblastic vasculitis. Intestinal or pulmonary hemorrhage may occur, and 7–9% percent of the cases will develop chronic renal sequelae. Salicylates are effective for the arthritis. Other treatment is directed at the symptoms. Steroids are not particularly effective.

❑❑ **A child has painful swollen joints along with a spiking high fever, shaking chills, signs of pericarditis, and a pale erythematous coalescing rash on the trunk, palms, and soles. Hepatosplenomegaly is found. What is the diagnosis?**

Systemic juvenile rheumatoid arthritis. Arthrocentesis is necessary to eliminate the possibility of septic arthritis. The rheumatoid factor and the antinuclear antibody usually are negative; one-fourth of patients will proceed to have joint destruction. This is the least common of the three types of JRA.

❑❑ **What treatment besides aspirin is effective in preventing the complications of Kawasaki disease?**

Intravenous immunoglobulins can reduce the incidence of coronary artery aneurysms to less than 5%.

☐☐   **Which joint is typically involved in the most common form of juvenile rheumatoid arthritis?**

The most common of the three forms of JRA usually involves the knee and does not lead to joint destruction. Reiter's syndrome, iridocyclitis, and inflammatory bowel disease all may be associated with this particular form of the disease.

☐☐   **A child has posttraumatic tenderness at the end of a long bone. A joint effusion is the only radiographic finding. What is the appropriate management?**

Immobilization and subsequent orthopedic evaluation for possible separation of the epiphysis from the metaphysis (i.e., Salter-Harris type I fracture).

☐☐   **A patient presents with pain along the radial aspect of the wrist extending into the forearm. What is the diagnostic test of choice?**

Finkelstein's test confirms the diagnosis of deQuervain's tenosynovitis, an overuse inflammation of the extensor pollicis brevis and the abductor pollicis where they pass along the groove of the radial styloid. The test is performed by instructing the patient to make a fist with the thumb tucked inside the other fingers. The test is positive for this condition if pain is reproduced when the examiner gently deviates the fist in the ulnar direction.

☐☐   **What autoimmune disease produces lesions that are sometimes urticarial in appearance yet are not pruritic?**

Erythema multiforme.

☐☐   **What disease classically produces erythematous plaques with dusky centers and red borders resembling a bulls-eye target?**

Erythema multiforme. This disease can also produce non-pruritic urticarial lesions, petechiae, vesicles, and bullae.

☐☐   **Which drugs are most commonly implicated in toxic epidermal necrolysis?**

Sulfonamides and sulfones, phenylbutazone and related drugs, barbiturates, other antiepileptic drugs, and antibiotics.

☐☐   **What is the appropriate management for TEN?**

Admit for management similar to that required for extensive second-degree burns. The mortality of TEN can be as high as 50% because of fluid loss and secondary infections.

☐☐   **What can cause erythema multiforme?**

EM can be triggered by viral or bacterial infections, by drugs of nearly all classes, and by malignancy.

☐☐   **What is the most common cause of allergic contact dermatitis?**

Toxicodendron species, such as poison oak, poison ivy, and poison sumac are responsible for more cases of contact dermatitis than all the other allergens combined.

☐☐   **Why does scratching spread poison oak and poison ivy?**

The antigenic resin contaminates the hands and fingernails and is thereby spread by rubbing or scratching. A single contaminated finger can produce more than 500 reactive groups of lesions.

☐☐   **How is the antigen of poison oak or poison ivy inactivated?**

Careful washing with soap and water destroys the antigen. Special attention must be paid to the fingernails, otherwise the antigenic resin can be carried for weeks.

❏❏ **What underlying illnesses should be considered in a patient with nontraumatic uveitis?**

Collagen vascular diseases, sarcoid, ankylosing spondylitis, Reiter's syndrome, tuberculosis, syphilis, toxoplasmosis, juvenile rheumatoid arthritis, and Lyme disease.

❏❏ **What is the probable diagnosis of a patient with myalgias, arthralgias, headache, and an annular erythematous lesion accompanied by central clearing?**

Stage I Lyme disease with the classic lesion of Erythema Chronicum Migrans (ECM). The primary lesion occurs at the site of the tick bite.

❏❏ **What rheumatologic ailments produce pulmonary hemorrhage?**

Goodpasture's disease, systemic lupus erythematosus, Wegener's granulomatosis, and nonspecific vasculitides.

❏❏ **What rheumatologic ailments can produce acute airway obstruction?**

Relapsing polychondritis and rheumatoid arthritis.

❏❏ **What infectious agents may produce a chronic smoldering arthritis with sterile aspiration cultures?**

Tuberculosis and fungal infections. A synovial biopsy may be required to confirm the diagnosis.

❏❏ **Which immune cells are responsible for adaptive immunity?**

Antigen specific immunity is the responsibility of the B and T lymphocytes.

❏❏ **Which are the only complement fixing immunoglobulins?**

IgG and IgM.

❏❏ **Which is the major protective Ig of external secretions?**

IgA.

❏❏ **Which Ig is the major host defense against parasites?**

IgE.

❏❏ **What are the two main functions of T cells?**

To signal B cell to make antibody and kill virally infected or tumor cells

❏❏ **What type of infections are newborns most susceptible to and why?**

Gram negative organisims. Since there is no passive transfer of IgM, which are heat stable opsonins, the opsoninization process is impaired.

❏❏ **So then, why aren't infants more susceptible to gram positive organisms?**

Passively transferred IgG serves as effective opsonins.

❏❏ **Why is the vaccine containing HiB polysaccharide ineffective in children under 2 years of age?**

It is not immunogenic! Infants cannot produce antibody to polysaccharide antigen unless it is conjugated to a protein carrier.

❏❏ **Peak mass of the thymus is reached at what time during development?**

Just before puberty.

❑❑   **What test would you order to exclude and/or diagnose the most common hypoglobulinemia?**

Quantification of Serum IgA.

❑❑   **12 month old infant with repeated pneucoccal pneumonia is found to have an immunoglobulin concentration of IgA, IgM, and IgE of <100 mg/dl and a lymph node biopsy demonstrating hypoplasia with absent germinal centers and rare plasma cells. Which viral vaccine would you be most cautious with administration?**

Hepatitis and polio vaccine. In children with Bruton's agammaglobulinemia viral infections such as hepatitis, polio, and echovirus can be fatal.

❑❑   **Blood products given to an individual with selective IgA deficiency must be prepared in what way?**

Washed (5x in normal saline) normal donor erythrocytes or blood products. 44% of IgA deficient patients have auto IgA antibody, which when present may precipitate anaphylaxis and death with transfusion of unprepared donor cells.

❑❑   **X-linked agammaglobulinemia and CVID are most susceptible to which infections?**

Pyogenic bacterial infections, most notably *S. aureus*, *H. influenzae*, *S. pnuemoniae*.

❑❑   **What four infectious agents are most commonly associated with asplenic individuals?**

S. pneumoniae, Neisseria sp., H. influenzae and, Salmonella sp.

❑❑   **Which disorder is considered the most severe of the recognized immunodeficiences?**

SCID

❑❑   **Fatality of hereditary angioedema can occur due to what condition?**

Edema of the larynx.

❑❑   **Acute neutrophilia occurs during what physiologic events?**

Physical exercise, and other epinephrine-induced reaction such as a panic response.

❑❑   **Reactive leukocytosis resembling a leukemia-like picture can occur in what clinical scenarios?**

Sepsis, systemic mycotic or protozoan, hepatic failure, diabetic acidosis, and azotemia.

❑❑   **What is the definition of neutropenia?**

Absolute Neutrophil Count (ANC) < 1500 cell/ml

❑❑   **What percent neonates born to eclamptic mothers have transient neutropenia?**

50%

❑❑   **What nutritional deficiencies may precipitate neutropenia?**

Vitamin B12, Folic Acid, and Copper.

❑❑   **Neutropenia and bacterial infection may herald the onset of?**

Overwhelming sepsis.

❑❑   **What is the prognosis of Chediak-Higashi syndrome?**

Affected persons may die at any time as illness frequently progresses to an accelerated phase characterized by lymphadenopathy, hepatosplenomegaly, pancytopenia, hemmorhage of GI and brain. This accelerated phase if often precipitated by lymphotrophic viral infections such as Epstein-Barr.

❑❑ **Would prophylactic antibiotics be indicated for this condition?**

No. Prevention with antibiotics has not been shown to be useful in this condition.

❑❑ **What is the most common inherited disorder of phagocyte function?**

Chronic Granulomatosus Disease (CGD).

❑❑ **Name the typical organisms isolated in culture of infected sites in patients with CGD .**

S. aureus, Klebsiella, Aerobacter, E. coli, Shigella, Samonella, Psuedomonas, S. marcescens, C. albicans, and *Aspergillus.*

❑❑ **Briefly explain the cellular basis for the Type I hypersensitivity reaction (Wheal and flare) and give a clinical example.**

This immediate type or anaphylactic hypersensitivity is mediated by circulating basophils and mast cells which become activated by cross-linking of IgE on their membrane surface. The prototypic IgE mediated disease is ragweed hay fever. Other, sometimes fatal anaphylactic reactions are the classic insect venom, or food induced allergies.

❑❑ **Briefly explain the cellular basis for the Type II hypersensitivity reaction (cytotoxic) and give a clinical example.**

These immune interactions involve integral cellular antigen components and IgG and IgM antibody formation to these "foreign" antigen determinants. The classic example is immune mediated hemolysis such as that seen in transfusion reactions or Hemolytic disease of the newborn.

❑❑ **Which hypersensitivity reaction is responsible for a majority of the glomerulopathies?**

90% of glomerulonephritis is Type III or immune complex disease.

❑❑ **What is a prototypic DTH type IV reaction?**

Contact allergy such as chemical induced contact dermatitis or poison ivy.

❑❑ **In taking a history when one suspects allergy, what are some of the most important components to include?**

History of exposure to potential allergens, frequency, duration, location, and progression of symptoms, seasonal symptoms, onset of symptoms, relieving factors (medication, diurnal variation, change in location), and nature of symptoms (dry vs. productive cough, clear vs. purulent sputum).

❑❑ **What test is most cost effective, sensitive, and specific in the diagnosis of allergy?**

In vivo skin testing.

❑❑ **What in vitro tests may be useful in the diagnosis of allergic conditions?**

WBC with differential, Ig serum content, RAST, leukocyte histamine release test.

❑❑ **A patient has a 5 mm "wheal and flare" reaction to ragweed, but denies seasonal allergic symptoms. What does this indicate?**

The patient has been exposed to the allergen, but may not be allergic.

❑❑ **What effects of corticosteroids are likely after two hours?**

Fall in peripheral eosinophils and lymphocytes.

❏❏ **What effects of corticosteroids are likely after six to eight hours?**

Improvement in pulmonary function in asthmatics and hyperglycemia.

❏❏ **What is the most common adverse effect on chronic systemic corticosteroid use?**

Suppression of linear growth.

❏❏ **What infections are children receiving chronic steroids particularly susceptible to?**

Disseminated varicella and *Pneumocystis carinii.*

❏❏ **What is the preferred dosing regimen of prednisone or prednisolone to lessen the hypothalmic-pituitary-adrenal axis suppressive effect?**

It is recommended that alternate day regimen given as a single dose between 6:00 and 8:00 am. If daily dosing is required, then administer a single dose between 6:00 and 8:00 am.

❏❏ **What patients are not good candidates for immunotherapy desensitization?**

Patients with atopic dermatitis and food allergy.

❏❏ **What is the prognosis of allergic rhinitis?**

90% of children 8 to 11 years later will still have persistent symptoms.

19% of children will develop asthma or wheezing.

❏❏ **What constitutes triad asthma?**

The syndrome of nasal polyps, asthma, and aspirin intolerance comprise triad asthma.

❏❏ **The most likely cause of foul-smelling, unilateral, blood-tinged, purulent discharge from a child's nose?**

Foreign body.

❏❏ **The most effective treatment of allergic rhinitis?**

Topical use of corticosteroid such as beclomethasone nasal spray.

❏❏ **What is the prognosis of childhood asthma?**

50% of all asthmatic children are symptom free within 10-20 year. In mild asthma, the remission rate is 50%, with only 5% experiencing severe disease. 95% of children with severe childhood asthma, however, become asthmatic adults.

❏❏ **Is *cor pulmonale* resulting from sustained pulmonary hypertension a common complication of asthma?**

No.

❏❏ **Define extrinsic asthma.**

Asthmatic exacerbation following environmental exposure to allergens such as dust, pollens, and dander.

❏❏ **Define intrinsic asthma.**

Asthmatic exacerbation not associated with an increase in IgE.

❏❏ **Does a child with asthma require a chest x-ray?**

Every child with an exacerbation does not require a chest x-ray, however it may be necessary to rule out other respiratory diagnosis.

❑❑ **Aside from albuterol, what other medications are used for asthmatic attack?**

Depending on severity, all or none of the following may be used: Oral steroids, nebulized anticholinergic (i.e. Atrovent), subcutaneous terbutaline (specific B2 agonist), and theophylline. The current treatment protocol changes frequently as new research is hot in this area.

❑❑ **What are the historical risk factors for status asthmaticus?**

Chronic steroid-dependent asthma, prior ICU admission, prior intubation, recurrent ER visits in past 48 hours, sudden onset of severe respiratory, poor therapy compliance, poor clinical recognition of attack severity, and hypoxic seizures.

❑❑ **What percent of patients with atopic dermatitis have elevated serum IgE levels?**

80%.

❑❑ **Describe the diagnostic criteria of atopic dermatitis in infants?**

Must have three major features namely, family history, extensor eczematous or lichenified dermatitis, and evidence of puritus. Patients must also have three minor features namely, chronic scaling of scalp, postauricular fissures, ichthyosis, xerosis, or hyperlinear palms.

❑❑ **Describe the clinical manifestation of urticaria?**

Well-circumscribed, erythematous raised skin lesions.

❑❑ **What is most common form of urticaria caused by physical factors?**

Cold urticaria.

❑❑ **What is the most effective treatment for control of urticaria?**

0.5 mg/kg Hydroxyzine (Atarax).

❑❑ **What substances can induce pseudoallergic anaphylaxis?**

Iodinated radiocontrast media, opiates, D-tubocurarine, thiamine, aspirin, and captopril.

❑❑ **When do most anaphylactic reactions occur?**

Within the first 30 minutes after initial exposure.

❑❑ **What are typical initial symptoms of an anaphylactic reaction?**

A tingling sensation around the mouth, followed by a warm feeling and tightness in the chest or throat.

❑❑ **What is standard treatment of an anaphylactic reaction?**

Aqueous epinephrine 1: 1000 at 0.1 ml/kg with maximum dosage of 0.3 ml for a child.

❑❑ **Which vaccines must be avoided by patients who have a severe allergy to eggs?**

Influenza and yellow fever vaccines.

❑❑ **What is the major cause of serum sickness?**

Drug allergy, particularly to penicillin.

❑❑ **Are atopic individuals at an increased risk for developing adverse drug reactions?**

No. However, they may suffer a more severe reaction if they do acquire a drug allergy.

❑❑ **What is the most common manifestation of an adverse drug reaction?**

Cutaneous eruption with urticarial, exanthematous, and eczematoid occur predominantly.

□□   **What test may be used to identify an anaphylactic hypersensitivity to penicillin?**

Skin testing with benzylpenicilloyl-polylysine (BPL PrePen) identifies a majority of children who are at risk.

□□   **Can you give a cephalosporin to someone who is allergic to penicillin?**

The right answer is, of course, no. However, this is very arbitrary depending on the severity of the allergy, and the efficacy of alternate medications. In general, the cross-reactivity is only about 5%, so they are fairly safely used in these patients.

□□   **When treatment with penicillin is absolutely necessary, which route of desensitization is the safest?**

Oral.

□□   **What is the most sensitive and specific sign of an infectious disease in an immunocompromised host?**

Fever.

□□   **Anti dsDNA antibodies are most indicative for what disease?**

Systemic lupus erythematosus.

□□   **Anti Ro(SSA) and La(SSB) are associated with what disease?**

Neonatal lupus syndrome.

□□   **The presence of antineutrophil cytoplasmic antibodies (c-ANCA) with a diffuse staining pattern in serum immunofluorescence is most commonly associated with what disease?**

Wegener's Granulomatosus.

□□   **The staining pattern described above may be associated with what other diseases?**

Kawasaki's disease and HIV.

□□   **The presence of anti phospholipdid antibodies with patients who have either primary or secondary antiphopholipid syndromes are at increased risk for what pathological events?**

Risk of thrombic events, thrombocytopenia, hemolytic anemia, stroke, chorea, transverse myelitis, and vascular heart disease.

□□   **In which two subgroups of JRA is joint destruction more likely?**

RA factor positive polyarticular, and systemic-onset JRA.

□□   **What percent of the above patients develop severe arthritis?**

>50%.

□□   **What are the most common manifestations of Juvenile Rheumatoid Arthritis (JRA)?**

High intermittent fever, rheumatoid rash, arthralgia or myalgia (during febrile episodes), and persistent arthritis of greater than six weeks duration.

□□   **What is the overall prognosis of JRA patients?**

At least 75% of patients with JRA will have long term remissions without significant residual deformity or loss of function

□□   **What pharmacological treatment is not indicated in the treatment of JRA?**

Corticosteroids.

☐☐   **How does ankylosing spondylitis differ from rheumatoid arthritis?**

Ankylosing spondilitis is characterized by involvement of the sacroiliac joints and lumbodorsal spine, predilection for males, occurrence of aortitis, familial incidence, RF negative, and lack of rheumatoid nodules or incidence of acute iridocyclitis.

☐☐   **What is the triad of Reiter's disease?**

Arthritis, conjunctivitis, urethritis (or cervicitis).

☐☐   **Reiter's disease may occur following infection with which microbial agents?**

Shigella, Yersinia, Enterocolitica, Camphylobacter, and *Chlamydia*.

☐☐   **What percent of children with inflammatory bowel disease have articular manifestations of the disease?**

10%.

☐☐   **Which therapies are most effective for children afflicted with rheumatological disease?**

Physical and occupational therapies.

☐☐   **What are the most frequent early symptoms of SLE in children?**

Fever, malaise, arthritis or arthralgia, and rash .

☐☐   **What is the best screening test for SLE?**

ANA should be demonstrable in all patients with active SLE.

☐☐   **What hematologic conditions are seen with patients who have SLE?**

Anemia, thrombocytopenia, and leukopenia occur frequently.

☐☐   **What neurologic disorders, if present, serve as diagnostic criteria for SLE?**

Seizures and psychosis.

☐☐   **What pharmacologic agents are most commonly associated with drug induced lupus?**

Anticonvulsants, antihypertensive, and isoniazid.

☐☐   **List the major causes of SLE mortality.**

Nephritis, central nervous system complications, infection, pulmonary lupus, and myocardial infarction.

☐☐   **When is anticoagulation therapy indicated in SLE?**

Patients with the persistent presence of antiphospholipid antibodies (because of the risk of venous or arterial thrombosis), migraine, recurrent fetal loss, TIA, stroke, avascular necrosis, transverse myelitis, pulmonary hypertension or embolus, livedo reticularis, leg ulcers, or thrombocytopenia.

☐☐   **What is the most effective means of diagnosing vasculitis in children?**

Clinical diagnosis is most reliable.

☐☐   **List the potentially fatal manifestations of Henoch-Schonlein syndrome.**

Acute renal failure; GI complications, such as hemorrhage, intussusception, and bowel infarction; and CNS involvement, which may precipitate seizures, paresis, or coma.

☐☐   **What clinical manifestations are seen in most patients with Henoch-Schonlein syndrome?**

Dermatological manifestations, which will be present in all patients. However, skin lesions are extremely varied. The classic lesion begins as a small wheal or erythematous maculopapule, which becomes petechial or pupuritic. The palpable purpural lesions will progress from red to purple to rusty color as they age.

❏❏   **Aside from the skin rash, what are the three most common manifestations of Henoch-Schonlein syndrome?**

Arthritis, 67%; GI complaints, 50%; and renal involvement, 25%-50%.

❏❏   **What test is most useful for recognizing coronary vascular disease, dilation, or aneurysmal formation?**

Two dimensional echocardiogram.

❏❏   **List the possible complications of Kawasaki's disease during the acute phase of the illness.**

Arthritis, myocarditis, pericarditis, mitral insufficiency, CHF, iridocyclitis, meningitis, and sterile pyuria.

❏❏   **Which form of vasculitis may be seen after infection with Hepatitis B?**

Polyarteritis nodosa.

❏❏   **What side effects might one see only rarely with the administration of IV gamma globulin?**

Anaphylaxis, chills, fever, headache, and myalgia.

❏❏   **Which tissue biopsy is most helpful for diagnosing Polyarteritis nodosa, but is rarely employed?**

Testicular biopsy.

❏❏   **T/F: Erythema nodosum is most common in children less than six years old.**

False. This disease is rarely seen before the age of six. It progressively increases in frequency up to the third decade in life.

❏❏   **Behcet syndrome is characterized by recurrent oral and genital ulcers and ocular inflammation. What additional symptoms are associated with a particularly poor prognosis?**

CNS abnormalities, such as cranial nerve palsies and psychosis.

❏❏   **The combination of pain, tenderness, and swelling of the costosternal junction is referred to as what syndrome?**

Tietze syndrome, or costochondritis.

❏❏   **What inflammatory conditions might one expect with secondary amyloidosis?**

JRA, cystic fibrosis, inflammatory bowel disease, and chronic infections such as tuberculosis.

GENITOURINARY AND RENAL

One's work may be finished someday, but one's educations, never.
- Alexandre Dumas

☐☐   **As of March, 1999, what is the American Academy of Pediatrics recommendation regarding routine circumcision?**

"Circumcision is not essential to a child's well-being at birth, even though it does have some potential medical benefits. These benefits are not compelling enough to warrant the AAP to recommend routine newborn circumcision. Instead, we encourage parents to discuss the benefits and risks of circumcision with their pediatrician, and then make an informed decision about what is in the best interest of their child," according to Carole Lannon, M.D., MPH, FAAP, chair of the AAP's Task Force on Circumcision. In other words, No to routine, though as always, the patient preference supercedes normally.

☐☐   **What is the <u>most</u> <u>common</u> cause of acute renal failure?**

Acute tubular necrosis. Acute tubular necrosis occurs after a toxic or an ischemic injury to the kidneys caused from shock, surgery, or rhabdomyolysis.

☐☐   **Why is surgical correction of cryptorchidism important?**

Cryptorchidism is when a testicle does not descend into the scrotum and is retained either in the abdominal cavity or in the inguinal canal. This condition can cause infertility in the affected testicle and will increase the risk of cancer in that testicle. Surgical correction is required to inhibit infertility, but the procedure has no bearing on the future development of testicular cancer. Surgery must be performed before the age of 5 to preserve fertility.

☐☐   **What is the most important feature for distinguishing between testicular torsion and epididymitis?**

The rate of the onset of pain. Torsional pain begins instantaneously at maximum intensity, whereas epididymal pain grows steadily over hours or days. Clinically, elevation of the scrotum will relieve pain related to epididymitis, but is not effective with torsional pain.

☐☐   **What is the <u>most</u> <u>common</u> cause of epididymitis?**

1) Prepubertal boys: Coliform bacteria
2) In men younger than 35: Chlamydia or Neisseria gonorrhea.
3) Older than 35: Coliform bacteria

☐☐   **What does epididymitis in childhood suggest?**

Obstructive or fistulous urinary defects. Epididymitis is rare in children.

☐☐   **What is the significance of the "blue dot" sign?**

This is pathognomonic of torsion of the appendix testis or epididymis. With transillumination of the testis, a blue reflection occurs. When detected early, a patient with torsion of the appendages will experience intense pain near the head of the epididymis or testis that is frequently associated with a palpable tender nodule. If normal flow to the affected testis can be confirmed by a testicular ultrasound, immediate surgery can be avoided. Most appendages will calcify or degenerate within 10 to 14 days without harm to the patient.

☐☐   **What is the treatment of epididymitis for children?**

1. In patients less than 40 years old, the most common pathogens that cause epididymitis are Chlamydia and gonorrhea. Treatment thereby includes ceftriaxone IM and doxycycline PO.

2. In prepubertal children, the common pathogens are coliform bacteria, and should be treated with TMP-SMX.

☐☐   **What 4 clinical findings are indicative of acute glomerulonephritis (GN)?**

1) Oliguria.
2) Hypertension.
3) Pulmonary edema.
4) Urine sediment containing red blood cells, white blood cells, protein, and red blood cell casts.

☐☐   **What is the differential diagnosis for rapidly progressive GN?**

1) Polyarteritis Nodosa (PAN): A systemic necrotizing vasculitis affecting primarily medium and small caliber arteries that can occur from infancy to old age. The peak incidence occurs at approximately 60 years of age. Ninety percent of patients with PAN will have renal involvement.

2) Systemic Lupus Erythematosus (SLE): An autoimmune disorder resulting, in part, from a necrotizing vasculitis of primarily small vessels which is complicated by direct immunoglobulin deposition in glomeruli. The mortality rate is 18-58%, depending on the histologic type.

3) Henoch-Schönlein Purpura: Another systemic necrotizing vasculitis of small vessels. Patients present with a nephritic syndrome without edema or hypertension or with hematuria.

4) Hemolytic Uremic Syndrome (HUS): Patients present with microangiopathic hemolytic anemia, thrombocytopenia, and renal dysfunction. The onset is rapid. It occurs in children about 1 week after a gastroenteritis or an URI. HUS may occur in adults, most commonly complicating pregnancy or the post partum period. Acute renal failure develops in 60% of children with HUS and usually resolves in weeks with only supportive therapy.

5) Thrombotic Thrombocytopenic Purpura: This condition is closely related to HUS with a higher occurrence in young adults. It is associated with fevers, more neurologic problems, and less renal involvement (i.e., usually with hematuria and proteinuria). The prognosis is much worse as compared to HUS with a 75% three-month mortality rate.

☐☐   **Which syndrome is characterized by a rapidly progressive, antiglomerular basement membrane antibody-induced GN that is preceded by pulmonary hemorrhage and hemoptysis?**

Goodpasture's syndrome.

☐☐   **What is the most common cause of hematuria?**

Lesions of the bladder or lower urinary tract. When hematuria originates in a kidney, the probable causes are polycystic kidney disease and nephropathy.

☐☐   **What are some causes of false-positive hematuria?**

Food coloring, beets, paprika, rifampin, phenothiazine, Dilantin, myoglobin, or menstruation.

☐☐   **A urinalysis reveals red cell casts and dysmorphic RBCs in the urine. What is the probable origin of hematuria?**

Glomerulus.

❑❑   **A 4 year old boy presents with a painless mass in his scrotum that fluctuates in size with palpation. The mass transilluminates. What is the diagnosis?**

This is probably a communicating hydrocele. An inguinal-scrotal ultrasound should distinguish hydrocele from bowel and a testicular nuclear scan should rule out the possibility of testicular torsion.

❑❑   **What is the composition of the <u>most</u> <u>common</u> kidney stones?**

Calcium oxalate (65%), followed by magnesium ammonium phosphate (struvite) (20%), calcium phosphate (7.5%), uric acid (5%), and cystine (1%)

❑❑   **A urinary pH of 7.3 is conducive to the formation of what kind of stones?**

Struvite and phosphate stones. Alkalotic urine actually inhibits the formation of uric acid and cystine stones. Conversely, struvite and phosphate stones are inhibited by a more acidic urine.

❑❑   **Which type of stone formation is caused by a genetic error?**

Cysteine stones. These stones are produced because there is an error in the transport of amino acids that results in cystinuria.

❑❑   **Where is kidney stone formation most likely to occur?**

In the proximal portion of the collecting system.

❑❑   **What is the five year recurrence rate for kidney stones?**

50%. The ten year recurrence rate is 70%.

❑❑   **What percent of patients spontaneously pass kidney stones?**

80%. This is largely dependent on size. 75% of stones less than 4 mm pass spontaneously, while only 10% of those larger than 6 mm pass spontaneously. Analgesics and increased fluid intake aid in outpatient management of kidney stones.

❑❑   **What is the <u>most</u> <u>common</u> cause of nephrotic syndrome in children?**

Minimal change disease is the most common cause in children.

❑❑   **Name some common nephrotoxic agents/substances.**

Aminoglycoside, NSAIDs, contrast dye, and myoglobin.

❑❑   **What is the definition of oliguria? Of anuria?**

Oliguria is defined as a urine output of less than 500 mL/day. Anuria is associated with a urine output of less than 100 mL/day.

❑❑   **What is the initial treatment for priapism?**

Terbutaline, 0.25–0.5 mg subcutaneously.

❑❑   **What is the <u>most</u> <u>common</u> origin of proteinuria?**

Pathology of the glomerulus. Other origins are tubular pathology or over production of protein.

❑❑   **When are symptoms related to renal insufficiency displayed?**

When 90% of the nephrons have been destroyed. Hypertension, diabetes mellitus, glomerulonephritis, polycystic kidney disease, tubulointerstitial disease, and obstructive uropathy are all causes of chronic renal failure.

❑❑   **If a urine dipstick is positive for blood yet the UA on the same urine is negative for RBCs, what is the probable disease?**

Rhabdomyolysis. Severe muscle damage can result in free myoglobin in the blood. Very high levels can lead to acute renal failure.

☐☐   **What is the <u>most</u> <u>common</u> neoplasm in men under 30?**

Seminomas. This is also the most common type of testicular neoplasm. The peak incidence is between the ages of 20-40 with a smaller peak occurring below the age of 10. Ninety to ninety five percent of these cancers are germinal tumors. However, only 60-70% are germinal in children. Cryptorchidism is a significant risk factor for this cancer.

☐☐   **What is the best tumor marker for testicular cancer?**

Placental alkaline phosphatase (PLAP). Seventy to ninety percent of patients with testicular cancer have elevated PLAP. Other tumor markers are alpha-fetoprotein and beta-human chorionic gonadotropin.

☐☐   **Testicular torsion is <u>most</u> <u>common</u> in which age group?**

14 year olds. Two-thirds of the cases occur in the second decade. The next most common group is newborns.

☐☐   **T/F: Testicular torsion frequently follows a history of strenuous physical activity or occurs during sleep.**

True.

☐☐   **T/F: Forty percent of patients with testicular torsion have a history of similar pain in the past that resolved spontaneously.**

True.

☐☐   **What is the definitive diagnostic test for testicular torsion?**

Emergent surgical exploration. Although radionuclide imaging and Doppler ultrasonography may be helpful, they are time-consuming, and their accuracy is operator-dependent. The warm ischemia time for testicular salvage may be as short as four hours. Therefore, after the diagnosis is made, immediate urologic consultation and surgical exploration are necessary.

☐☐   **What is the definitive treatment for testicular torsion?**

Bilateral orchiopexy in which the testes are surgically attached to the scrotum.

☐☐   **What is the <u>most</u> <u>common</u> cause of urinary tract infections (UTI)?**

E. coli (80%). *E. coli* is also the most common cause of pyelonephritis and pyelitis due to its ascension from the lower urinary tract. *Staphylococcus saprophyticus* accounts for 5-15% of the UTI cases.

☐☐   **Which patients with UTIs are candidates for single dose or short-course (i.e., 3 days) antibiotic therapy with trimethoprim-sulfamethoxazole?**

Non-pregnant females without risk factors for subclinical pyelonephritis, such as prolonged symptoms, recurrent UTIs, diabetes mellitus, urinary tract abnormalities, or recurrent pyelonephritis. Follow up within 1 week is a mandatory for these patients.

☐☐   **Varicoceles are <u>most</u> <u>common</u> in which part of the scrotum?**

The left. Varicoceles are a collection of veins in the scrotum. These patients have a higher incidence of infertility, presumably because of the increased temperature of the testes surrounded by the warm blood of the varicocele. Incidentally, the left testes is the first to descend and also hangs lower than the right in the majority of men. Hernias are also more common on the left side too.

☐☐   **What is the <u>most</u> <u>common</u> renal tumor in children?**

Wilm's tumor. This occurs in children under 5 years of age.

❏❏   **A second trimester ultrasound is performed on a pregnant female and it demonstrates oligohydramnios, nonvisualization of the bladder, and absent kidneys. What disorder should be suspected?**

Bilateral renal agenesis (Potter's Syndrome).

❏❏   **What tumor in children is associated with horseshoe kidneys?**

Wilms tumor.

❏❏   **What is the gold standard laboratory test for diagnosing a urinary tract infection?**

Urine culture.

❏❏   **A newborn presents with a palpable abdominal mass. What is the most common cause?**

A hydronephrotic kidney.

❏❏   **What is the difference between primary and secondary nocturnal enuresis?**

Primary enuresis is when the child never has a period of nighttime continence, while secondary nocturnal enuresis is a developing condition in a formerly dry child following a significant emotional event.

❏❏   **How do you treat nocturnal enuresis?**

Reassure the parents that the problem is self-limiting and advise them not to invoke punitive measures that may adversely affect the psychological development of the child.

❏❏   **What is hypospadias?**

A congenital penile deformity resulting from incomplete development of the distal or anterior urethra.

❏❏   **What is the most common congenital anomaly of the penis?**

Hypospadias.

❏❏   **What anomalies are associated with agenesis of the penis?**

Anal, rectal, and renal anomalies.

❏❏   **What is phimosis?**

An inability to retract the prepuce at an age when it should normally be retracted.

❏❏   **What is a paraphimosis?**

A condition where a phimotic prepuce is retracted behind the coronal sulcus and this retraction cannot be reduced.

❏❏   **What are the complications of cryptorchidism?**

Infertility, tumor development in the undescended testes, hernias, and torsion of the cryptorchid testes.

❏❏   **In a patient with cryptorchidism what is the risk of developing a malignant testicular tumor in the third to fourth decade of life?**

20-44%.

❏❏   **What is the most common tumor which develops in an undescended testes?**

Seminoma (60%).

❏❏   **What are the findings in a patient with testicular torsion?**

The scrotum is swollen, tender and difficult to examine. The cremasteric reflex is absent.

❏❏   **What is a varicocele?**

Dilatation of the pampiniform venous plexus due to valvular incompetence of the spermatic vein.

❏❏   **What are the complications of circumcision?**

Hemorrhage, infection, dehiscence, denudation of the shaft, glandular injury, and urinary retention.

❏❏   **What is balanitis?**

Infection of the prepuce most often due to mixed flora.

❏❏   **Gross hematuria of renal origin has what characteristics?**

The color is generally brown or cola-colored and may contain red blood cells casts.

❏❏   **A 7-year-old male presents with sensorineural hearing loss, cataracts, and recurrent microscopic hematuria. What is the most likely diagnosis?**

Alports syndrome.

❏❏   **A 5-year-old child presents with sudden onset of gross hematuria, edema, hypertension, and renal insufficiency two weeks after a sore throat, what is the most likely diagnosis?**

Acute post-streptococcal glomerulonephritis.

❏❏   **What are the complications of acute post-streptococcal glomerulonephritis?**

Hyperkalemia, hypertension, hyperphosphatemia, hypocalcemia, acidosis, seizures, uremia, and volume overload.

❏❏   **What is the prognosis for a patient with post-streptococcal glomerulonephritis?**

95% of children will completely recover within one month.

❏❏   **What are the most common causes of nephrotic syndrome between six months and one year of age?**

Idiopathic nephrotic syndrome or drug-induced nephrosis.

❏❏   **An 11-year-old female presents with a purpuric rash on the buttocks and lower extremities, arthralgias, and abdominal pain. What is the most likely diagnosis?**

Henoch-Schonlein purpura.

❏❏   **What is the most common form of systemic vasculitis in children?**

Anaphylactoid (Henoch-Schonlein purpura).

❏❏   **What is the most common cause of acute renal failure in young children?**

Hemolytic-uremic syndrome.

❏❏   **A 4-year-old presents with irritability, weakness, lethargy, dehydration, edema, petechiae, and hepatosplenomegaly ten days after an episode of gastroenteritis. Laboratory results reveal a low platelet count and hemoglobulin level, what is the most likely diagnosis?**

Hemolytic-uremic syndrome.

❏❏   **What are the complications of hemolytic uremic syndrome?**

Fluid overload, anemia, acidosis, hyperkalemia, congestive heart failure, hypertension, and uremia.

❏❏   **A patient presents with a flat nose, recessed chin, epicanthal folds, low-set abnormal ears, club feet and bilateral renal agenesis. What is the likely diagnosis?**

Potter's syndrome.

❏❏   **A patient presents with proteinuria on routine urinalysis, which is absent, after obtaining a voiding specimen from the same patient upon awakening in the morning, what is the most likely diagnosis?**

Postural (orthostatic) proteinuria.

❏❏   **What is postural (orthostatic) proteinuria?**

Significant proteinuria in the upright position with normal or slightly increased serum protein.

❏❏   **What are the characteristics of the nephrotic syndrome?**

Edema, hyperlipidemia, hypoproteinemia, and proteinuria.

❏❏   **What is the treatment for children with nephrotic syndrome due to minimal change disease?**

Corticosteroid therapy.

❏❏   **What is renal tubular acidosis?**

A clinical state of systemic hyperchloremic acidosis due to impaired urinary acidification.

❏❏   **What is proximal renal tubular acidosis (RTA)?**

A renal disorder resulting in reduced proximal tubular reabsorption of bicarbonate due to deficient carbonic anhydrase production.

❏❏   **What are the most common causes of chronic renal failure in a child under 5 years of age?**

Anatomic abnormalities of the kidneys.

❏❏   **What are the most common causes of chronic renal failure in children greater than 5 years of age?**

Glomerulonephritis, hemolytic uremic syndrome, or hereditary disorders (Alport syndrome, cystic disease).

❏❏   **What are the mechanisms behind anemia of chronic renal failure?**

Decreased erythropoietin production, low grade hemolysis, bleeding, decreased erythrocyte survival, inadequate iron intake, inadequate folic acid intake, and inhibition of erythropoiesis.

❏❏   **What are the causes of hypertension in a patient with chronic renal failure?**

Sodium and water overload and excessive renin production.

❏❏   **At what age does the GFR approximate adult values (correcting for body surface area)?**

3 years old

❏❏   **What is the formula for calculating the clearance of a substance?**

Cs (ml/min)=(Us(mg/ml)xV(ml/min))/Ps (mg/ml) (where Cs is clearance of the substance; Us is concentration of substance in urine; V is urine flow rate; and Ps is concentration of substance in plasma).

❏❏   **A child complains of "red urine". What foods can cause this?**

Beets, blackberries and red food coloring.

❏❏   **What are the four most common causes of recurrent gross hematuria in the absence of trauma?**

Acute PSG, IgA nephropathy, familial nephritis (Alport syndrome), and idiopathic.

❐❐   **What is the prognosis of a child with Berger nephropathy?**

Most patients do not have significant renal damage and only supportive therapy is recommended. However, about 1/3 of the patients will develop progressive disease (note: this disorder is also known as IgA nephropathy).

❐❐   **A 13 year old boy presents with gross hematuria and some hearing loss. What is your diagnosis?**

Alports syndrome.

❐❐   **What is the most common cause of gross hematuria in children?**

IgA nephropathy.

❐❐   **What is the classic presentation of post-streptococcal glomerulonephritis (PSG)?**

Sudden development of gross hematuria, hypertension, edema and renal insufficiency following a throat or skin infection with group A B-hemolytic streptococcus. Patients frequently also have generalized complaints of fever, malaise, lethargy, abdominal pain, etc.

❐❐   **How early in the development of "strep throat" will antibiotic therapy decrease the risk for PSG?**

Antibiotics have not been found to decrease the risk for PSG.

❐❐   **What lab test best confirms PSG as the diagnosis?**

Anti-DNAse B antibody titer

❐❐   **What is the most common form of lupus nephritis?**

Diffuse proliferative nephritis (WHO class IV). Unfortunately, this is also the most severe form.

❐❐   **The biopsy of the kidney from a 14 year old boy with nephrotic syndrome shows increased mesangial cells and, on immunofluorescence, C3 deposits in the mesangium. What is the boy's diagnosis and prognosis?**

This child has membranoproliferative glomerulonephritis (a type of chronic glomerulonephritis). Prognosis is poor, with many patients progressing to end-stage renal failure.

❐❐   **What is the most common manifestation of Goodpasture disease?**

Hemoptysis. These patients usually develop pulmonary hemorrhage before any signs of renal failure develop.

❐❐   **HUS most commonly follows infection with what organism?**

E. coli (O157:H7). The disease is usually a sequelae to a bout of gastroenteritis caused by this organism.

❐❐   **What is the diagnostic triad for HUS?**

Microangiopathic anemia, acute renal failure, and thrombocytopenia ($20k\text{-}100k/mm'$).

❐❐   **What is the prognosis for patients with acute renal failure secondary to HUS?**

Over 90% survival with many patients eventually recovering normal renal function.

❐❐   **What is the role of corticosteroids in the treatment of HUS?**

None.

❐❐   **What is the best medical management of HUS?**

Heparin and frequent peritoneal dialysis along with aggressive management of hematological manifestations.

❏❏   **The mother of a 2 month old male infant is concerned that she cannot retract the foreskin. Should you circumcise at this point?**

No. More than 85% of uncircumcised males can retract the foreskin by the 3rd year. Before this time it is not a concern.

❏❏   **Why is chronic dialysis therapy to be avoided in children?**

Dialysis for end stage renal disease (ERSD) in children is associated with failure to thrive, social maladaption, lack of sexual maturity, and chronic encephalopathy.

❏❏   **Name two causes of ESRD with patients less than 5 years old.**

Congenital and obstructive uropathy.

❏❏   **What is the most common cause of ESRD in children 13-17 years old?**

Glomerulopathies.

❏❏   **What is the diagnostic triad of the nephrotic syndrome (we told you once already)?**

Edema, hyperlipidemia, and proteinuria with hypoproteinemia.

❏❏   **What is the most common cause of the nephrotic syndrome in children?**

Idiopathic nephrotic syndrome, of which the most common type is minimal change disease.

❏❏   **What is the most common cause of acute scrotal pain in patients less than 6 years old?**

Testicular torsion.

❏❏   **How is renal tubular acidosis (RTA) classified?**

Into one of three types: Type 1-distal RTA, Type II-proximal RTA, or Type IV- mineralocorticoid deficiency. There is no type III.

❏❏   **What are the mechanisms for the different types of RTA?**

In Type I, there is a deficiency in the secretion of the hydrogen ion by the distal tubule and collecting duct. The mechanism for Type II is a decrease in the bicarbonate reabsorption in the proximal tubule.

❏❏   **Which isolated form of RTA will be most likely to lead to renal failure?**

Distal (Type I), though most cases of Type I RTA have an excellent prognosis.

❏❏   **What is Fanconi syndrome?**

Phosphaturia (with hypophosphatemia), renal glycosuria, and generalized aminoaciduria.

❏❏   **Why do patients with Fanconi syndrome commonly present with rickets?**

This is due to both hypophosphatemia and metabolic acidosis which, among other things, is believed to decrease the conversion of vitamin D to its active metabolite.

❏❏   **What is the most common presentation of idiopathic nephrotic syndrome?**

Edema, frequently in conjunction with anorexia, diarrhea and abdominal pain.

❏❏   **What percentage of kidney transplants donated from a relative (usually a parent) are still functional after three years?**

75-80%

❑❑   **Children with horseshoe kidneys are at increased risk of developing what tumor?**

Wilms tumor.

❑❑   **Are circumcised males more, less, or equally likely to develop urinary tract infection when compared to their uncut counterparts?**

Less

❑❑   **A urinary tract infection due to what organism may lead to hyperammonemia?**

Proteus.

❑❑   **What is the definitive diagnostic test for suspected acute pyelonephritis?**

CT. However, this is hardly used as a good H&P and less expensive tests are usually sufficient to make the diagnosis.

❑❑   **Aside from the cost factor, why should you be hesitant to order a CT scan on a child with suspected pyelonephritis?**

To protect the gonads from radiation, especially in the females. The ovaries can become cancerous from a relatively small amount of radiation.

❑❑   **Why should you order an ultrasound for a child with acute febrile urinary tract infection?**

To rule out an obstruction

❑❑   **A concerned mother asks you whether it is common for her 5 year old son to still be wetting his bed at night. What should you tell her?**

Not to be concerned, as about one-fifth of children his age have this problem. 15-20% of children stop having this problem each year.

❑❑   **The above mentioned mother is not relieved to find she and her son have to "wait it out". "Isn't there something you can do to make it better now?", she asks. What is your response?**

You can prescribe desmopressin nasal spray, which will temporarily ease the condition, but time is still the main factor in treatment.

❑❑   **What is the cause of primary vesicoureteral reflux?**

This is due to a congenital defect in which the valve at the vesicoureteral junction is patent or incompetent.

❑❑   **How do you grade a vesicoureteral reflux?**

There are 5 grades: I-no dilatation, II-no dilatation, but reflux reaches upper collecting system, III-ureter dilated and there may be blunting of the calyceal fornices, IV-ureter is grossly dilated, V-all details of calyces are lost and the entire ureter is grossly dilated and tortuous.

❑❑   **A newborn child has his urethral opening on the ventral side of the glands. What are some common abnormalities frequently seen concomitantly with this condition?**

Inguinal hernias and undescended testes.

❑❑   **What is the treatment for paraphimosis?**

As the glans edema and venous engorgement can lead to arterial compromise, this is a true emergency. First, try to manually compress the edema, after which the foreskin may be successfully reduced. If this does not work, a superficial vertical incision of the constricting band (after local anesthetic) will decompress the gland. Obviously, this procedure should be performed by a urologist or emergency medicine physician.

❑❑   **A child is born with cryptorchidism. What are the likely sequelae of this condition?**

Infertility (though early surgical correction decreases the risk of this), and malignant testicular cancer later in life in about 30-40% of patients (early surgery will do nothing to alter this).

❑❑   **You are at home barbecuing a fine steak on a sunny day when a neighbor comes running to you with his little boy, who is grabbing his groin area and crying in agony. You examine the boy and it looks as if it could be testicular torsion. What do you do?**

Flip your steak, then try manual detorsion. In right testicular torsion, the testis is rotated clockwise and the left testis counterclockwise. Thus, you need to reverse the directions. Obviously, this is a surgical emergency and this should be done while preparations for hospital transport is arranged.

HEMATOLOGY
AND ONCOLOGY

"A new scientific truth does not triumph by convincing its opponents and making them see the light, but rather because its opponents eventually die, and a new generation grows up that is familiar with it."
- Max Planck (1858-1947)

□□   **Which types of blood loss are indicative of a bleeding disorder?**

1) Spontaneous bleeding from many sites.
2) Bleeding from non-traumatic sites.
3) Delayed bleeding several hours after trauma.
4) Bleeding into deep tissues or joints.

□□   **Mucocutaneous bleeding, including petechiae, ecchymoses, epistaxis, GI, GU, or menorrhagia are indicative of what coagulation abnormality?**

Qualitative or quantitative platelet disorders.

□□   **Bleeding into joints or potential spaces (i.e., retroperitoneum), as well as delayed bleeding, suggests what type of bleeding disorder?**

Coagulation Factor Deficiency.

□□   **What is primary hemostasis?**

It is the platelet interaction with the vascular subendothelium that results in the formation of a platelet plug at the site of injury.

□□   **What 4 components are required for primary hemostasis?**

1) Normal vascular subendothelium (collagen).
2) Functional platelets.
3) Normal von Willebrand factor (connects the platelet to the endothelium via glycoprotein Ib).
4) Normal Fibrinogen (connects platelets to each other via glycoprotein IIB-IIIA).

□□   **What is the final end-product of secondary hemostasis (coagulation cascade)?**

Cross-linked fibrin.

□□   **What is the principle physiologic activator of the fibrinolytic system?**

Tissue plasminogen activator (tPA). tPA is released from endothelial cells and converts plasminogen, adsorbed in the fibrin clot, to plasmin. Plasmin degrades fibrinogen and fibrin monomer into fibrin degradation products (FDPs, aka fibrin split products) and cross-linked fibrin into D-dimers.

□□   **Below what platelet count is spontaneous hemorrhage likely to occur?**

$< 10,000/mm^2$.

□□   **It is generally agreed that most patients with active bleeding and platelet counts $< 50,000/mm^2$ should receive platelet transfusion. How much will the platelet count be raised for each unit of platelets infused?**

$10,000/mm^2$.

❑❑　　**What groups of patients with thrombocytopenia would be unlikely to respond to platelet infusions?**

Those with platelet antibodies (ITP or hypersplenism).

❑❑　　**What is the only coagulation factor not synthesized by hepatocytes?**

Factor VIII.

❑❑　　**What are the clinical complications of DIC?**

Bleeding, thrombosis, and purpura fulminans.

❑❑　　**What three laboratory studies would be most helpful in establishing the diagnosis of DIC?**

1) Prothrombin time—prolonged.
2) Platelet count—usually low.
3) Fibrinogen level—low.

❑❑　　**What are the most common hemostatic abnormalities in patients infected with HIV?**

Thrombocytopenia and acquired circulating anticoagulants (causes prolongation of aPTT).

❑❑　　**What is the pentad of Thrombotic Thrombocytopenic Purpura (TTP)?**

1) Fever.
2) Thrombocytopenia.
3) Neurologic symptoms.
4) Renal insufficiency.
5) Microangiopathic hemolytic anemia (MAHA).

❑❑　　**What is the most common inherited bleeding disorder?**

von Willebrand Disease.

❑❑　　**What is the most common hemoglobin variant?**

Hemoglobin S (Valine substituted for glutamic acid in the sixth position on the ß-chain).

❑❑　　**What types of clinical crises are seen in patients with sickle-cell disease?**

1) Vasoocclusive (thrombotic).
2) Hematologic (sequestration and aplastic).
3) Infectious.

❑❑　　**What is the most common type of sickle-cell crisis?**

Vasoocclusive (average: 4 attacks/year).

❑❑　　**What percentage of patients with sickle-cell disease have gallstones?**

75% (only 10% are symptomatic).

❑❑　　**What is the only type of vasoocclusive crisis that is painless?**

CNS crisis (most commonly cerebral infarction in children and cerebral hemorrhage in adults).

❑❑　　**What are the mainstays of therapy for a patient in sickle-cell crisis?**

1) Hydration.
2) Analgesia.
3) Oxygen (only beneficial if patient is hypoxic).

4) Cardiac monitoring (if patient has history of cardiac disease or is having chest pain).

❑❑   **What is the <u>most</u> <u>common</u> human enzyme defect?**

Glucose-6-phosphate Dehydrogenase Deficiency (G-6-PD).

❑❑   **What drugs should be avoided in patients with G-6-PD Deficiency?**

1) Drugs that induce oxidation.
2) Sulfa.
3) Antimalarials.
4) Pyridium.
5) Nitrofurantoin.

❑❑   **What is the single most useful test in ascertaining the presence of hemolysis and a normal marrow response?**

The reticulocyte count.

❑❑   **What is the <u>most</u> <u>common</u> morphologic abnormality of red cells in hemolytic states?**

Spherocytes.

❑❑   **What is the <u>most</u> <u>common</u> clinical presentation of TTP (Thrombotic thrombocytopenic purpura)?**

Neurologic symptoms including headache, confusion, cranial nerve palsies, coma, and seizures.

❑❑   **In a child 6 months to 4 year of age with an antecedent URI, the findings of fever, acute renal failure, microangiopathic hemolytic anemia (MAHA), and thrombocytopenia are suggestive of what disorder?**

Hemolytic Uremic Syndrome.

❑❑   **What is the <u>most</u> <u>common</u> worldwide cause of hemolytic anemia?**

Malaria.

❑❑   **By how much will the infusion of one unit of PRBcs raise the hemoglobin and hematocrit in a 30 kg patient?**

<u>Hemoglobin</u>: 1 g/dL.
<u>Hematocrit</u>: 3%.

❑❑   **What are the 5 contents of cryoprecipitate?**

1) Factor VIII C.
2) von Willebrand Factor.
3) Fibrinogen.
4) Factor XIII.
5) Fibronectin.

❑❑   **What is the first step in treating all immediate transfusion reactions?**

Stop the transfusion.

❑❑   **What type of immediate transfusion reaction is not dose-related and can often be completed following patient evaluation and treatment with diphenhydramine?**

Allergic transfusion reaction.

❑❑   **What infection carries the highest risk of transmission by blood transfusion?**

Hepatitis C (1:3,300 units).

❑❑   **What is the currently approved emergency replacement therapy for massive hemorrhage?**

Type-specific, uncrossmatched blood (available in 10-15 minutes). Type O negative, whereas immediately life-saving in certain situations, carries the risk of life-threatening transfusion reactions.

❑❑   **In current practice, which blood components are routinely infused along with PRBCs in a patient receiving a massive transfusion?**

None. The practice of routinely using platelet transfusion and FFP is costly, dangerous, and unwarranted.

❑❑   **What is the only crystalloid fluid compatible with PRBCs?**

Normal saline.

❑❑   **Vitamin K dependent factors of the clotting cascade include:**

X, IX, VII and II. Remember 1972.

❑❑   **What is von Willebrand's disease?**

It is an autosomal dominant disorder of platelet function. It causes bleeding from mucous membranes, menorrhagia, and increased bleeding from wounds. Patients with von Willebrand's disease have less (or dysfunctional) von Willebrand's factor.

❑❑   **What lab abnormalities does DIC cause?**

Increased PT, elevated fibrin split products, decreased fibrinogen and thrombocytopenia.

❑❑   **What factors are deficient in Classic hemophilia, Christmas disease, and von Willebrand's disease, respectively?**

Classic hemophilia: Factor VIII.

Christmas disease: Factor IX.

Willebrand's disease: Factor VIIIc + von Willebrand's cofactor.

❑❑   **Which pathway involves factors VIII and IX?**

Intrinsic pathway.

❑❑   **What effect does deficiency of factors VIII and IX have on PT and on PTT?**

Deficiency leads to increase in PTT.

❑❑   **What pathway does the PT measure, and what factor is unique to this pathway?**

Extrinsic and factor VII, respectively.

❑❑   **How may hemophilia A be clinically distinguished from hemophilia B?**

Hemophilia A is not clinically distinguishable from Christmas disease (Hemophilia B).

❑❑   **Which blood product is given when the coagulation abnormality is unknown?**

FFP.

❑❑   **The most frequently encountered platelet disorder of childhood is:**

Idiopathic thrombocytopenic purpura

❑❑   **The characteristic bone marrow finding in ITP is:**

Increased or normal megakaryocytes

❑❑   **Potential treatment modalities for ITP include:**

Gamma globulin or steroids

❏❏   **How do gamma globulin and steroids work in the treatment of ITP?**

They block the uptake of antibody-coated platelets by splenic macrophages.

❏❏   **Under what circumstances is a bone marrow aspirate crucial in the diagnosis and treatment of ITP?**

If treatment with steroids is planned, a bone marrow aspirate must be performed to rule out leukemia. Steroid treatment can delay the diagnosis of an occult leukemia.

❏❏   **The most common cause of neutropenia found in the evaluation of a febrile child is:**

Viral illness

❏❏   **The most likely diagnosis in a child with poor growth, hepatosplenomegaly, pallor, hemoglobin of 4.0 gm/dL, and an MCV of 60 is:**

Thalassemia major

❏❏   **Ethnic groups with a high incidence of α thalassemia gene include those from which geographic areas?**

- Countries bordering the Mediterranean
- Southeast Asia

❏❏   **Why is the pulse oximetry reading normal in a patient with cyanosis and methemoglobinemia?**

Because pulse oximetry devices measure oxygen saturation of that hemoglobin available for saturation, blood oximetry levels will be low in this condition. pO2 is normal.

❏❏   **List drugs and other substances implicated in causing methemoglobinemia in children:**

Sulfa antibiotics, quinones, phenacetin, benzocaine, nitrites, aniline dyes, and naphthalene (moth balls).

❏❏   **Oxygen binding of hemoglobin is severely impaired in methemoglobinemia because of what change in heme iron?**

More heme iron is present in the ferric rather than ferrous state.

❏❏   **The definitive test for diagnosing sickling disorders is:**

Hemoglobin electrophoresis

❏❏   **Alternatives for treating bleeding in a patient with Factor VIII deficiency and an inhibitor are:**

- Children with low inhibitor titers and minor hemorrhage may respond to Factor VIII
- Factor IX concentrates
- Plasmapheresis and factor replacement
- High dose Factor VIII (>100 units/kg)

❏❏   **In vonWillebrands Disease there is a decrease in or a defect of what protein?**

VonWillebrandís factor (vWF) which, when combined with factor VIII procoagulant protein (factor VIII:C), forms factor VIII.

❏❏   **Typical lab findings in vonWillebrands Disease include:**

- Normal platelet count
- Normal pro-time
- Normal or increase partial thromboplastin time

- Increased bleeding time

❑❑ **There is simultaneous activation of coagulation and fibrinolysis in what pathologic condition?**

Disseminated Intravascular Coagulation

❑❑ **The predominant symptom in DIC is:**

Bleeding

❑❑ **Common ischemic complications of DIC include:**

- Renal failure
- Seizures/coma
- Pulmonary infarcts
- Hemorrhagic necrosis of the skin

❑❑ **The most common familial and congenital abnormality of the red blood cell membrane is:**

Hereditary spherocytosis

❑❑ **The usual pattern of inheritance for hereditary spherocytosis is:**

Autosomal dominant but it may be autosomal recessive and there is a high rate of new mutations.

❑❑ **The most common molecular defect in hereditary spherocytosis is an abnormality in what protein?**

Spectrin

❑❑ **Complications of hereditary spherocytosis include:**

- Hyperbilirubinemia in newborn period
- Hemolytic anemia
- Gallstones
- Susceptibility to aplastic and hypoplastic crises secondary to viral infections

❑❑ **How is the diagnosis of hereditary spherocytosis made?**

- Blood smear
- Splenomegaly
- Family history
- Osmotic fragility test

❑❑ **Treatment of hereditary spherocytosis may include:**

Splenectomy

❑❑ **A cure for thalassemia major is possible with:**

Bone marrow transplant

❑❑ **A 4 month old African American male is given trimethoprim-sulfamethoxazole for otitis media and 24 hours later develops a severe hemolytic anemia. What is the most likely cause?**

G-6-PD deficiency

❑❑ **G-6-PD deficiency is prevalent in what ethnic groups?**

Greek, southern Italians, Sephardic Jews, Filipinos, south Chinese, African Americans and Thai's.

□□   A 15 year old female has cervical adenopathy and supraclavicular nodes. The patient has had fevers which last several days, followed by afebrile periods lasting several days. The most likely malignancy would be?

Hodgkin's Disease. The recurrent fevers and adenopathies hint at this diagnosis. Diagnosis would be obtained by lymph node biopsy.

□□   At what is age is a sickle cell patient at greatest risk for sepsis?

Six months to 3 years.

□□   Why is the patient from the previous question considered at high risk during this age?

Because there is limited protective antibody, and splenic function is decreased or completely absent.

□□   What are some of the signs and symptoms of central nervous system infarction secondary to sickle cell vaso-occlusion?

Mild, fleeting TIA-like symptoms, seizures, hemiparesis, coma, death.

□□   What are the signs and symptoms of splenic sequestration crisis?

Pallor, weakness, lethargy, disorientation, shock, decreased level of consciousness, and an enlarged spleen.

□□   What is the most common cause of aplastic crisis in patients with hemolytic anemia?

Parvovirus B19 infection.

□□   What percentage of hemoglobins A and F are found in a normal term infant?

Hemoglobin A: 30%

Hemoglobin F: 70%

□□   The amount of hemoglobin F declines to < 2% by what age?

6-12 months.

□□   Normal red blood cell life span is:

120 days

□□   What factors contribute to the pathophysiology of chronic disease anemia?

Decreased red cell life span (hyperactive reticuloendothelial system), hypoactive bone marrow, erythropoietin production inadequate for degree of anemia, and an abnormality of iron metabolism.

□□   A patient receiving a transfusion of packed red cells abruptly develops fever, chills, chest pain, dyspnea and tachycardia. What is the most likely cause?

Acute hemolytic transfusion reaction due to ABO incompatibility.

□□   Which factors contribute to physiologic anemia during infancy?

Abrupt cessation of erythropoiesis with onset of respiration, low erythropoietin levels (made in the liver during the neonatal period), decreased half life and increased volume of distribution of erythropoietin, shortened survival of fetal rbc, and expansion of the infant's blood volume with rapid weight gain during the first three months.

□□   At what age does the physiologic anemia of infancy peak?

2-3 months in full term infants; 3-6 weeks in prematures.

□□   Which deficiencies cause megaloblastic anemia in children?

Folic acid and/or vitamin B12.

❐❐   **Which test assesses the absorbtion rate of vitamin B12?**

The Schilling test.

❐❐   **T/F: Infants absorb the iron from cows milk more efficiently than that of breast milk.**

False. Iron is absorbed 2-3 times more efficiently from breast milk.

❐❐   **Iron deficiency anemia in an older child should prompt an investigation for what?**

Blood loss

❐❐   **A hemophiliac presents with a headache after minor head trauma. What should your management include?**

CT of the brain, and factor replacement

❐❐   **What is the most common cancer in children?**

Acute lymphoblastic leukemia.

❐❐   **Define the drug regimen MOPP.**

Mechlorethamine, Oncovin, Prednisone, and Procarbazine.

❐❐   **What is the MOPP regimen of drugs used to treat?**

Hodgkin's lymphoma.

❐❐   **A patient with chronic myelocytic leukemia, who is on busulfan therapy, comes to the ER complaining of shortness of breath. What should you suspect?**

Pulmonary fibrosis, a toxicity of busulfan.

❐❐   **What is the mechanism of action for methotrexate?**

It inhibits the enzyme dihydrofolate reductase.

❐❐   **What is the drug of choice for treating a Wilms' tumor?**

Actinomycin D.

❐❐   **Childhood cancer is a leading cause of death. How does it rank?**

Childhood cancer is only exceeded by trauma as a leading cause of death in the 1-15 year-old population.

❐❐   **Which chemotherapeutic agents are associated with pulmonary fibrosis?**

Bleomycin, BCNU, and Busulfan are commonly associated with pulmonary fibrosis. Cyclophosphamide and Methotrexate are rarely implicated.

❐❐   **What is the most common extracranial solid tumor in the pediatric patient?**

Neuroblastoma. It accounts for about 10% of all pediatric malignancies.

❐❐   **Most cases of neuroblastoma are diagnosed by what age?**

Eighty-five percent of cases are diagnosed before the age of five years, the median age of diagnosis is two years.

❐❐   **The most common form of childhood malignancy is?**

Leukemia. Approximately 2,500 children a year are affected annually in the United States.

❏❏   **Which genetic disorders increase the incidence of leukemia?**

Down's syndrome, Fanconi anemia and ataxia-telangiectasis.

❏❏   **What are the most frequent sites of osteosarcoma involvement?**

The femur, tibia, and humerus. Usually this tumor is found in the metaphysis of long bones.

❏❏   **After osteosarcoma, what is the most frequent bone tumor in children and adolescents?**

Ewings sarcoma. This tumor accounts for about 30% of all primary bone tumors.

❏❏   **A 2 year old male has a seborrheic rash, chronically draining ears, and loose teeth. What is your diagnosis?**

Histiocytosis X.

❏❏   **What is the most common pediatric liver tumor of childhood?**

The hepatoblastoma. The second most common is hepatocellular carcinoma.

❏❏   **A 7 year old female in Tanner stage 3 has lower abdominal pain of unknown etiology, and a 4 cm abdominal mass. What is the most likely diagnosis?**

An ovarian tumor.

❏❏   **What is the origin of most testicular childhood tumors?**

Germ cell. Germ cell tumors account for 35% to 45% of childhood testicular tumors.

❏❏   **Urinary catecholamine metabolite levels are useful in diagnosing which common pediatric malignancy?**

Neuroblastoma. The most useful metabolites are vanillylmandelic acid and homovanillic acid.

❏❏   **A three year old girl is brought in for a mass protruding from her vaginal area. There are no signs of abuse. What is the most likely diagnosis?**

Sarcoma botryoides. Adenocarcinoma is more common in adolescents.

❏❏   **A 3 year old male presents with proptosis and periorbital ecchymosis. What is the most likely malignancy?**

Neuroblastoma. Occasionally, these patients are mistaken for battered children.

❏❏   **A 14 year old male presents with a history of headache, morning vomiting and ataxia. What is your diagnosis?**

A posterior fossa tumor. The most likely tumor to occur at this age is a medulloblastoma.

❏❏   **A 6 year old male is diagnosed and treated for intussusception. What tumor is associated with this?**

After the age of 5, it would be unusual to have an intussusception without a lead point. The most likely malignancy would be a non-Hodgkin's lymphoma.

❏❏   **How does cryptorchism effect the risk of testicular malignancy?**

The risk is 30-50 times greater than in a normal testicle. About one-eighth of testicular tumors develop in cryptorchid testes.

❏❏   **How common is Hodgkin's disease during childhood?**

Children less than 10 years of age constitute 4% of all cases of Hodgkin's disease. Patients between the ages of 11 to 16 years of age constitute another 11%.

❏❏   **What are the second most common neoplasms during childhood?**

Primary central nervous system tumors. These account for 20% of all cancers of childhood.

❏❏   **Which pediatric brain tumor has the worst prognosis?**

A brain stem Glioma. Children typically die within two years of presentation.

❏❏   **EBV has been associated with which malignancies?**

Nasopharyngeal carcinoma, Burkitt lymphoma and Hodgkin's lymphoma. Hepatocellular carcinoma is associated with Hepatitis B.

❏❏   **A leukemia patient is exposed to Varicella, which he has never had. What is the best course of action?**

Varicella immune globulin within three days of exposure.

❏❏   **What percentage of neuroblastoma patients have metastatic disease at the time of their diagnosis?**

75%. The usual sites are lymph nodes bone marrow, liver, skin, orbit and bone.

❏❏   **What is the most common thyroid tumor in childhood?**

Papillary adenocarcinoma. This accounts for about three-quarters of malignant thyroid tumors.

❏❏   **A 2 year old male is brought in by his mother because he has a flank mass. He is hypertensive and polycythemic. Urineanalysis reveals hematuria. What is your diagnosis?**

Wilms tumor. Typically, the mass is noted by the patient's primary caregiver. Hypertension, hematuria, and (less commonly) polycythemia may be seen.

❏❏   **A 15 year old male complains of tibial pain after playing football. X-ray shows an "onion skin" appearance of the tibia. What condition is patient likely to have?**

Ewing Sarcoma. The onion skin appearance is characteristic of this tumor.

❏❏   **What are the most common sites of involvement of a rhabdomyosarcoma?**

The head and neck regions. Other areas that can be involved are the genitourinary tract, the extremities, and the trunk.

❏❏   **What is the leading cause of death from leukemia?**

Infection. The second leading cause is hemorrhage.

❏❏   **What percentage of children with acute lymphoblastic leukemia are cured by conventional chemotherapy?**

70%.

❏❏   **What is the disease-free survival rate of patients with ALL after BMT?**

15%-65%, with relapse rates of 30%-70%.

❏❏   **Define Graft Versus Host Disease (GVHD)?**

Engraftment of immunocompetent donor cells into an immunocompromised host, resulting in cell mediated cytotoxic destruction of host cells if an immunologic incompatibility exists.

❏❏   **When does acute GVHD present and what are the typical manifestations?**

Acute GVHD typically occurs about day 19 (median) just as the patient begins to engraft and is characterized by erythroderma, cholestatic hepatitis, and enteritis.

❑❑   **What is the clinical definition of chronic GVHD (cGVHD)?**

As early as 60-70 days status post engraftment, patients exhibit signs of a systemic autoimmune process, manifesting as Sjogren syndrome, systemic lupus erythrematosus, scleroderma, primary bililary cirrhosis, and recurrent infections with encapsulated bacteria, fungus, or viruses.

❑❑   **What is the mechanism of action of cyclosporine?**

It selectively inhibits the translation of IL-2 mRNA by helper T-cells, thus attenuating the T-cell activation pathways.

❑❑   **In what time period, post-operatively, is a transplant patient at greatest risk for acute rejection?**

During the first 3 months.

DERMATOLOGY

"Adventure is worthwhile in itself."
- Amelia Earhart

☐☐ **A 16 year old slender female with no history of diabetes or other endocrine problem is found to have acanthosis nigricans on routine examination. What might you want to work her up for?**

Underlying malignancy. Acanthosis nigricans is often a marker for malignancy, especially of the GI tract. It is the velvety brown hyperpigmentation and thickening of the flexures common in the axilla and the groin. It is also associated with obesity, diabetes, and endocrine disorders.

☐☐ **What are Beau lines?**

Transverse grooves in the nailbed caused by the disruption of the nailbed matrix secondary to systemic illness. Illness can actually be dated by these lines as nails grow 1 mm/month.

☐☐ **Candida albicans infections of the skin are <u>most</u> <u>commonly</u> located where?**

In the intertriginous areas (i.e., in the folds of the skin, axilla, groin, under the breasts, etc.) Candida albicans appears as a beefy red rash with satellite lesions.

☐☐ **Patients with untreated orbital or central facial abscesses are at risk for developing what serious complication?**

Cavernous sinus thrombosis.

☐☐ **A mother is worried that her 5 year old will get chicken pox because she was playing with her neighbor who was diagnosed with chicken pox and had crusty lesions all over his body. If this was the only day she played with the neighbor will she develop chicken pox too?**

No. Chicken pox is only contagious 48 hours before the rash breaks out and until the vesicles have crusted over.

☐☐ **What are the <u>most</u> <u>common</u> causes of allergic contact dermatitis?**

Poison ivy, poison sumac, poison oak, ragweed, topical medications, nickel, chromium, rubber, glue, cosmetics, and hair dyes.

☐☐ **A mother brings her 14 year old boy to you a week after you prescribed ampicillin for his pharyngitis. Mom says he developed a rash over his torso, arms, legs, and even the palms of his hands. On examination the patient has a erythematous, maculopapular rash in the places described. What might the child have other than pharyngitis?**

Infectious mononucleosis. In almost 95% of patients with Epstein Barr viruses that are treated with ampicillin, a rash will develop. The rash and subsequent desquamation will last about a week.

☐☐ **What is the <u>most</u> <u>common</u> bullous disease?**

Erythema multiforme. The typical erythema multiforme lesion is the iris lesion (a gray center with a red rim). These lesions are symmetrical and most frequently found on the distal extremities spreading proximally. Patients may also have plaques, papules, and bullous lesions. The disease is most common in children and young adults.

❑❑   What is the <u>most</u> <u>common</u> cause of erythema multiforme?

Repetitive minor herpes simplex infections (90%). Drug reactions are the second most common cause for erythema multiforme. The rash generally erupts 7–10 days after a bout of herpes.

❑❑   What is the <u>most</u> <u>common</u> location of erythema nodosum?

The shins. They can also be found on the extensor surfaces of the forearms. Erythema nodosum are erythematous subcutaneous nodules which result from inflammation of subcutaneous fat and small vessels.

❑❑   A patient presents with a raised, red, small, and painful plaque on the face. On exam, a distinct, sharp, advancing edge is noted. What is the cause?

Erysipelas is caused by group A streptococci. When the face is involved, the patient should be admitted.

❑❑   What type of reaction is erythema multiforme?

Hypersensitivity. Bullae are subepidermal, the dermis is edematous, and a lymphatic infiltrate may be present around the capillaries and venules. In children, infections are the most important cause; in adults, drugs and malignancies are more common causes. EM is often seen during epidemics of adenovirus, atypical pneumonia, and histoplasmosis.

❑❑   What is the <u>most</u> <u>common</u> cause of erythema nodosum in the Western world?

Drug reactions - most commonly due to sulfonamides. Erythema nodosum is also associated with the following systemic diseases: fungal infection, inflammatory bowel disease, sarcoidosis, streptococcal infection, and tuberculosis.

❑❑   What are the causes of exfoliative dermatitis?

Chemicals, drugs, and cutaneous or systemic diseases. Usually scaly erythematous dermatitis involves most or all of the surface skin. It can be recognized by erythroderma with epidermal flaking or scaling. Acute signs and symptoms may include low-grade fever, pruritus, chills, and skin tightness. The chronic condition may produce dystrophic nails, thinning of body hair, and patchy hyperpigmentation or hypopigmentation. Cutaneous vasodilation may result in increased cardiac output and high-output cardiac failure. Splenomegaly suggests leukemia or lymphoma.

❑❑   Your neighbor brings her 4 year old little girl to you because she has a "disgusting" rash. The child's face is patched with vesiculopustular lesions covered in a thick, honey-colored crust. Just two days ago, these lesions were small red papules. Diagnosis?

Impetigo contagiosa. This is most common in children and usually occurs on exposed areas of skin. Treat by removing the crusts and cleansing the bases and prescribing systemic antibiotics (erythromycin, cephalosporin, or dicloxacillin).

❑❑   What is the <u>most</u> <u>common</u> organism responsible for the above child's infection?

50–90% of impetigo contagiosa cases are caused by *Staphylococcus aureus* alone. *α-hemolytic streptococcus* is the second most common infecting agent, being the sole affecting agent in 10% of cases or coinfecting with *staphylococcus aureus*.

❑❑   What is the Koebner phenomenon?

The development of plaques in areas where trauma has occurred. Just a scratch can trigger the development of a plaque. This is most common in patients with psoriasis and lichen planus.

❑❑   A patient of yours has dysplastic nevus syndrome. She comes to you depressed because her aunt has just been diagnosed with melanoma. What is her risk of developing melanoma too?

100%. People with familial dysplastic nevus syndrome have a genetic disposition for melanoma. If diagnosis is made in the family, then the remaining members who also have the above syndrome will inevitably develop melanoma too.

❏❏ **Differentiate between pigmented and dysplastic nevi.**

Pigmented nevi are benign moles that are uniform in appearance. They are most common in sun exposed areas. Pigmented nevi are suspicious and warrant biopsy if they grow suddenly, change color, bleed, or begin to hurt. Dysplastic nevi are not uniform in appearance and they are frequently larger than 5–12 mm in diameter. 50% of malignant melanomas originate from the melanocytes in moles.

❏❏ **How should steroids be prescribed in a patient with poison ivy?**

Prednisone 40–60 mg q d tapered over 2 to 3 weeks. Short courses may result in rebound.

❏❏ **How may the *Toxicodendron* species be recognized?**

Poison oak and ivy have leaves with 3 leaflets per leaf. They also have U- or V-shaped leaf scars. The milky sap becomes black when exposed to air.

❏❏ **How quickly will people react to the *Toxicodendron* antigen?**

Contact dermatitis typically develops within 2 days of exposure; cases have been reported as quickly as 8 hours to as long as 10d. Lesions appear in a linear arrangement of papulovesicles or erythema. Fluid from vesicles does not contain antigen and does not transmit the dermatitis.

❏❏ **What is the <u>most</u> <u>common</u> cause of secondary pyodermia?**

Like impetigo and ecthyma, this superinfection of the skin is caused predominantly by *Staphylococcus aureus* (80–85%). Other responsible organisms are *Streptococcus, Proteus, Pseudomonas,* and *E. coli..*

❏❏ **A 17 year old female comes to your office complaining of a rash over her elbows and her knees. On examination you find that she has several clearly demarcated erythematous plaques that are covered with silvery scales that can be removed with scraping. These lesions are on her extensor surfaces only in the areas previously mentioned. Examination of her nails reveals pitting in the nailbed. What is her prognosis?**

Psoriasis is an intermittent disease that may spontaneously disappear or may be life long. There may be associated arthritis in the distal interphalangeal joints; otherwise, the disease is limited to the skin and nails. Treatment is with hydration of the skin and topical mid-potency steroids.

❏❏ **A 12 year old female comes to your office complaining of intense itching in the webs between her fingers that worsens at night. On close examination you see a few small squiggly lines 1 cm x 1 mm where the patient has been scratching herself. Diagnosis?**

Scabies. Scabies are due to the mite *Sarcoptes scabiei* var. *hominis.* Scabies are spread by close contact; therefore, all household contacts should also be treated.

❏❏ **A 16 year old patient presents to your office complaining of greasy, red, scaly, plaques in her eyebrows, eyelids and nose that are spreading to the naso-labial folds. What patient population is this disease more likely to occur in?**

The above patient has seborrheic dermatitis. This can occur in anyone but is also a common problem in patients with HIV and Parkinson's disease. The infant form of the disease is "cradle cap."

❏❏ **What are the 2 distinct causes of toxic epidermal necrolysis (scalded skin syndrome)?**

(1) Staphylococcal and (2) drugs or chemicals. Both begin with appearance of patches of tender erythema followed by loosening of the skin and denuding to glistening bases.

Staphylococcal scalded skin syndrome is commonly found in children younger than 5 and is due to toxin that cleaves within the epidermis under the stratum granulosum.

❑❑   **What areas does Staphylococcal scalded skin syndrome (SSSS) usually affect?**

The face around nose and mouth, neck, axillae, and groin. Disease commonly occurs after upper respiratory tract infections or purulent conjunctivitis. Nikolsky's sign is present when lateral pressure on the skin results in epidermal separation from the dermis.

❑❑   **How can SSSS be distinguished from scalded skin syndrome caused by drugs or chemicals?**

In drug or chemical etiologies, the skin separates at the dermoepidermal junction. This drug-induced TEN carries up to 50% mortality as a result of fluid loss and secondary infection. On microscopic exam of SSSS, intraepidermal cleavage occurs, and a few acantholytic keratinocytes can be seen. In non-staphylococcal type, cellular debris, inflammatory cells, and basal cell keratinocytes are present.

❑❑   **What is the treatment of SSSS?**

Oral or IV penicillinase-resistant penicillin, baths of potassium permanganate or dressings soaked in 0.5% silver nitrate, and fluids. Corticosteroids and silver sulfadine are contraindicated.

❑❑   **A patient presents with fever, myalgias, malaise, and arthralgias. On exam, findings include bullous lesions of the lips, eyes, and nose. The patient indicates eating is very painful. What should the family be told about the patient's prognosis?**

Stevens-Johnson syndrome has a mortality of 5–10% and may have significant complications including corneal ulceration, panophthalmitis, corneal opacities, anterior uveitis, blindness, hematuria, renal tubular necrosis, and progressive renal failure. Scarring of the foreskin and stenosis of the vagina can occur. Treatment in a burn unit is supportive; steroids may provide symptomatic relief; however, they are not of proven value and may be contraindicated.

❑❑   **What is the most common cause of Stevens-Johnson syndrome?**

Drugs, most commonly sulfa drugs. Other causes are responses to infections with *Mycoplasma pneumonia* and herpes simplex virus. The disease is self-limiting but severely uncomfortable.

❑❑   **A patient who was born with a diffuse capillary hemangioma in the distribution of the ophthalmic division of the trigeminal nerve will have what neurological findings?**

Epilepsy (usually generalized seizures), mental retardation, and/or hemiparesis. This is Sturge-Weber syndrome. The patient is born with a hemangioma of the ophthalmic nerve and ipsilateral angiomas of the pia matter and cortex (most commonly in the parieto-occipital area).

❑❑   **Tinea capitis is most commonly seen in what age group?**

Children aged 4–14. This is a fungal infection of the scalp that begins as a papule around one hair shaft and then spreads to other follicles. The infection can cause the hairs to break off, leaving little black dot stumps and patches of alopecia. Trichophyton tonsurans is responsible for 90% of the cases. Wood's lamp examination will fluoresce only Microsporum infections, which are responsible for the remaining 10%. This is also called "ringworm of the scalp."

❑❑   **What are the 3 most common causes of acute urticaria?**

1) Medicine.
2) Arthropod bites.
3) Infection.

Urticaria, also known as hives, is a localized swelling due to a cytokine mediated increase in vascular permeability.

❏❏   **What is the <u>most</u> <u>common</u> location of verrucae vulgaris?**

This is the common wart. It is usually located on the back of the hands or fingers and is caused by HPV.

❏❏   **What foods cause acne?**

There is no evidence that any particular foods cause acne.

❏❏   **Does stress exacerbate acne?**

Yes, though the mechanism is unclear.

❏❏   **What is the causative agent of acne?**

Propionubacterium acnes, and the resulting obstruction and inflammatory response.

❏❏   **How effective are alcohol cleaning pads at preventing acne?**

There is no evidence to suggest they are effective at all.

❏❏   **Can prolonged treatment with systemic antibiotics be used to treat acne?**

Yes.

❏❏   **An 16 year old male complains of persistent acne on the forehead. What should you tell him?**

That this is most likely due to greasy hair preparations (Pomade acne). Changing, or stopping those products should improve symptoms.

❏❏   **What is the most effective medication for acne?**

Tretinoin (Retin-A)

❏❏   **Does cleansing of the face with soap and water decrease the incidence of comedones on an adolescent face?**

No. It may decrease surface lipids so the skin looks cleaner, but surface lipids are not involved in comedone generation.

❏❏   **What organism is the most common cause of bullous impetigo?**

Coagulase positive *Staph. aureus*.

❏❏   **What is the best treatment for impetigo?**

Bactroban topical lotion.

❏❏   **What is the treatment for atopic dermatitis?**

Oral antihistimines, topical steroids, emollients, and avoidance of irritants.

❏❏   **Elevations of which immunoglobulin is common in atopic dermatitis?**

IgE

❏❏   **Of gels, creams, lotions, and ointments, which has the highest fat content?**

Ointment >cream > gel > lotion. The more fat, the greater the lubricating effect.

❏❏   **What are the two main organisms responsible for Tinea Capitus?**

Microsporum canis and Trichophyton tonsurans. Of these two, T. tonsurans is the most contagious.

❏❏   **How do you make the diagnosis of Tinea Versicolor?**

Examination under a Wood's lamp would show yellow fluorescence. Also, a KOH prep is useful in confirming diagnosis.

❏❏   **What is the recommended therapy for Tinea Capitis?**

Oral Griseofulvin (15-20 mg/kg/day) and shampooing twice a week with 2.5% Selenium Sulfide.

❏❏   **If you want to sound more sophisticated while writing your H&P on a child with Tinea Capitis and a tender, fluctuant mass, what would you call it?**

A kerion.

❏❏   **What is the causative agent of Tinea Versicolor?**

Pityrosporum orbiculare (Malassezia furfur), a fungus.

❏❏   **Patients with what conditions are more likely to develop vitiligo?**

Diabetes, Addison's disease, thyroid disorders and pernicious anemia.

❏❏   **Which areas of the body are normally most affected by vitiligo?**

Areas that are normally hyperpigmented (i.e. face, areolae) and areas subject to friction (i.e. hands, elbows).

❏❏   **What is telogen effluvium?**

Significant hair loss seen after significant stress (severe illness, surgery, tumor therapy, etc.).

❏❏   **What is the drug of choice for head lice?**

Permethrin (Nix)

❏❏   **How fast does human hair grow?**

1 cm per month.

❏❏   **Where is the best place to get a scraping to rule out scabies?**

The web spaces between the fingers and toes.

❏❏   **What is the treatment of choice for scabies?**

5% Permethrin cream.

❏❏   **What is the hair loss pattern of seborrheic dermatitis?**

Localized.

❏❏   **Viewing a Giemsa stain of a scraping of a newborn infant with irregular blotchy yellow papules, you notice eosinophils. What is the diagnosis?**

Erythema toxicum.

❏❏   **What is the life expectancy of the newborn that develops erythema toxicum three days after his birth?**

Normal. This is a benign and self-limited disease that is extremely common in the neonate.

❏❏   **A child is brought to your office for the first time. You notice that the child is clearly ataxic. You suspect ataxia-telangiectasia. Where would you expect the dermatological lesions to first present?**

Bulbar conjunctiva, bridge of nose, ears, and the anterior chest.

❏❏   **What is the Auspitz sign?**

When, after removal of a psoriatic scale, you notice multiple distinct bleeding points.

❏❏ **Is childhood psoriasis usually bilaterally symmetrical?**

Yes.

❏❏ **Psoriatic arthritis classically attacks which joints?**

The DIPs of hands and feet.

❏❏ **Are freckles inherited?**

Yes, they are inherited in an autosomal dominant pattern.

❏❏ **Are freckles a risk factor for the development of melanoma?**

Yes.

❏❏ **An 11 year old female presents with a maculopapular rash on trunk and upper legs. The rash is in lines along the long axis of the ovoid lesions. The patient states that 1 week ago, she had only 1 lesion which was round and "about as wide as a golf ball". What is your diagnosis?**

Pityriasis rosea.

❏❏ **What is the distribution of the rash in pityriasis rosea?**

"Christmas tree" pattern with parallel rows of lesions on the trunk.

❏❏ **What maneuver can you perform to diagnose urticaria pigmentosa?**

The Darier sign - stroking the lesion, which releases histamine from mast cells leading to urticarea.

❏❏ **Is there a role for topical steroids in acute severe sunburn?**

Yes. It may relieve pain and inflammation.

❏❏ **Patients on which antibiotic are most likely to have a photoallergic drug reaction?**

Tetracycline and sulfonamides.

❏❏ **A 17 year old girl complains that she can't wear gold earring without developing a localized rash. This is true not only in her earlobes, but also in all the pierced body parts (nose, navel, and eyebrows). What is her allergy to?**

Nickel, which is commonly found in some jewelry. She would have to wear either stainless steel or pure gold to avoid the allergy.

❏❏ **In a child with scalded skin syndrome (SSS), you notice that pressing on the blister enlarges it laterally. What is the name of this phenomenon?**

Nikolsky sign-A sign of epidermal fragility.

❏❏ **Can you develop Rhus dermatitis from physical contact with someone who already has the condition?**

Not unless they have not yet washed off the allergen.

❏❏ **What is the treatment for scalp lesions of seborrheic dermatitis?**

Antiseborrheic shampoo (i.e. tar, selenium sulfide).

GENETICS

"There lives more faith in honest doubt, believe me, than in half the creeds."
- Alfred Lord Tennyson

☐☐ **What are the four types of major mutant gene inheritance?**

(1) Dominant, (2) heterozygous recessive, (3) homozygous recessive, and (4) x-linked recessive.

☐☐ **What does a "dominant " mutation mean?**

A single mutant gene of a pair is dominant if it alone can cause abnormality. The chance of inheriting this mutant gene is 50%.

☐☐ **What does a "heterozygous recessive" mutation mean?**

A single mutant gene which causes no evident abnormality. The individual with this gene is called a heterozygous carrier.

☐☐ **What does "homozygous recessive" mean?**

When both genes of a pair are mutant the abnormal effect is expressed. The parents are usually carriers and have a 25% chance of having an affected offspring.

☐☐ **What are the defects seen in the DiGeorge syndrome?**

Hypoplasia to plasia of thymus (immunity problems), hypoplasia to plasia of the parathyroids (hypocalcemia and seizures), and cardiac anomalies.

☐☐ **Prenatal exposure to cocaine has been associated with what anomolies?**

Microcephaly, genitourinary abnormalities.

☐☐ **What are some effects of alcohol on the fetus?**

Effects may include: prenatal and postnatal growth deficiency, mental retardation (average IQ 63), microcephaly, short palpebral fissures, maxillary hypoplasia, short nose, smooth philtrum with thin and smooth upper lip, altered palmar creases, and VSD.

☐☐ **What are some effects of Dilantin on the fetus?**

Mild to moderate prenatal growth deficiency, borderline to mild mental retardation, wide anterior fontanelle, broad depressed nasal bridge, short nose, bowed upper lip, low set hairline, small nails, and strabismus.

☐☐ **What is Kartanger Syndrome?**

Fetus inversus, sinusitis, bronchiectasis and immotile sperm. Etiology is autosomal recessive.

☐☐ **What is the mode of inheritance for Albinism?**

Autosomal recessive.

☐☐ **What is the mode of inheritance for Cystic Fibrosis?**

Autosomal recessive (4% of US whites).

❑❑ **What is the mode of inheritance for Hemoglobin SS (sickle cell anemia)?**

Autosomal recessive (8% of US blacks).

❑❑ **What is the mode of inheritance for Tay-Sachs disease?**

Autosomal recessive (3% US Askkenazi Jews).

❑❑ **What is the mode of inheritance for neurofibromatosis?**

Autosomal dominant.

❑❑ **What is the mode of inheritance for all types of polycystic kidneys?**

Autosomal dominant.

❑❑ **What is the mode of inheritance for retinoblastoma?**

Autosomal dominant.

❑❑ **What is the mode of inheritance for Ocular Albinism?**

X-linked recessive.

❑❑ **What is the mode of inheritance for Red-Green Color blindness?**

X-linked recessive.

❑❑ **What is the mode of inheritance for nephrogenic diabetes insipidus?**

X-linked recessive.

❑❑ **What is the mode of inheritance for glucose-6-phosphate dehydrogenase deficiency?**

X-linked recessive (effects 10-14% of black Americans).

❑❑ **What is the mode of inheritance for Duchenne muscular dystrophy?**

X-linked recessive.

❑❑ **What is the mode of inheritance for Factor VIII Deficiency (Hemophilia A)?**

X-linked recessive.

❑❑ **What is the mode of inheritance for Factor IX deficiency?**

X-linked recessive.

❑❑ **What is the mode of inheritance for Hunter Syndrome?**

X-linked recessive.

❑❑ **What is the mode of inheritance for Vitamin D resistant rickets?**

X-linked dominant.

❑❑ **Name some clinical features of Trisomy-21 (Down's Syndrome).**

Mental retardation, hypotonia, flat occiput, epicanthal folds, Simean crease, gap between 1st and 2nd toes, endocardial cushion defects, and Brunsfield spots (speckled iris).

❑❑ **Name some clinical features of Trisomy-18.**

Mental retardation, chypertonia, low birth weight, prominant occiput, micrognathia, malformed ears, FSD and PDA, cleft lip, T.E.F., flexion deformities of fingers and rocker bottom feet.

❑❑ **Name some clinical features of Trisomy-13.**

Mental retardation, seizures, microcephaly, cleft lip and/or palate, microphthalmia, polydactyly, and simean crease.

☐☐   **What is the incidence of Down's Syndrome?**

1:800 (correlated with maternal age).

☐☐   **What is the incidence of Trisomy 13?**

1:20,000.

☐☐   **What is the incidence of Trisomy 18?**

1:800

☐☐   **What type of cancer is more common in individuals with Down's Syndrome?**

Acute leukemia (mostly lymphoblastic type).

☐☐   **Deletion of 5p chromosome results in what syndrome?**

Cri-du-Chat Syndrome. The characteristic cry disappears in late infancy. Infants have mental retardation, microcephaly, low set ears, low birth weight, and partial syndactyly.

☐☐   **What is the karyotype of Turner Syndrome?**

45, X (45XO). Incidence is 1:10,000 for female births. Analysis of the products of spontaneous abortion reveal 45X karyotype to be the most common chromosomal alteration.

☐☐   **What are some common clinical features of Turner Syndrome?**

Short stature, streak gonads, and primary amenorrhea.

☐☐   **What is the stereotype of Klinefelter Syndrome?**

Two or more X chromosomes and one or more Y chromosomes (usually 47 XXY).

☐☐   **What are some common clinical features of Klinefelter Syndrome with 47XXY?**

Mental retardation is only 10%. 100% of affected males are infertile (impaired spermiogenesis), with 99% having small testes.

☐☐   **What is "Fragile X" syndrome?**

Syndrome of mental retardation with macroorchidism in males.

☐☐   **What are some effects seen in Fetal Rubella Syndrome?**

Growth deficiency, microcephaly (with mental retardation), deafness, cataracts, PDA., thrombocytopenia, jaundice, and pneumonia. (Cultures of the rubella virus may be present up to 3 years.)

CARDIOVASCULAR

"Life is short, the Art is long, opportunity fleeting, experience delusive, judgment difficult"
-Hippocrates

❏❏   **Name three possible causes of an enlarged heart, poor myocardial function and dysrhythmia in a pediatric patient?**

Etiologies include myocarditis, congenital heart disease, heart failure, septic shock, endocardial fibroelastosis, anomalous left coronary artery from the pulmonary artery, Pompe's disease, medial necrosis of the coronary arteries, cardiomyopathy, pericarditis, rheumatic fever, systemic lupus erythematosus, rheumatoid arthritis, and ulcerative colitis.

❏❏   **What are some causes of SVT in children?**

Pericarditis, MI, pre-excitation syndromes, mitral valve prolapse, rheumatic heart disease, pneumonia, and ethanol.

❏❏   **What is the mechanism that _most_ _commonly_ produces SVTs?**

Reentry. Another common cause is abnormal automaticity (i.e., ectopic foci).

❏❏   **What are the key feature of Mobitz I (Wenckebach) 2^0 AV block?**

A progressive prolongation of the PR interval until the atrial impulse is no longer conducted. If symptomatic, atropine and transcutaneous/transvenous pacing is required.

❏❏   **What is Mobitz II 2^0 AV block, and how is it treated?**

A constant PR interval in which one or more beats fail to conduct. Treat with atropine and transcutaneous/transvenous pacing.

❏❏   **A patient presents to the hospital 1 month after placement of a mechanical prosthetic valve with fever, chills, and a leukocytosis. Endocarditis is suspected. Which type of bacterium is _most_ _common_?**

Staphylococcus aureus or *Staphylococcus epidermidis*.

❏❏   **A patient presents with a history of episodic elevations in BP. She complains of headache, diarrhea, and skin flushing. What is the diagnosis?**

Pheochromocytoma.

❏❏   **What maneuvers will increase hypertrophic cardiomyopathy murmurs?**

Valsalva, standing, and amyl nitrate.

❏❏   **What maneuvers will decrease hypertrophic cardiomyopathic murmurs?**

Handgrip, squatting, and leg elevation in the supine patient.

❏❏   **What is the _most_ _common_ cause of myocarditis in the US?**

Viruses. Other causes include post viral myocarditis, an autoimmune response to recent viral infection, bacteria (diphtheria and tuberculosis), fungi, protozoan (Chagas' disease), and spirochetes (Lyme disease).

❏❏   What is the <u>most</u> <u>common</u> cause of mitral stenosis?

Rheumatic heart disease. The most common initial symptom is dyspnea.

❏❏   A mid systolic click with a late systolic crescendo murmur is indicative of what cardiac disease?

Mitral valve prolapse.

❏❏   Is mitral valve prolapse (MVP) more common in males or in females?

Females have a stronger genetic link to the disease. Only 2-5% of the population has symptomatic MVP.

❏❏   What is the hallmark sign of mitral valve prolapse?

A midsystolic click sometimes accompanied by a late systolic murmur. MVP is largely a clinical diagnosis. An ECG is performed to assess the degree of prolapse. Other clinical findings include a laterally displaced diffuse apical pulse, decreased S1, split S2, and a holosystolic murmur radiating to the axilla.

❏❏   What is the percentage of patients with palpitations who also have cardiac disease?

50%.

❏❏   A 15-year-old patient presents with splinted breathing and sharp, precordial chest pain that radiates to the back. The pain increases with inspiration and is mildly relieved by placing the patient in a forward sitting position. What does the ECG look like?

The patient probably has pericarditis. The ECG reveals intermittent supraventricular tachycardias, ST-segment depression in VR and V1. ST-segment elevation in all other leads, PR depression, and T-wave inversion may arise.

❏❏   What is the <u>most</u> <u>common</u> cause of pericarditis?

Idiopathic. Other causes are MI, post viral syndrome, aortic dissection that has ruptured into the pericardium, malignancy, radiation, chest trauma, connective tissue disease, uremia, and drugs (i.e., procainamide or hydralazine).

❏❏   What physical finding is usually indicative of acute pericarditis?

Pericardial friction rub. The rub is best heard at the left sternal border or apex with the patient in a forward sitting position. Other findings include fever and tachycardia.

❏❏   Acute pyogenic pericarditis is <u>most</u> <u>commonly</u> caused by which organisms?

Staphylococcus and *Haemophilus influenza.*

❏❏   What is the treatment for pericarditis without effusion?

A 2 week treatment of aspirin q 4 hours is recommended if no contradictions exist and if effusion is not present. Ibuprofen, indomethacin, or colchicine are other alternatives. The use of corticosteroids is controversial, as recurrent pericarditis is common when doses are tapered.

❏❏   Which anomalies of the great vessels result in airway obstruction?

1) Right aortic arch with or without a left ligamentum arteriosum
2) Double aortic arch
3) Anomalous innominate or left carotid artery
4) Aberrant right subclavian
5) Anomalous left pulmonary artery

❏❏   When measuring a pulsus paradoxus, what is considered a normal difference in systolic BP (with inspiration versus expiration)?

8-10 mmHg.

☐☐   **Which congenital heart lesions commonly present with cyanosis in an infant's first day of life?**

All the abnormalities that start with a **T**: Tetralogy of Fallot, Transposition of the great vessels, Total anomalous pulmonary circulation, Truncus arteriosus, and Tricuspid valve atresia.

☐☐   **What is the usual presentation of children with a ventricular septal defect?**

A systolic murmur in the first days of life with no signs related to their condition. They usually resolve spontaneously.

☐☐   **How do infants with atrial septal defects usually present?**

The majority of these children are totally asymptomatic, and the defect usually is not diagnosed until they are school age.

☐☐   **A short PR interval and a delta wave are characteristic of what cardiac anomaly?**

Wolff-Parkinson-White (WPW) syndrome. This is due to a reentry phenomenon along the Bundle of Kent.

☐☐   **Which patients with mitral valve prolapse (MVP) should receive prophylactic antibiotics to protect against subacute bacterial endocarditis?**

Patients with MVP and a systolic murmur.

☐☐   **How does the size of a VSD correlate with the risk of infective endocarditis?**

It doesn't. The risk is independent of size.

☐☐   **What is Eisenmenger syndrome?**

A right-to-left or bidirectional cardiac shunt secondary to development of high pulmonary resistance. Commonly from an obstructive pulmonary vascular disease. This is usually seen in patients with VSD, but can occur with ASD, PDA, or other communication between aorta and pulmonary artery.

☐☐   **A 16-year-old boy comes to your office for a pre-participation sports physical. What three findings during the physical exam can help you identify those patients at risk for sudden cardiac arrest?**

Presence of dysrhythmia, a pathologic murmur, and marfanoid features.

☐☐   **What test can be used to identify vasovagal neuroregulatory syncope as the cause of syncope in children with a history of "falling out"?**

The tilt-table test.

☐☐   **What test can be used to differentiate congenital heart disease from primary pulmonary parenchymal disease in a newborn with cyanosis?**

The hyperoxia test.

☐☐   **On a chest x-ray of a child, what bony abnormality would lead you to suspect coarctation of the aorta?**

Bilateral rib notching, due to increased flow through internal mammary arteries.

☐☐   **What are the common cardiac complications of Kawasaki disease?**

Coronary artery aneurysm and thrombosis, myocarditis, MI, and valvular insufficiency.

☐☐   **What are the common cardiac complications of juvenile rheumatoid arthritis?**

Pericarditis and (rare) myocarditis.

❑❑   **What are the common cardiac complications of Marfan syndrome?**

Aortic and mitral insufficiency, MVP, and dissecting aortic aneurysm.

❑❑   **What are the common cardiac complications of sickle cell anemia?**

High output cardiac failure, cardiomyopathy and cor pulmonale.

❑❑   **What congenital cardiac diseases will present with increased pulmonary markings on a chest x-ray?**

Transposition of the great arteries and total anomalous pulmonary venous return (also known as the "Snowman effect").

❑❑   **In classifying a heart murmur's intensity, what differentiates a III from a IV?**

The absence (III) or presence (IV) of a thrill.

❑❑   **What is the murmur of an ASD?**

Mid-systolic rumbling murmur best heard at the lower left sternal border.

❑❑   **Describe the most common 'innocent' murmur?**

Medium-pitched, "musical" or vibratory systolic ejection murmur best heard at LLSB without radiation.

❑❑   **How common is an 'innocent' murmur?**

Very. Up to 30% of children have one, with peak incidence between 3-7 years of age.

❑❑   **What is the test of choice to examine for the presence of vegetations in a child with endocarditis?**

Transesophageal echocardiography (TEE).

❑❑   **What is the most common cardiac malformation?**

VSD. This accounts for about 25% of all heart diseases. Prognosis depends largely on size of the defect - if small it may close spontaneously (usually before 4 years of age).

❑❑   **A 10-year-old child with a history of VSD is about to have an impacted tooth removed. What antibiotic should he be given prophylactically to prevent endocarditis?**

Amoxicillin 50 mg/kg one hour before the procedure and 25 mg/kg six hours after the first dose. If the patient has a penicillin allergy, use erythromycin 20 mg/kg one hour before and 10 mg/kg six hours after the first dose.

❑❑   **What is the treatment of choice for a patent ductus arteriosus (PDA)?**

Surgical ligation and division, regardless of age.

❑❑   **What compound constricts the ductus arteriosus right after birth?**

Oxygen, which is a vasoconstrictor. (Of course you knew that)

❑❑   **When is it most effective to administer indomethacin to newborns with patent ductus arteriosus?**

During the first 24-48 hours of life, with a second and third dose at 12 and 36 hours, following the initial dose.

❑❑   **What percentage of patent ductus arteriosi that were initially closed with indomethacin reopen?**

25%. It is more likely to reopen if therapy is started beyond the first week of life.

❑❑   **How does squatting help children with hypoxia secondary to their TOF?**

It increases their systemic vascular resistance.

❑❑   **What test confirms the clinical suspicion of PDA?**

2-D echocardiogram detects up to 90% .

❑❑   **What is the most common indication for pacemaker installation in children?**

Symptomatic bradycardia (i.e. Stokes-Adams attacks).

❑❑   **A 3-year-old child presents with premature atrial contractions (PACs). Should this be a cause of concern?**

No, they are usually benign, except in children less than 1 year old, or those on digitalis.

❑❑   **Name the anomalies found in TOF.**

Pulmonary stenosis, VSD, dextroposition of aorta with septal override and RVH.

❑❑   **What are the most common complications of TOF prior to correction?**

Cerebral thromboses, brain abscess, bacterial endocarditis and CHF.

❑❑   **Arteriography shows a communication between the pulmonary artery and pulmonary vein. What's your diagnosis?**

Osler-Weber-Rendu syndrome. This is the most common form of a pulmonary AV fistula.

❑❑   **What medication has been shown to decrease the fever and discomfort associated with acute attacks of Kawasaki syndrome?**

High dose aspirin therapy.

❑❑   **What laboratory findings differentiate Kawasaki disease from measles?**

Children with Kawasaki syndrome tend to have an increased WBC count and ESR.

❑❑   **What congenital cardiac defects are commonly seen in children with Down's syndrome?**

Endocardial cushion defect, ASD, VSD.

❑❑   **What congenital cardiac defects are commonly seen in infants with fetal alcohol syndrome?**

ASD, VSD.

❑❑   **What congenital cardiac defects are commonly seen in patients with autosomal dominant polycystic kidney disease?**

Mitral valve prolapse (MVP).

❑❑   **What is the 5-year survival rate of infants and children who undergo a complete heart transplantation?**

70-85% with immunosuppressive agents.

❑❑   **What is the primary cause of congestive heart failure (CHF) in infancy and childhood?**

Congenital heart disease.

❑❑   **What diseases lead to a pulsus paradoxus greater than 20 mm Hg?**

Cardiac tamponade, asthma, CHF.

❏❏   **What does a high pulsus paradoxus indicate?**

Circulatory compromise.

❏❏   **What are the classic presenting features of pericarditis in children?**

Positional sharp substernal chest pain, abdominal pain, tachycardia, tachypnea, dyspnea, fever, friction rub.

❏❏   **What are the potential complications from pericarditis?**

Myocarditis, pericardial effusion, pericardial tamponade.

❏❏   **What is the mortality rate from myocarditis?**

35%

❏❏   **What are the findings in an infant with acute CHF?**

1. Irritability
2. Poor feeding
3. Lethargy
4. Failure to thrive
5. Tachycardia
6. Tachypnea
7. Hyperactive precordium
8. Gallop rhythm
9. Rales
10. Hepatomegaly

Peripheral edema and neck vein distention are noted only in older children.

❏❏   **What condition in children is infective endocarditis most often associated with?**

Congenital heart disease (40% of cases).

❏❏   **A patient is diagnosed with infective endocarditis, she has a history of recent dental surgery, what is the most likely organism?**

Streptococcal viridans.

❏❏   **In a previously healthy child without congenital heart disease, what is the most common cause of infective endocarditis?**

Staphylococcus aureus.

❏❏   **In what percentage of cases of bacterial endocarditis will blood cultures be positive?**

90%.

❏❏   **A child presents with chest pain and a new murmur, which cardiac conditions should be suspected?**

Hypertrophic obstructive cardiomyopathy and aortic stenosis.

❏❏   **Describe the Jones criteria (major) for diagnosing rheumatic fever.**

Carditis, polyarthritis, chorea, erythema marginatum, and subcutaneous nodules.

❏❏   **Which of the major criteria is most commonly seen?**

Polyarthritis.

❏❏   **Describe the rash present in rheumatic fever.**

Non-pruritic, fine, lacey in appearance with central blanching and a serpiginous pattern.

❏❏   **What is the most common cardiac defect in children and adolescents with rheumatic heart disease?**

Mitral insufficiency.

❏❏ **What are the cardiac complications of Kawasaki disease?**

Myocarditis and coronary artery aneurysms.

❏❏ **What percent of untreated patients with Kawasaki's disease will develop coronary artery aneurysms?**

15% to 25%. The coronary artery damage can lead to thrombosis or sudden death after acute symptoms have resolved.

❏❏ **What is the most common dysrhythmia seen in the pediatric age group?**

Supraventricular tachycardia (SVT)

❏❏ **What is the most common cause of SVT in infants?**

Congenital heart disease (30%). Other causes include fever, infection, or drug exposure (20%), and unknown etiology (50%).

❏❏ **Twenty-five percent of SVT is associated with what syndrome?**

Wolf-Parkinson-White.

❏❏ **What problem can occur by using digoxin to treat SVT in a patient with the WPW syndrome?**

Digoxin can shorten the refractory period in the bypass tract and enhance conduction in the accessory pathway, leading to a rapid ventricular response and ventricular fibrillation.

❏❏ **What are the most common causes of atrial fibrillation and flutter?**

Congenital heart disease, rheumatic fever, dilated cardiomyopathy, hyperthyroidism.

❏❏ **Why should atrial flutter be treated in a patient with congenital heart disease?**

Because this patient's risk of sudden death is four times higher than normal.

❏❏ **By what age should a child's ECG resemble an adults?**

> 3 years of age.

❏❏ **What are the possible etiologies for ventricular tachycardia?**

Electrolyte imbalance, metabolic disturbances, cardiac tumors, drugs, cardiac catheterization or surgery, congenital heart disease, cardiomyopathies, prolonged QT syndrome, and idiopathic.

❏❏ **What is the treatment for premature atrial contractions (PACs)?**

No treatment is required in an asymptomatic patient but frequent PACs should be evaluated to rule out myocarditis.

❏❏ **When should premature ventricular contractions (PVCs) be treated?**

Treat those that cause, or are likely to cause, hemodynamic compromise.

❏❏ **What are the characteristics of a nonpathologic murmur?**

Low-grade, short, occur early in systole.

❏❏ **In the pre-term infant, what is the most common cause of congestive heart failure?**

Persistent patent ductus arteriosus.

❏❏ **What is the most common cause of cardiac chest pain in an infant or child?**

Anomalous pulmonary origin of a coronary artery.

❏❏   **What are the most reliable respiratory characteristics of congenital cyanotic cardiac disease?**

Tachypnea and increased depth of respiration in the presence of cyanosis without respiratory distress that does not respond to 100% oxygen, suggesting a right to left shunt.

❏❏   **What is the most common atrial septal defect seen and what does it involve anatomically?**

Most often involves the fossa ovalis, is midseptal, and is of the ostium secundum type.

❏❏   **What other cardiac abnormality is most commonly associated with an atrial septal defect?**

Mitral valve prolapse in 10-20% of patients with ostium secundum atrial septal defect.

❏❏   **What are the most notable cardiac ausculatatory findings in children with atrial septal defects?**

Normal or split first heart sound, accentuation of the tricuspid valve closure sound, a midsystolic pulmonary ejection murmur and a wide, fixed split second heart sound.

❏❏   **What non-cardiac problem is most common in children with an atrial septal defect?**

Respiratory infections. They must be treated promptly to avoid the unlikely but severe consequences of infective endocarditis.

❏❏   **What is the most common clinical symptom of patients with atrial septal defect, regardless of age?**

Exertional dyspnea and fatigue.

❏❏   **What percentage of congenital heart defects do AV septal defects account for? (These are also known as endocardial cushion defects and AV canal defects.)**

4-5%

SURGERY

"Practice all the operations, performing them with each hand and both together – for they are both alike- your object being to attain ability, grace, speed, painlessness, elegance, and readiness."
- Hippocrates

□□   **What is the most common acute surgical condition of the abdomen?**

Acute appendicitis.

□□   **Why would you order a chest x-ray in a case of acute abdomen (no one said anything about an "acute chest")?**

An upright chest x-ray can more easily show air under the diaphragm, an indication of a ruptured viscous. In addition, subdiaphragmatic abscesses or pancreatitis can cause pleural effusions that are evident on chest x-ray. Lastly, lower lobe pneumococcal pneumonia can present as abdominal pain.

□□   **A 16 year old boy comes into your office complaining of increasing difficulty breathing since he woke up this morning. You listen to the lungs and they sound normal. What should you be concerned about?**

Spontaneous pneumothorax. Remember, the classic patient with a spontaneous pneumothorax is a young, skinny, athletic male. In most circumstances, the pneumothorax is fairly small and is often times not heard – even after you've seen the films.

□□   **If you suspect a spontaneous pneumothorax, what type of xray should you order?**

PA and Lateral of the chest. The classic teaching is that expiratory views are more sensitive, but new studies in radiology literature does not support this. Regular films will also give better views for other etiologies.

□□   **What might the abdominal films reveal on a patient with appendicitis?**

Sentinel loops with air fluid levels in the RLQ, a gas filled appendix or a fecalith (pathognomonic). A barium enema may show a partially filled appendix, a mass effect on the medial/inferior boarder of the cecum, and mucosal changes on the terminal ileum.

□□   **What is the most common cause of appendicitis?**

Fecaliths. Fecaliths are found in 40% of uncomplicated appendicitis cases, 65% of cases involving gangrenous appendices that have not ruptured, and in 90% of cases involving ruptured appendices. Other causes of appendicitis include lymphoid tissue hypertrophy, inspissated barium, foreign bodies, and strictures.

□□   **How does retrocecal appendicitis most commonly present?**

Dysuria and hematuria (due to the proximity of the appendix to the right ureter). Poorly localized abdominal pain, anorexia, nausea, vomiting, diarrhea, mild fever, and peritoneal signs are also frequently common.

□□   **What percentage of acute abdomens with a pre-operative diagnosis of appendicitis actually had appendicitis as a postoperative diagnosis?**

85%. Other postoperative diagnoses commonly include acute mesenteric lymphadenitis, PID, epiploic appendicitis, ruptured graafian follicle, acute gastroenteritis, and twisted ovarian cysts.

☐☐   **What is the characteristic temporal sequence of the following signs and symptoms of appendicitis?**

Anorexia, abdominal pain, and vomiting are the order of occurrence in 95% of patients with acute appendicitis.

☐☐   **Differentiate between McBurney's point, Rovsing's sign, the obturator sign, and the psoas sign.**

McBurney's point—Point of maximal tenderness in a patient with appendicitis. Location is 2/3 of the way between the umbilicus and the iliac crest on the right side of the abdomen.
Rovsing's sign—Palpation of LLQ causes pain in the RLQ.
Obturator sign—Internal rotation of a flexed hip causes pain.
Psoas sign—Extension of the right thigh causes pain. This is also indicative of an inflamed appendix.

☐☐   **What is the rate of appendiceal rupture in the pediatric population?**

The pediatric population has a rupture rate of 15–50%, and an associated mortality rate of 3%.

☐☐   **What is the most common organism in wound infections?**

Staphylococcus.

☐☐   **A patient who develops a reddish-brown exudate within 6 hours of an appendectomy most likely has a wound with what type of infection?**

Clostridium. Necrotizing fasciitis, dehiscence, and sepsis may result if not treated promptly.

☐☐   **What is the appropriate bolus for a dehydrated child who weighs 15 Kg?**

300 ml (20 ml/kg).

☐☐   **What is the formula for determining the average daily fluid requirements for a patient?**

100 cc/kg/day for the first 10 kg   (or 4 cc/kg/hr)

50 cc/kg/day for the next 10 kg   (or 2 cc/kg/hr)

20 cc/kg/day for the next 10 kg.   (or 1 cc/kg/hr)

☐☐   **So using the above formula, how much fluid per day should be given to a 32 kg child?**

(100 x 10) + (50 x 10) + (20 x 12)= 1000 + 500 + 240 = 1740 cc per day

☐☐   **Normal saline and Ringer's lactate have how many mEq/L of sodium, respectively?**

154 mEq/L, 130 mEq/L.

☐☐   **Matching transplants:**

1. Autograft   a. Donor and recipient are genetically the same.
2. Heterotrophic   b. Donor and recipient are the same person.
3. Isograft   c. Donor and recipient are of the same species.
4. Orthotopic   d. Donor and recipient belong to different species.
5. Allograft   e. Transplantation to a normal anatomical position.
6. Xenograft   f. Transplantation to a different anatomical position.

Answers: (1) b, (2) f, (3) a, (4) e, (5) c, and (6) d.

☐☐   **What transplant organ can be preserved the longest?**

The kidney. Kidneys can be preserved in cold storage for up to 48 hours, the pancreas and liver for 8 hours, and the heart for 4 hours. Viability can be extended by using cold storage solutions, such as Collins solution and UW-Belzer solution.

☐☐ **What is the most common cause of bleeding in a postoperative patient?**

Poor local control.

☐☐ **At what point of airway obstruction will inspiratory stridor become evident?**

70% occlusion.

☐☐ **What is Kehr's sign?**

A pain in the left shoulder, made worse in Trendelenburg. This is a sign of splenic injury. It is only present in 50% of such cases. In addition to the patient's history and physical exam, peritoneal lavage will determine bleeding in the peritoneum if the spleen is bleeding. This is not organ specific but leads to laparotomy, which is organ specific.

☐☐ **What postoperative complication does a patient most likely have if he has a fever and shoulder pain occuring four days after a splenectomy?**

Subphrenic abscess. This can cause fever and irritation to the diaphragm and the branch of the phrenic nerve that innervates it.

☐☐ **Which organisms are most commonly responsible for overwhelming postsplenectomy sepsis?**

Encapsulated organisms: pneumococcus (50%); meningococcus (12%); E. Coli (11%); H. Influenza (8%); staphylococcus (8%); and streptococcus (7%).

☐☐ **What is a sentinel loop?**

A distended loop of bowel seen on x-ray that lies near a localized inflammatory process. This is a clue to an underlying inflammatory process adjacent to the distended bowel. It can often be seen in pancreatitis or appendicitis.

☐☐ **What is the sensory innervation to the nipple, umbilicus, and perianal region?**

Nipple: T4.
Umbilicus: T10.
Perianal: S2–4.

☐☐ **Matching:**

1) Neuropraxia   a) Damage to the axon, no damage to the sheath.
2) Axonotmesis   b) Temporary loss of function, no damage to axon.
3) Neurotmesis   c) Damage to axon and sheath.

Answers: (1) b, (2) a, and (3) c.

☐☐ **A 16 year old female fears she has cancer in both breasts. Her breasts are lumpy with mild swelling. She has a greenish-yellow discharge from her nipples and is sore in the upper outer quadrants of her breasts, and she says the pain usually begins one week before menstruation, and disappears when her menses is over. Does she have breast cancer?**

Probably not. These symptoms indicate fibrocystic breast changes, which are not a premalignant syndrome.

☐☐ **What is the most common non-cystic breast tumor?**

Fibroadenomas. These small, painless, mobile round tumors are most common in women under the age of twenty-five.

☐☐   What is the most common tumor in the first year of life?

Wilm's tumor. Hepatoma is second.

☐☐   What is the average age of diagnosis of Wilm's tumors?

3 years old. Cure rates are as high as 90% in patients with no metastasis.

☐☐   What are the most common sites of secondary malignancies in patients who have had Wilm's tumors?

Hepatocellular carcinoma, leukemia, lymphoma, and soft tissue sarcoma. 1–2% of patients with Wilm's tumors will develop secondary malignancies.

☐☐   Pheochromocytomas produce what?

Catecholamines. Symptoms include increased blood pressure, perspiration, heart palpitations, anxiety, and weight loss.

☐☐   Vanillylmandelic acid, normetanephrine, and metanephrine found in the urine are indicative of what illness?

Pheochromocytoma.

☐☐   Where are the majority of pheochromocytomas located?

90% are found in the adrenal medulla. The remaining 10% are found in other tissues originating from neural crest cells.

☐☐   What is the pheochromocytoma rule of 10's?

10% are malignant, 10% are multiple or bilateral, 10% are extra-adrenal, 10% occur in children, 10% recur after surgical removal, and 10% are familial.

☐☐   What is the most common benign tumor of the liver?

Cavernous hemangiomas.

☐☐   Hepatic cancer most commonly metastasizes to what organ?

The lung (bronchiogenic carcinoma).

☐☐   Surgery is curative for liver cancer in what percentage of resectable asymptomatic tumors?

> 70% of children without cirrhosis. If the patient has cirrhosis and a tumor < 2 cm, then surgery is curative 70% of the time. If the patient has cirrhosis and a tumor > 3 cm, then cure rates are only 10%.

☐☐   What is the two year survival rate for patients who have had liver transplants to cure liver cancer?

25–30%.

☐☐   In what types of tumors will α-fetoprotein (AFP) be elevated?

Primary hepatic neoplasms and endodermal sinus or yolk sac tumors of the ovaries and testes. AFP is present in 30% of patients with primary liver cancer.

☐☐   What is the most common cause of portal hypertension?

Intrahepatic obstruction (90%). Cirrhosis is the most common cause of intrahepatic obstruction. Other causes of portal hypertension are increased hepatopetal flow without obstruction (i.e., fistulas), and extrahepatic outflow obstruction.

❏❏   **What is the most commonly isolated organism in pyogenic hepatic abscesses?**

E. coli or other Gram-negative bacteria. The source of such bacteria is most likely infection in the biliary system.

❏❏   **What clinical sign can help in the diagnosis of cholecystitis?**

Pain on inspiration with palpation in RUQ. This is called Murphy's sign. As the patient breaths in, the gallbladder is lowered in the abdomen and comes in contact with peritoneum just below the examiner's hand. An inflamed gallbladder will be greatly aggravated by this event, and the patient will discontinue her deep breath.

❏❏   **What is the difference between cholelithiasis, cholecystitis, choledocholithiasis, and cholangitis?**

Cholelithiasis: The existence of gallstones in the gallbladder.

Cholecystitis: The inflammation of the gallbladder secondary to gallstones.

Choledocholithiasis: The existence of gallstones in the common bile duct that have migrated from the gallbladder.

Cholangitis: The inflammation of the common bile duct often secondary to bacterial infection or choledocholithiasis.

❏❏   **Which ethnic group has a proportionately larger number of people with symptomatic gallstones?**

Native Americans. By the age of 60, 80% of Native-Americans with previously asymptomatic gallstones will develop symptoms, as compared to only 30% of Caucasian-Americans, and 20% of African-Americans.

❏❏   **What percentage of patients with cholangitis are also septic?**

50%. Chills, fever, and shock can occur.

❏❏   **After a cholecystectomy, can gallstones reform?**

Yes. They can recur in the bile ducts.

❏❏   **Where do most hernias occur?**

In the groin (75%). Incisional and ventral hernias account for 10%, and umbilical hernias count for 3%.

❏❏   **The majority of inguinal hernias in infants and children are what kind of hernias?**

Indirect inguinal hernias.

❏❏   **Differentiate between reducible, incarcerated, strangulated, Richter, and complete hernias.**

Reducible: The contents of the hernia sac return to the abdomen spontaneously, or with slight pressure, when the patient is in a recumbent position.

Incarcerated: The contents of the hernia sac are irreducible and cannot be returned to the abdomen.

Strangulated: The sac and its contents turn gangrenous.

Richter: Only part of the hernia sac and its contents becomes strangulated. This hernia may spontaneously reduce and be overlooked.

<u>Complete</u>: An inguinal hernia that passes all the way into the scrotum.

❑❑   **What are the boundaries of Hesselbach's triangle?**

The triangle is medial to the inferior epigastric artery, superior to the inguinal ligament, and lateral to the rectus sheath. Hesselbach's triangle is the site through which direct hernias pass.

❑❑   **A direct hernia is due to a weakness in what tissue?**

The transversalis fascia, which composes the floor of the Hesselbach triangle.

❑❑   **Indirect inguinal hernias occur secondary to what defect?**

A failure of the processus vaginalis to close. The resulting hernia can then pass through the inguinal ring.

❑❑   **What is the most common hernia in females?**

Direct hernias. Indirect hernias are the most common hernias overall (i.e., in both sexes combined).

While femoral hernias are more common in females than in males, they are still not as common as direct hernias.

❑❑   **Of all the hernias in the groin area, which type will most likely strangulate?**

A femoral hernia. Femoral hernias occur in the femoral canal, an unyielding space between the lacunar ligament and the femoral vein.

❑❑   **Which is more common, sliding or paraesophageal hiatal hernias?**

Sliding hiatal hernias, which account for 95% of hiatal hernias.

❑❑   **What are the signs and symptoms of intestinal obstruction in a newborn?**

Maternal polyhydramnios, abdominal distention, failure to pass meconium, and vomiting.

❑❑   **A newborn's vomit will be stained with bile if the obstruction is distal to what anatomical structure?**

The ampulla of Vater.

❑❑   **What are the common causes of neonatal obstruction?**

Annular pancreas, Hirshsprung's disease, intestinal atresia, malrotation and volvulus or peritoneal bands, meconium plug, small left colon syndrome, and stenosis.

❑❑   **What is the double bubble sign?**

The appearance of the distended stomach and duodenum on x-ray in a patient with duodenal obstruction. This is classically seen in duodenal atresia of the newborn. It is commonly associated with Down's Syndrome.

❑❑   **What is the most common cause of obstruction in children?**

Hernia.

❑❑   **What is the most common site of intestinal obstruction secondary to gall stones?**

The terminal ileum. 55–60% will have associated air in the biliary tree.

❑❑   **What is Rendu-Osler-Weber syndrome?**

Hereditary hemorrhagic telangiectasias found in the small intestine.

❑❑   **If blood is recovered from the stomach after an NG tube is inserted, where is GI bleeding likely?**

Above the ligament of Treitz.

❏❏ **What is the major cause of death in patients with Hirshsprung's disease?**

Enterocolitis.

❏❏ **Is Hirshsprung's disease more common in males or females?**

Males. The ratio is 5:1.

❏❏ **What is the Meckel's diverticulum rule of 2's?**

2% of the population has it, it is 2 inches long, it is 2 feet from the ileocecal valve, it most commonly occurs in children under 2, and is symptomatic in 2%.

❏❏ **Rectal bleeding in a patient with Meckel's diverticula is most likely due to what condition?**

Ulceration of ectopic gastric mucosa.

❏❏ **Cellulitis of the umbilicus in a pediatric patient with an acute abdomen is most likely due to what condition?**

A perforated Meckel's diverticulum.

❏❏ **What is the difference in prognosis between familial polyposis and Gardner's disease?**

Although both are inheritable conditions of colonic polyps, Gardner's disease rarely results in malignancy, while familial polyposa virtually always results in malignancy.

❏❏ **What percentage of patients with familial polyposis will go on to develop carcinoma of the colorectum?**

100%. Due to the imminent development of cancer, these patients are advised to have total colectomies and ileostomies.

❏❏ **A patient complains of severe pain with defecation, constipation, and blood streaked stools, which contain bloody discharge following bowel movements. What is the diagnosis, and what is the most common place this will be found?**

Anal fissure. 90% of anal fissures are found in the posterior midline. If fissures are found elsewhere in the anal canal, anal intercourse, TB, carcinoma, Crohn's disease, or syphilis should be considered.

❏❏ **What are some extraintestinal manifestations of ulcerative colitis?**

Ankylosing spondylitis, sclerosing cholangiitis, arthralgias, ocular complications, erythema nodosum, aphthous ulcers in the mouth, thromboembolic disease, pyoderma gangrenous, nephrolithiasis, and cirrhosis of the liver.

❏❏ **What is the most frequent site of carcinoid tumors?**

The appendix accounts for 50% of carcinoid tumors. The second most common site is the small bowel (the ileum).

❏❏ **What is the most common tumor of the testes?**

Malignant lymphoma.

❏❏ **What is the most common germinal tumor of the testes?**

Seminoma (40%). The overall survival rate for seminomas is 85%, as hematogenous spread does not occur until late in the disease. Other germinal tumors are embryonic cell carcinoma (25%), teratocarcinoma (25%), and choriocarcinoma. Germinal cell tumors of the testes are the most common malignant tumors of the testes.

❑❑   **In what age group is torsion of the testicles most common?**

Adolescents.

❑❑   **What is the maximum amount of time a testes can remain torsed without irreversible damage being done?**

4–6 hours.

❑❑   **What lab value is indicative of bony metastasis?**

Increased alkaline phosphatase.

❑❑   **What is the most sensitive indicator of shock in children?**

Tachycardia.

❑❑   **What is the initial fluid bolus that should be given to children in shock?**

20 ml/kg..

❑❑   **What is the most common long bone fractured?**

The tibia.

❑❑   **Describe a common patient with a slipped capital femoral epiphysis.**

Obese boy, 10–16 years old. Groin or knee discomfort increases with activity; he may have a limp. Often bilateral. The slip is best seen on a lateral view.

❑❑   **What is the most common ankle injury?**

75% of ankle injuries are sprains with 90% of these involving the lateral complex. 90% of lateral ligament injuries are anterior talofibular.

❑❑   **What is the most helpful physical exam test for anterior talofibular ligament injury?**

Anterior drawer test. > 3 mm of excursion might be significant (compare sides); > 1 cm is always significant.

❑❑   **Which bone is most commonly fractured at birth?**

The clavicle.

❑❑   **What type of Salter-Harris fracture has the worst prognosis?**

Type V—compression injury of the epiphyseal plate.

❑❑   **Which is the more sensitive test used to determine an anterior cruciate ligament tear in the knee: the anterior drawer test or the Lachman test?**

Lachman test. While the knee is held at 20° flexion and the distal femur is stabilized, the lower leg is pulled forward. Greater than 5 mm anterior laxity compared to the other knee is evidence of an anterior cruciate ligament tear.

❑❑   **What is "nursemaid's elbow"?**

Subluxation of the radial head. During forceful retraction, some fibers of the annular ligament that encircle the radial neck become trapped between the radial head and the capitellum. On presentation, the arm is held in slight flexion and pronation.

❑❑   **Why "tap" a knee with an acute hemarthrosis?**

Relieve pressure and pain and see if fat globules are present indicating a fracture.

❏❏   **What are the most common lower extremity injuries to bone in children?**

Tibial and fibular shaft fractures, usually secondary to twist forces.

❏❏   **What are the differences between avulsion of the tibial tubercle and Osgood-Schlatter disease?**

Both occur at the tibial tubercle. Avulsion presents with acute inability to walk, lateral view of the knee is most diagnostic; treatment is surgical. Osgood-Schlatter's has vague history of intermittent pain, is bilateral in 25% of cases, has pain with range of motion but not with rest; treatment is symptomatic and not surgical.

❏❏   **What is a toddler fracture?**

Common cause of limp or refusal to walk in this age group is a spiral fracture of the tibia, without fibular involvement.

❏❏   **What is the most common Salter-Harris class fracture?**

Type II. A triangular fracture involving the metaphysis and an epiphyseal separation.

❏❏   **Why is maintenance of core body temperature more difficult in a small child?**

A child has a larger surface are to volume ration, and is therefore more susceptible to heat loss.

❏❏   **Is surgery an effective way to decrease the incidence of complications in children with duodenal hematomas?**

No.

❏❏   **What is the most likely cause of a subdural hematoma with retinal hemorrhages in a child?**

Child abuse.

❏❏   **A small child reportedly fell 4 feet from a bed, and landed directly on her head. Is this history consistent with a subdural hematoma?**

No.

❏❏   **In a child with loss of pulses distal to a fracture site, what is the first step in management?**

Gentle attempt to realign the limb. In children with non-penetrating trauma loss of pules are more likely to be caused by spasm, pressure on or kinking of a vessel then from actual vessel injury.

❏❏   **What is the weakest portion of a child's bone?**

The physis.

❏❏   **What is the major concern with injury to the physis?**

The potential for subsequent growth arrest.

❏❏   **What is the most common physeal injury?**

The distal radius.

❏❏   **What is a Type I Salter-Harris fracture?**

A separation of the epiphysis from the metaphysis. Usually caused by avulsion or shearing forces. Prognosis is good.

❏❏   **What is a Type II Salter-Harris fracture?**

A fracture through the physis which exits the metaphysis. Prognosis is good.

❑❑   **What is a Type III Salter-Harris fracture?**

A fracture through the physis which exits the epiphysis into the articular surface. Much worse prognosis that Types I & II. ORIF is often required.

❑❑   **What is a Type IV Salter-Harris fracture?**

A fracture extending through the metaphysis, physis and epiphysis. Carries a high rate of premature physeal arrest.

❑❑   **What is a Type V Salter-Harris fracture?**

A crushing injury of the physis. Often difficult to pick up radiographically. Usually diagnosed retrospectively after growth arrest occurs.

❑❑   **What is the most common cause of painful hip in older children?**

Transient synovitis. It can be difficult to distinguish from septic arthritis.

❑❑   **What percent of pediatric burns are inflicted?**

16-20%.

❑❑   **What are some of the proposed etiologies of acute osteomyelitis in children?**

Possible mechanisms include transient bacteremia, trauma, malnutrition, and recent illness.

❑❑   **What are some possible findings in a child with a septic hip joint?**

The hip may be held in external rotation and flexed. Any motion of the joint will be very painful.

❑❑   **What bacterial pathogens are associated with osteomyelitis in children?**

Staph aureus is the most common (40-80% of cases), H. influenza type b (especially in unimmunized children less than 3 years old). Less common: S. pneumoniae, S. pyogenes, Salmonella, Brucella, Kingella, Serratia, coagulase negative Staph and Neisseriae (the latter two occasionally associated with sepsis and osteomyelitis in neonates). Pseudomonas must be considered, especially with puncture wounds to the foot (especially through a gym shoe); N. gonorrhea must be considered in sexually active patients.

❑❑   **Are x-rays helpful in diagnosing osteomyelitis?**

X-rays done within the first week may be negative; periosteal reaction and bony destruction take about 10-14 days to become radiographically evident.

❑❑   **What is the treatment of osteomyelitis in children? Of a septic joint?**

Pending culture results, treatment with broad-spectrum antibiotics including coverage for S. aureus is recommended; neonates should also be covered for group B strep, and gram negative coliforms; treatment for osteomyelitis associated with puncture wounds should provide coverage for Pseudomonas. Treatment for a septic joint should also provide coverage for H. flu type b (incidence of this has decreased as immunization for H. flu increases). Primary treatment for a septic joint is irrigation and drainage of the joint in the operating room, obtaining cultures prior to starting antibiotics. Sexually active patients should be covered for N. gonorrhea.

❑❑   **What is toxic synovitis?**

It is a noninfectious inflammatory condition that is seen in children approximately 3-7 years old, often involves the hip, and may follow a viral upper respiratory infection. It may be confused with a septic hip (which must be ruled out first) or Legg-Calve-Perthes. There may be decreased medial rotation of the hip in flexion, and some decreased abduction and extension. The child may have low grade fever, but unlike a septic hip, the CBC and ESR are usually normal, the child does not appear toxic, and has better range of motion of the hip. Ultrasonography can help to visualize a distended capsule as distinguished from synovial thickening which may be seen in Perthes' disease. Aspiration of the hip may be required to distinguish synovitis from a septic joint. It is treated with bed rest, anti-inflammatories, and the patient should be re-evaluated to assure resolution of symptoms has occurred.

☐☐   What is a physis?

A cartilaginous growth plate which appears lucent on x-ray; also called the epiphyseal growth plate.

☐☐   What is an epiphysis?

A secondary ossification center at the ends of long bones, which is separated by the physis from the remainder of the bone.

☐☐   What is an apophysis?

A secondary bone growth center at the insertion of tendons onto bones; it does not participate in a joint. Traction on immature apophyses may cause a variety of painful conditions.

☐☐   What is a metaphysis?

The flared portion at the ends of a bone next to the physis, where the calcified cartilage from the physis is replaced by encochondral bone.

☐☐   What is a diaphysis?

The shaft of a long bone.

☐☐   What is equinus?

Plantar flexed position or deformity of the foot so that the person walks on their toes.

☐☐   What is a valgus deformity? Varus deformity?

Valgus deformity is angulation of an extremity at a joint with the more distal part angled away from the midline. Varus deformity is angulation of an extremity at a joint with the more distal part angled toward the midline.

☐☐   What are some common terms used in describing orthopedic findings?

Pes: refers to the foot
Genu: refers to the knee
Coxa: refers to the hip
Cubitus: refers to the elbow
Talipes: a general term for foot deformities
Cavus: abnormally arched foot
Dislocation: complete loss of contact between
Planus: flat two joint surfaces
Subluxation: incomplete loss of contact between two joint surfaces

☐☐   Are dislocations and sprains more common in children or adults?

Dislocations and ligamentous injuries are uncommon in prepubertal children as the ligaments and joints are quite strong as compared to the adjoining growth plates. Excessive force applied to a child's joint is more likely to cause a fracture through the growth plate than a dislocation or sprain.

☐☐   Can fractures result in overgrowth or undergrowth of the involved bone?

Both. Fractures involving the growth plate may result in arrest of growth and severe shortening or uneven arrest of growth leading to angular deformities. Fractures can also result in overgrowth as some fractures stimulate growth at the physis of the fractured bone.

☐☐   What findings comprise the shaken baby syndrome?

Retinal hemorrhage, subdural hematoma, and rib fractures.

☐☐   What is an antalgic limp?

It is a painful limp characterized by a shortened stance phase to decrease time on the affected extremity.

☐☐   What is a Trendelenberg gait?

It is a non-painful limp, indicative of underling hip instability or muscle weakness, characterized by an equal stance phase between the involved and uninvolved side. The child will attempt to shift the center of gravity over the involved side for improved balance.

☐☐   What are some causes (according to age) of painful limping?

Antalgic gait may be caused by: (1-3 year old): infection, occult trauma, or neoplasm; (4-10 year old): infection, transient synovitis of the hip, Legg-Calve-Perthes disease, rheumatologic disorder, trauma, or neoplasm; (11+ year old): slipped capital femoral epiphysis, rheumatologic disorder, trauma. It may also be seen in sickle cell disease.

☐☐   What are some causes of Trendelenberg gait?

(1-3 year old): hip dislocation, neuromuscular disease
(4-10 year old): hip dislocation, neuromuscular disorder

☐☐   What are some intrauterine factors that may predispose to DDH?

Breech position, first born (smaller, more constraining uterus), or anything else that restricts fetal movement

☐☐   What is the Ortolani maneuver?

Gentle abduction with the hip in flexion while lifting up on the greater trochanter which results in reduction of a dislocated hip with an palpable "clunk" as the femoral head slips over the posterior rim of the acetabulum.

☐☐   What is the Barlow maneuver?

Adduction of the hip in flexion while pushing down gently on the femoral head, in a dislocatable hip, will cause dislocation as the femoral head slips out of the acetabulum.

☐☐   What is the most sensitive indicator of hip disease?

Decreased internal rotation of the hip.

☐☐   What makes the blood supply to the capital femoral epiphysis vulnerable?

The retinacular vessels lie on the surface of the femoral neck and are intracapsular; they enter the epiphysis from the periphery and are subject to damage from trauma, joint infection, and other vascular insults.

☐☐   What is Legg-Calve-Perthes disease (LCPD)?

It is an idiopathic avascular necrosis of the capital femoral epiphysis in a child (usually male) aged 2-12 years (mean: 7 years). Male to female ratio: 4-5:1

☐☐   What is the treatment of LCPD?

The treatment is directed at maintaining the femoral head within the acetabulum which acts as a mold for the re-ossifying femoral head. The treatment goal is to prevent femoral head deformity and osteoarthritis. Treatments may be surgical or non-surgical.

☐☐   What are some clinical manifestations of LCPD?

Antalgic gait, muscle spasm (with restricted abduction and internal rotation), proximal thigh atrophy, thigh pain, and mild shortness of stature.

□□   **What is the most common adolescent hip disorder?**

Slipped capital femoral epiphysis (SCFE).

□□   **What is SCFE?**

It is an inferior and posterior slippage of the head of the femur off the femoral neck. Slips can be either chronic or acute. It most typically presents in summer months, and is coincident with increased physical activity.

□□   **SCFE typically occurs in which individuals?**

Obese adolescents with delayed skeletal maturation or in tall, thin children after a recent growth spurt. If a slip occurs before the age of ten, endocrine disorder or systemic disorder should be suspected. It is seen in males much more commonly than females.

□□   **Is SCFE bilateral or unilateral?**

The disease usually presents unilaterally with thigh, knee, or groin pain and a limp. Up to 30-40% of children with one slip will develop bilateral disease eventually and must be followed for this possibility.

□□   **What is the treatment of SCFE?**

SCFE is one of the few pediatric orthopedic emergencies. Weight bearing must cease to prevent a partial slip from becoming complete (complete slips carry an increased risk of vascular compromise and aseptic necrosis). The treatment is surgical by performing an epihysiodesis of the capital femoral epiphysis with in situ pinning with cannulated screws.

□□   **What are the two major complications of SCFE?**

Osteonecrosis (secondary to damage to the retinacular vessels) and chondrolysis (degeneration of the articular cartilage) of the hip.

□□   **What are growing pains?**

They are nighttime thigh and calf pains most commonly seen in 4-10 year olds with symmetric limb pains unaccompanied by systemic symptoms such as fever or weight loss. Although termed growing pains, they are usually not seen in adolescents who undergo a faster rate of growth than younger children.

□□   **What is the VATER association?**

Vertebral anomalies
Imperforate Anus
TracheoEsophageal fistula
Radial dysplasia (clubhand)
Renal abnormalities.

□□   **Is back pain in children common?**

No, it is unusual and frequently due to organic causes. Etiologies include inflammatory diseases, rheumatologic diseases, developmental diseases, mechanical trauma, and neoplastic diseases.

□□   **What types of tumors may be found in children who have back pain?**

Tumors may involve the vertebral column or the spinal cord. Benign tumors include osteoid osteomas, osteoblastoma (giant osteoid osteoma-greater than 20 mm), solitary bone cysts, and eosinophilic granuloma. Malignant tumors may be osseous (osteogenic or Ewing's sarcoma), neurogenic (neuroblastoma), or metastatic.

□□   **What is torticollis?**

It refers to twisted, or wry, neck, where the head is tipped to one side, with the occiput rotated toward the shoulder. Etiologies include soft tissue trauma, rotary subluxation of the cervical spine, dystonic reactions, muscular causes (e.g. viral myositis), osseous causes, neurogenic causes, and Sandifer syndrome (Gastroesophageal reflux, iron deficiency anemia, vomiting, and a head-tilting trait).

☐☐   **What is a ganglion?**

It is a fluid-filled cyst at the wrist where a defect in the joint capsule allows herniation of the synovium. If the synovium ruptures, fluid collects in the soft tissue where it gets walled off by fibrous tissue. They are benign and tend to disappear over time.

☐☐   **Which carpal bones form the articular surface of the hand?**

The scaphoid and lunate bones.

☐☐   **What is polydactyly?**

Extra digits which may be simple skin tags and digit remnants which do not have palpable bone within or complex varieties which require formal amputation.

☐☐   **What is syndactyly?**

It is fusion of one digit to its neighbor. It may be bony or cutaneous.

☐☐   **Where is syndactyly most often seen?**

It is most often seen between the third (long) and fourth (ring) fingers and the second and third toes.

☐☐   **What is clinodactyly?**

It is curving of a digit, most often the fifth digit and may be directed either radially or in an ulnar direction. It often results from hypoplasia of the middle phalanx and is usually a minor anomaly.

☐☐   **What causes trigger finger?**

Thickening of the tendon of the flexor hallucis longus (in the thumb) or the flexor digitorum longus (of the fingers) in the flexor sheath causing a flexion deformity (triggering). This may be a fixed deformity.

☐☐   **What are the three regions of the foot?**

The hindfoot (the calcaneus and the talus), the midfoot (the navicular, the cuboid, and the three cuneiform bones), and the forefoot (the matatarsals and toes).

☐☐   **What is the joint between the calcaneus and the talus?**

The talocalcaneal or subtalar joint.

☐☐   **What congenital deformity causes "rocker-bottom" foot?**

Congenital vertical talus (congenital convex pes valgus); it may be idiopathic, but is often associated with an underlying neurologic or orthopedic disorder or syndrome.

☐☐   **What is hammer toe?**

It is a flexion deformity at the PIP of the toe with extension at the metatarsophalangeal joint.

☐☐   **What is mallet toe?**

It is a flexion deformity at the distal interphalangeal joint which usually requires release of the flexor digitorum longus tendon.

☐☐   **What is genu varum?**

Bow-legs. It may be physiologic (secondary to intrauterine positioning) or due to asymmetric growth, dysplasia, or metabolic disorders.

□□ **What is a Baker cyst?**

A popliteal or Baker cyst is a benign, fluid-filled cyst of the popliteal space caused by outpouchings of the knee joint capsule or bursae between the gastrocnemius and semimembranosus tendons. Most are idiopathic and resolve spontaneously.

□□ **An adolescent boy presents with pain over the tibial tubercle after athletic activity and presents with a tender prominent tibial tubercle. What is the diagnosis?**

Osgood-Schlatter disease; complete resolution of symptoms over 1-2 years is expected as physeal closure of the tubercle occurs. Symptomatic care with rest, anti-inflammatories, and non-steroidal medication is the usual treatment.

□□ **What is bony dysplasia?**

Dysplasias of bone (and cartilage) refers to a variety of conditions involving metaphyses, diaphyses, epiphyses, and cartilage usually associated with short stature. As a group, they are common and associated with a high rate of stillbirths and early postnatal deaths. Most are genetically based, but some drugs (e.g. warfarin) or Vitamin K deficiency may also cause dysplasia. Some examples include epiphyseal dysplasias, metaphyseal dysplasias, metaphyseal dysostosis, hypochondroplasia, achondroplasia, oteogenesis imperfecta, and diaphyseal dysplasia.

□□ **What is achondroplasia?**

It is a pure autosomal dominant skeletal spondylometaphyseal dysplasia.

□□ **What are some of the features of achondroplasia?**

Short trunk and limbs, large cranium with frontal bossing, flattened nasal bridge, hypoplasia of the maxilla, relative mandibular prognathism moderate brachydactyly, wide hands, with hypotonia noted in infancy.

□□ **What are some of the non-skeletal features that may be associated with achondroplasia?**

Dental malocclusion, recurrent otitis media, chronic serous otitis media, sleep apnea, and early child death may be seen secondary to cervical cord compression due to a small foramen magnum, and hydrocephalus secondary to obstruction of the foramen magnum.

□□ **What is the prognosis for children with achondroplasia?**

They usually have a normal life span except for the uncommon patient with hydrocephalus or spinal cord compressions.

□□ **When does limb bud development usually begin?**

It begins at four to five weeks of gestation. A thin ridge of ectoderm caps the limb buds and is the prerequisite for normal limb and finger development.

□□ **What is osteopenia?**

It refers to generalized decrease in bone mass. It may be due to decreased production of bone or increased resorption and is a feature of several inherited and acquired disorders of childhood.

□□ **What is osteoporosis?**

It is the clinical syndrome secondary to osteopenia, with increased susceptibility to fractures.

□□ **What is osteogenesis imperfecta?**

It is the most prevalent of the osteoporotic syndromes in children. It is the result of a variety of defects in the production of type I collagen, with mutations in one of the two genes for type I procollagen. It is divided into four types. Type II is usually lethal in the perinatal period and characterized by "crumpled bone" syndrome and beaded ribs. Approximately 50% are stillborn and most die of respiratory insufficiency. Type III and IV are rare.

☐☐   **What are some of the characteristics of Osteogenesis Imperfecta Type I?**

Characteristics include bones with thin cortices, osteoporosis, multiple bone fractures usually occurring between ages 2 and 3 years and continuing through early adolescence. Patients may present with hypermobile joints, kyphoscoliosis, joint dislocations, bowed limbs, increased capillary fragility, thin skin, and scleras which often appear blue. Most have hearing loss secondary to osteosclerosis. Type I-B patients have dentinogenesis imperfecta (dentin is rich in type I collagen). This condition is inherited as an autosomal dominant disorder.

☐☐   **Why do the sclerae appear blue in many patients with Osteogenesis Imperfecta?**

The thin sclerae allows for choroidal pigment to show through and this appears blue.

☐☐   **What are wormian bones (in most patients with Osteogenesis Imperfecta)?**

This refers to the wiggled markings seen on x-rays of the skull. Multiple small bony islands, separated by sutures, are seen.

☐☐   **What is osteopetrosis?**

It refers to conditions in which generalized increased bone density is found ("marble bone disease"). There are several different forms. Osteopetrosis with precocious manifestations is present at an early age and has a progressive course associated with early death.

☐☐   **What is Marfan syndrome?**

It is a syndrome characterized by tall, slim stature secondary to a defect in fibrillin (a major component of extracellular microfibrils contributing to the structural integrity of connective tissue). Patients may exhibit scoliosis, joint hyperextensibility, striae, pectus, hernias, aortic valve dilatation, and mitral valve prolapse, and a high incidence of upward dislocation of the lens of the eye.

☐☐   **What is rickets?**

It is a group of diseases secondary to mineral deficiency at the growth plate slowing growth with decreased bone age. It can be caused by vitamin D deficiency, renal tubular wasting of phosphate, or a miscellaneous group of conditions including: hypophosphatasia (deficiency of alkaline phosphatase), hyperphosphatasia, renal osteodystrophy (with hyperphosphatemia and secondary hypocalcemia). Rickets is characterized by generalized osteoporosis with curving of weight-bearing bones, fraying of metaphyses, and increased width of growth plates.

☐☐   **What drugs may be associated with rickets?**

Chronic use of anticonvulsants (especially a combination of phenytoin and phenobarbital) may contribute to rickets in a small number of children.

☐☐   **What is juvenile rheumatoid arthritis?**

It is a disease or group of diseases with chronic synovitis and extra-articular manifestations. By definition, it must be present for six weeks in children sixteen years of age or younger, after other causes have been ruled out. (Most post-infectious arthritis is gone by six weeks.). It may be monoarticular or pauciarticular (involving four or fewer joints). Knees are affected in approximately 75% of children with monoarticular JRA, with the elbow the next most commonly affected.

HEAD AND NECK

"If the profession does not recognize them, the public will learn of them and the law will insist on them."
- Joseph Lister, on his germ theory and doctrines of sterility

❑❑ **If you suspect rupture of the round or oval window in a patient that comes to you for acute hearing loss what test might you perform?**

Applying positive pressure to the tympanic membrane will cause the patient to have ipsilateral nystagmus if there is a rupture.

❑❑ **What systemic sexually transmitted disease is associated with sensorineural hearing loss?**

Syphilis. 7% of patients with idiopathic hearing loss test positive for treponemal antibodies.

❑❑ **What is the most common cause of odontogenic pain?**

Carious tooth. The offending tooth when percussed with a tongue blade will produce a sharp pain. The pain may be felt in the ear, throat, eyes, temple, or other side of the jaw.

❑❑ **A child falls and knocks out his front tooth. How would treatment differ if the child was age 3 versus age 13?**

With primary teeth, no reimplantation should be attempted because of the risk of ankylosis or fusion to the bone. However, with permanent teeth reimplantation should occur as soon as possible. Remaining periodontal fibers are a key to success. Thus, the tooth should not be wiped dry as this may disrupt the periodontal ligament fibers still attached.

❑❑ **A 18 year old presents with both his upper central incisors in hand after an altercation. How can you tell which is the right tooth and which is left?**

When looking at the facial (anterior) surface of the tooth, the sharper angle faces midline. So when replacing the teeth, the two sharp angles should be midline.

❑❑ **What is the best transport medium for an avulsed tooth?**

Hank's solution, a pH balanced cell culture medium, which can even help restore cell viability if the tooth has been avulsed for more than 30 minutes. Milk is an alternative, or the patient, if able to keep from aspiration, may place the tooth underneath his/her tongue.

❑❑ **A patient accidentally swallowed his crown while eating. He cannot afford another crown and wants to know if this one could be used again once it passes?**

Yes. It can be sterilized and replaced.

❑❑ **A three year old child presents with a unilateral purulent rhinorrhea. What is the most likely diagnosis?**

Nasal foreign body.

❑❑ **A child with a sinus infection presents with proptosis, a red swollen eyelid and an inferiolaterally displaced globe. What is the diagnosis?**

Orbital cellulitis and abscess associated with ethmoid sinusitis.

❏❏   **How do patients with retropharyngeal abscesses appear?**

Febrile, ill-appearing, stridorous, drooling, and in an opisthotonic position. These children may complain of difficulty swallowing, or may refuse to eat.

❏❏   **What is the most common organism to cause a retropharyngeal abscess?**

ß-hemolytic streptococcus.

❏❏   **A 16 year old female presents with dull right ear and jaw pain and a burning sensation in the roof of her mouth which is worse in the evening. She also hears a "popping" sound when she opens and closes her mouth. Exam reveals tenderness of the joint capsule. What is the diagnosis and treatment?**

TMJ syndrome. Treat with physiotherapy, analgesia, soft diet, muscle relaxants and occlusive therapy. Apply warm moist compresses 4–5 times daily for 15 minutes for 7–10 days.

❏❏   **A 14 year old diabetic male presents with pain, itching, and discharge from the right ear. The tympanic membrane is intact. What is the diagnosis?**

Otitis externa. Treat by suctioning ear and 1 week of antibiotic steroid otic solution. An ear wick may improve delivery of the antibiotic. Suspect malignant otitis externa in the diabetic patient.

❏❏   **A patient presents with ear pain and fluid-filled blisters on the tympanic membrane. What is the diagnosis?**

Bullous myringitis, commonly caused by Mycoplasma or viruses. Treat with erythromycin.

❏❏   **What is the most frequent cause of hearing loss?**

Cerumen impaction.

❏❏   **What would the physical finding be in unilateral sensory hearing loss?**

The patient will lateralize and have air conduction greater than bone conduction (i.e. normal Rinne test) indicating no conductive loss. The Weber test will lateralize to the normal ear. The most common cause of this is viral neuritis.

❏❏   **What is the most common organism which causes pediatric acute otitis media?**

Streptococcus pneumoniae, followed by Haemophilus influenzae and Moraxella catarrhalis.

❏❏   **What is the most common cause of sialoadenitis?**

Mumps.

❏❏   **What does grunting versus inspiratory stridor indicate?**

Grunting is specific for lower respiratory tract disease, such as pneumonia, asthma, or bronchiolitis.

Stridor localizes respiratory obstruction to the level at or above the larynx.

❏❏   **What is the most common cause of epiglottis?**

Hemophilus influenzae. (n.b. This has changed dramatically since the introduction of the H. flu vaccine, and this entity will likely be considered a very rare entity, and usually caused by Streptococcus).

❏❏   **A patient presents with an itching, tearing, right eye. On exam huge cobblestone papillae are found under the upper lid. What is the diagnosis?**

Allergic conjunctivitis.

❏❏   **In what age group are peritonsillar abscesses most common?**

Adolescents and young adults. Symptoms may include: ear pain, trismus, drooling, and alteration of voice.

□□   **What are the ocular manifestations of Lyme disease?**

Uveitis, keratitis, and optic neuritis.

□□   **What are the ocular manifestations of congenital rubella?**

Retinitis with fine, powdery retinal pigmentation (most common), cataract, glaucoma (10%), microphthalmos (10%), corneal edema, and iris atrophy.

□□   **What type of conjuntivitis is caused by adenovirus?**

Acute follicular conjunctivitis.

□□   **Are topical antivirals effective in the treatment of adenoviral keratoconjunctivitis?**

No.

□□   **How long from the onset of symptoms in the second eye do patients with adenoviral epidemic keratoconjunctivitis shed infectious virus?**

2 weeks.

□□   **What are the ocular signs of cat-scratch disease?**

Follicular conjunctivitis with granulomatous nodules on the palbebral conjuntiva, swollen preauricular or submandibular lymph nodes.

□□   **What is the most common cause of ophthalmia neonatorum in the U.S.?**

Chlamydia trachomatis.

□□   **What retinal involvement can be associated with infectious mononucleosis (Epstein-Barr Virus)?**

Macular edema, retinal hemorrhages, chorioretinitis, punctate outer retinitis, multifocal chorioretinitis and panuveitis.

□□   **What is the most common viral cause of neonatal keratoconjunctivitis?**

Herpes simplex.

□□   **How common is strabismus during the first few months of life?**

Strabismus during infancy occurs in approximately one-third of infants during the first six months of life.

□□   **What causes the appearance of pseudoesotropia?**

A wide nasal bridge and/or prominent epicanthal folds.

□□   **How can pseudoesotropia be differentiated from true esotropia?**

Using the corneal light reflex or alternate cover test when possible.

□□   **What can often be documented in parents of children with infantile esotropia?**

Reduced binocular vision. This has been suggested to be a subthreshold effect of the "gene(s)" that cause the disorder.

PSYCHOSOCIAL PEARLS

"Laughter is the best medicine. Next to sex, of course. And medicine."
- Vice Pope Doug

❏❏　　**In what percentage of cases of child sexual abuse is the abuser known by the child?**

90%.

❏❏　　**In what percentage of cases of child abuse is the mother also abused?**

50%.

❏❏　　**What are the <u>most</u> <u>common</u> ages for child physical abuse?**

Two-thirds of physically abused children are under the age of 3, and one-third are under the age of 6 months.

❏❏　　**In addition to an evaluation for child abuse, what laboratory studies should be done in the child with multiple bruises?**

CBC with differential, platelet count, PT, and UA.

❏❏　　**What are the clinical clues of domestic violence?**

Any evidence of injury during pregnancy or late entry into prenatal care. Also, look for injuries presenting after significant delay or in various stages of healing—especially to the head, neck, breasts, abdomen, or areas suggesting a defensive posture such as forearm bruises. Vague complaints or unusual injuries, such as bites, scratches, burns, or rope marks, as well as suicide.

❏❏　　**What is the <u>most</u> <u>common</u> cause of referral to child psychiatrists?**

Attention Deficit Hyperactivity Disorder. ADHD accounts for 30–50% of child psychiatric outpatients.

❏❏　　**The brother of a female patient with ADHD is at increased risk for what other disorders?**

Conduct, mood, anxiety, and antisocial disorders, substance abuse, and of course ADHD. Relatives of girls with ADHD are at higher risk of disorders than relatives of boys.

❏❏　　**What effect does ADHD have on sleep?**

ADHD causes restless sleep and decreases the time from the onset of sleep until actual REM sleep (REM latency).

❏❏　　**What are the side-effects of Ritalin?**

Ritalin (Methylphenidate) is a psychostimulant used to treat ADHD. Side-effects include depression, headache, hypertension, insomnia, and abdominal pain.

❏❏　　**Are the majority of affective disorder patients bipolar or unipolar?**

Unipolar (80%).

❏❏　　**What is the most frequent first episode of bipolar disease, mania or depression?**

Mania. Depression is rarely the first symptom. In fact, only 5–10% of patients that develop depression first go on to have manic episodes. 1/3 of manic patients never have a depressive episode.

❑❑ **First degree relatives of bipolar patients are at a greater risk for what mental illnesses?**

Unipolar disorders and alcoholism.

❑❑ **What is the most common clinical symptom of a patient with a borderline personality disorder?**

Chronic boredom. Other symptoms include: severe mood swings, volatile relationships, continuous and uncontrollable anger, and impulsiveness.

❑❑ **A patient presents to your office with parotid gland swelling and erosion of the enamel on her teeth. What findings might you expect to find in this patient?**

The patient described most likely has bulimia. Elevated serum amylase and hypokalemia are associated with bulimia.

❑❑ **List some common laboratory findings associated with eating disorders?**

Hyponatremia, hypokalemia, hypocalcemia, hypophosphatemia, anemia, hypoglycemia, starvation ketoacidosis, abnormal glucose tolerance, hypothyroidism due to low T3 levels, persistently elevated cortisol due to starvation, low FSH, LH and estrogens, and elevated growth hormone.

❑❑ **What is the prevalence of conduct disorder?**

10%. It is much more common in boys and is familial.

❑❑ **Children with conduct disorder are most likely to develop what adult disorder?**

About 40% will have some pathology as adults. The most common disorder is antisocial personality disorder.

❑❑ **What is conversion disorder?**

Internal psychological conflict that manifests itself as somatic symptoms. Voluntary motor or sensory function is affected. Examples include weakness, imbalance, dysphagia, and changes in vision, hearing, or sensation. These symptoms are not feigned or intentionally produced. They are also not fully explained by medical conditions.

❑❑ **What is the most familial of all psychiatric diseases?**

Idiopathic enuresis. If one parent had enuresis, there is a 44% chance that the child will have it. If both parents had enuresis then the likely hood increases to 77%.

❑❑ **By what age do most children stop wetting their beds?**

By age 4. Bed wetting after this age is considered enuresis.

❑❑ **What percentage of 4 year olds still have nocturnal enuresis?**

30%. 10% of 6 year olds still wet their beds.

❑❑ **What is the medical treatment for idiopathic enuresis?**

Desmopressin nose drops or imipramine. Most cases eventually resolve spontaneously.

❑❑ **How should a 12 year old who snorts and shouts obscenities uncontrollably be treated?**

Neuroleptics are very good at controlling Gilles de la Tourette syndrome. It develops in childhood with facial twitches, uncontrollable arm movements, and tics. The condition worsens in adolescence.

❑❑ **A 16 year old male presents to your office complaining of pleuritic pain, palpitations, dyspnea, dizziness and tingling in his arms and legs. What is the diagnosis?**

Hyperventilation syndrome. This is frequently associated with anxiety. The tingling is due to decreased carbonate in the blood.

❑❑   **A 17 year old male is brought to your office by a concerned friend. It appears the patient sleeps excessively, has been inhaling his food like there is no tomorrow, and is getting into fights at bars whenever he goes out. He also has been hypersexual, pursuing every female within a 5 mile radius. What is the diagnosis?**

No, this is not a description of every college guy you ever dated although the similarities are amazingly striking. This is the Kleine-Levin syndrome. It can be treated with stimulants.

❑❑   **A 6 year old boy consistently wets his pants. You tell the mother to reward dry periods with treats and praise. This will help reinforce desired behavior. What kind of conditioning is this?**

Positive operant conditioning. This principle was defined by Pavlov.

❑❑   **A 14 year old female comes to your office complaining of sudden episodes of palpitations, diaphoresis, lightheadedness, a fear of losing control, a sense of being choked, tremors, and paresthesias. What is the diagnosis?**

Panic disorder. Panic disorders need not be linked to any events. Though they are commonly associated with agoraphobia, social phobia, mitral prolapse, and late non-melancholic depression.

❑❑   **What percentage of patients with panic disorder also suffer from major depression?**

50%. Patients that suffer panic attacks generally have low self-esteem in addition to major depression.

❑❑   **What is the <u>most</u> <u>common</u> specific phobia exhibited during childhood?**

Animal phobia.

❑❑   **What are the signs and symptoms suggestive of an organic source of psychosis?**

Acute onset, disorientation, visual or tactile hallucinations, age less than 10, and evidence suggesting overdose or acute ingestion, such as abnormal vital signs, pupil size and reactivity, or nystagmus.

❑❑   **What is the difference between schizophrenia and schizophreniform disorder?**

Schizophreniform disorder implies the same signs and symptoms as schizophrenia, yet these symptoms have been present for less than 6 months. The impaired functioning in schizophreniform disorder is not consistent. Schizophreniform disorder is generally a provisional diagnosis with schizophrenia following.

❑❑   **What are the 5 criteria for a diagnosis of Schizophrenia?**

1) Psychosis.
2) Emotional blunting.
3) No affective features or episodes.
4) Clear consciousness.
5) The absence of coarse brain disease, systemic illness, and drug abuse.

❑❑   **Are first degree relatives of schizophrenics more likely to have schizoidia or schizophrenia?**

First degree relatives of schizophrenics are 3 times as likely to have schizoidia as schizophrenia.

❑❑   **A patient who is unable to express his anger, has few close friends, is indifferent to praise from others, is absent-minded, and is emotionally cold and aloof most likely has what kind of personality disorder?**

Schizoidia.

❑❑   **Separation anxiety has an average onset of what age?**

Age 9. These children fear leaving home, sleep, being alone, going to school and losing their parents. 75% develop somatic complaints in order to avoid attending school.

❑❑ **By what age are children aware of their own sex?**

18 months. By age 2–3, a child can answer the question as to whether he/she is a boy or a girl.

❑❑ **What psychiatric problems are associated with violence?**

Acute schizophrenia, paranoid ideation, catatonic excitation, mania, borderline and antisocial personality disorders, delusional depression, posttraumatic stress disorder, and decompensating obsessive/compulsive disorder.

❑❑ **Define the following:**

<u>Akathisia</u>: Internal restlessness. The patient feels as if he is "jumping out of his skin." Treatment is with propranolol.

<u>Echolalia</u>: Meaningless automatic repetition of someone else's words. This may occur immediately or even months after hearing the words.

<u>Catalepsy</u>: The patient maintains the same posture over a long period of time.

<u>Waxy flexibility</u>: The patient offers resistance to anyone trying to change his position, then gradually allows himself to be moved to a new posture, much like a clay figure.

<u>Stereotypy</u>: Patient goes through repetitive motions that have no goal.

<u>Verbigeration</u>: Verbal stereotypy. The patient repeats words over and over.

<u>Gegenhalten</u>: The patient resists external manipulation with the same force being applied.

GYNECOLOGY PEARLS

*"Somewhere on this globe, every ten seconds, there is a woman giving birth to a child.
She must be found and stopped."*

--Sam Stevenson, American comedian

❏❏　　**What is secondary amenorrhea?**

No menstruation for 6 months or more in a female who previously had regular menses.

❏❏　　**What is the <u>most</u> <u>common</u> cause of secondary amenorrhea?**

Yes, the obvious: pregnancy. The second most common cause is hypothalamic hypogonadism which can be due to weight loss, anorexia nervosa, stress, excessive exercise, or hypothalamic disease.

❏❏　　**Virtually all severe cases of dysfunctional uterine bleeding occur in what age group?**

Adolescent females shortly after the onset of menstruation.

❏❏　　**What is the <u>most</u> <u>common</u> benign breast tumor?**

Fibroadenoma. They are most common in young women (under 30). They are usually solitary, mobile masses with distinct borders.

❏❏　　**What are the rates of pregnancy with the following forms of birth control: (1) surgical sterilization, IUDs, or oral contraceptives; (2) coitus interruptus and rhythm method; (3) condoms; and (4) foams, jellies, sponges, or diaphragms?**

1) .2–2%, 2) 10%, 3) 12%, and 4), 18–20%.

❏❏　　**What predisposes a female to yeast infections?**

Diabetes, oral contraceptives, and antibiotics.

❏❏　　**What is the <u>most</u> <u>common</u> cause of vaginitis?**

Candida albicans.

❏❏　　**Female pseudohermaphroditism is <u>most</u> <u>commonly</u> due to what condition?**

Congenital adrenal hyperplasia. The defective adrenals cannot produce normal amounts of cortisol. These patients have normal XX chromosomes, but an excess of endogenous adrenal steroids has virilizing effects.

❏❏　　**What is the number one cause of UTIs?**

E. coli.

❏❏　　**A 16 year old female comes to you complaining of fever, aches and pains, and painful genital sores that looked like blisters 2 days ago until they popped and started hurting. What would you expect to find on culture of the vesicular fluid?**

This patient most likely has the herpes simplex virus, type 2. Tzanck smear or a culture will show multinucleated giant cells by Giemsa stain.

❐❐ **A mother comes to your office because she fears her 7 month old daughter's vagina is "closing up". Examination reveals midline fusion of the labia minora, obscuring the view of the introitus. What is the diagnosis?**

Labial adhesions or acquired attachment of the labia minora. This is thought to occur because of low levels of endogenous estrogen in preadolescent girls, resulting in a thin epithelial surface of the labia minora. This thin epithelial surface is prone to maceration and inflammation, leading to fusion of the edges.

❐❐ **What is the treatment for labial adhesions?**

Topical estrogen cream for 4-6 weeks, followed by application of an inert cream, such as zinc oxide, for an additional 2 weeks, to keep the healing surfaces apart. Expectant management is also acceptable, as this condition remits in early puberty; however, most caretakers will want their daughters treated.

❐❐ **What is primary dysmenorrhea?**

Primary dysmenorrhea is painful menses that is not attributable to any other cause, such as endometriosis, PID or structural pelvic disorders.

❐❐ **What is the etiology of primary dysmenorrhea?**

Primary dysmenorrhea is caused by endometrial prostaglandins that are secreted after ovulation, causing uterine contractions that can lead to myometrial ischemia and pain; this pain can last up to 48 hours after menses have begun.

❐❐ **What are the treatment options for primary dysmenorrhea?**

First line therapy consists of prostaglandin inhibitors such as NSAIDS (aspirin, ibuprofen, naproxen sodium-the latter two are more potent prostaglandin inhibitors). For the sexually active teen, oral contraceptives, which will inhibit ovulation, are another alternative, especially if NSAIDS fail to work.

❐❐ **What is the pathophysiology behind dysfunctional uterine bleeding (DUB)?**

DUB is due to anovulatory bleeding, caused by estrogen that is unopposed by progesterone. This causes the endometrium to undergo sporadic growth and sloughing without cyclic coordination. The amount of estrogen secreted by the ovaries varies and bleeding can occur because of a fall in estrogen (withdrawal bleeding) or when the endometrium outgrows its blood supply (breakthrough bleeding).

❐❐ **What is the most common cause of vaginitis in symptomatic, prepubertal girls?**

N. gonorrhoeae, followed less commonly by Shigella, Group A beta-hemolytic streptococcus, *c. trachomatis* and *trichomonas vaginalis*.

❐❐ **What is the most common cause of vaginitis in girls who are pubertal but not sexually active?**

C. albicans.

❐❐ **What is the most prevalent sexually transmitted disease among adolescent females?**

Human papilloma virus.

❐❐ **A teenage girl presents with milky, non-bloody discharge from her nipples. She is not pregnant. What is the diagnosis and etiology of the discharge?**

This patient has galactorrhea, which is most often caused by a pituitary adenoma that secretes prolactin. Galactorrhea can also be caused by certain drugs, such as phenothiazines, antihistamines, diazepam, cimetidine, metoclopramide, opiates (codeine, morphine), antihypertensive agents (verapamil) and tricyclic antidepressants. If amenorrhea is also present, thyroid disease should be suspected.

□□   **What are some of the clinical features of polycystic ovary syndrome (Stein-Leventhal syndrome)?**

Hirsutism, obesity, amenorrhea or infertility, and ovarian enlargement are some of the principal features; acanthosis nigricans and insulin resistance are seen in a small percentage of patients. However, many patients may not have all of these features.

□□   **What are the typical symptoms of "mittelschmerz" (ovulatory pain)?**

1) Sudden onset of right or left lower quadrant pain that occurs 2 weeks after the last menses (midcycle).
2) No evidence of intrauterine pregnancy.
3) A pelvic examination that reveals unilateral adnexal tenderness with no mass, no cervical motion tenderness, and no vaginal bleeding.
4) Pain that lasts only 24-36 hours.

PREVENTIVE PEARLS

"There are 3 types of untruths: Lies, Damned Lies, and Statistics."
- Disraeli

□□   **What infant immunization is most likely to cause a reaction in infants receiving standard immunizations?**

The pertussis component of the DTP. Minor reactions (local induration and pain, mild fever) occur in 75% of children who receive the vaccine. This is the most common reaction though reactions can be as severe as shock, encephalopathy and convulsions.

□□   **Differentiate between the Sabin and Salk vaccinations.**

Both prevent polio; the Sabin (OPV) is a live, attenuated trivalent poliovirus. The Salk (IPV) is an inactivated trivalent vaccine.

□□   **When is it appropriate to screen the population for a disease?**

When the disease is prevalent, when failure to catch the disease results in significant morbidity, when appropriate screening tests exist, or when therapy initiated due to the early detection will significantly alter the pattern of the disease.

□□   **Matching:**

1) Sensitive.
2) Specific.
3) Positive predictive value.
4) Negative predictive value.

a) Actual positives/total number of positive test results.
b) Actual positives/total number with the disease.
c) Actual negatives/total number without the disease.
d) Actual negatives/total number of negative test results.

Answers: (1) b, (2) c, (3) a, and (4) d.
Sensitivity = a/(a + c); Specificity = d/(b + d); Positive predictive value = a/(a + b); Negative predictive value = d/(c + d).

□□   **Give the equation for prevalence of a disease.**

Prevalence is the incidence of a disease multiplied by the duration of the disease.

□□   **Define crude death rate.**

Crude death rate = (deaths in 1 year/population in same year) x 1,000.

□□   **Define infant mortality rate.**

Infant mortality rate = (infant deaths in 1 year/live births in same year) x 1,000 (Infants = $\leq$1 year.).

□□   **Define fetal mortality rate.**

Fetal mortality rate = (stillbirths in 1 year/live births in same year) x 1,000.

□□   **Define neonatal death rate.**

Neonatal death rate = (the number of newborn deaths in 1 year/live births in same year) x 1,000. (Newborn = infant < 1 month).

❑❑   **Match the prevention with the example that fits.**

1) Primary prevention
2) Secondary prevention
3) Tertiary prevention

a) Tetanus booster shots every 10 years
b) Controlling blood sugar with appropriate diet and insulin
c) Identifying and treating a patient with asymptomatic diabetes mellitus.

Answers: (1) a, (2) c, and (3) b.

Primary prevention prevents a disease from ever occurring.
Secondary prevention prevents future problems if actions are taken during an asymptomatic period.
Tertiary prevention prevents further complications in a disease that is already present.

❑❑   **In the 1990s, what percentage of US households have 2 parents?**

25%.

❑❑   **What percentage of untreated group A *β-hemolytic streptococcal* infections will progress to rheumatic fever?**

3%. Increased incidence of the disease is noted in lower socioeconomic areas.

❑❑   **In what age group is post streptococcal glomerulonephritis <u>most</u> <u>common</u>?**

Peak incidence is between ages 3 and 7.

❑❑   **When should you first check a child's blood lead level?**

At 1–2 years. By this age, children are mobile and can easily find tasty paint chips and other lead based objects.

❑❑   **What is used to control outbreaks of meningococcal meningitis?**

Rifampin and ceftriaxone are used as chemoprophylaxis for contacts. A vaccine for groups A, C, Y, and W-135 is available and widely used even though most outbreaks are caused by strains A, B, C, and W-135.

❑❑   **Geographically, where is multiple sclerosis most prevalent?**

In the northern U.S. Migration to warmer climates does not seem to affect the disease. People born in the north will still have a higher incidence of the disease.

❑❑   **What percentage of obesity can be attributed to genetic causes?**

25–30%.

❑❑   **What percentage of obesity can be attributed to organic causes?**

1%.

❑❑   **Immunocompromised patients can safely be given which vaccines?**

Killed or inactivated vaccines are safe for immunocompromised patients. The vaccines listed below all fit that criteria.

1) Diphtheria
2) *H. Influenzae*
3) Influenza
4) Pneumococcal
5) Enhanced inactivated polio
6) Hepatitis
7) Pertussis
8) Tetanus

❑❑   **Which vaccines should immunocompromised patients avoid?**

Oral polio and MMR.

❑❑ **Aside from those who are immunocompromised, which patients should not receive live vaccines?**

Pregnant women should not receive live viruses, especially MMR (due to the tetragonic potential). Oral polio should be avoided in anyone in close contact with an immunocompromised person because of the virus's ability to spread.

❑❑ **Can you administer vaccinations to a patient who has a URI and a fever of 37.5°C?**

Yes. URI or gastrointestinal illness are not contraindications to vaccination. Fever may be as high as 38°C and the vaccine still administered. Likewise, use of antibiotics or recent exposure to illness is not a reason to delay vaccination.

❑❑ **How many millimeters indicate a positive reaction to the Mantoux skin test in a person with HIV?**

≥ 5 mm. In individuals with risk factors for TB, induration must be ≥ 10 mm. For those with no risk factors, induration must be ≥ 15 mm to be positive.

❑❑ **Influenza epidemics and pandemics are generally associated with which strain of influenza?**

Influenza A.

❑❑ **When should the influenza vaccine be given?**

In September or October, about 1–2 months before flu season begins. The vaccine, unlike amantadine, is protective against influenza A and B.

❑❑ **What is a contraindication to the administration of the influenza vaccine?**

A history of anaphylactic hypersensitivity to eggs or their products.

❑❑ **What is the number one cause of death for African-American males between the ages of 10 and 24?**

Firearm injury. The overall homicide rate for young men in the US is over 7 times that of the next developed country. For Hispanic males, the rate is 10 times higher; for African-American males, the rate is over 30 times higher than in comparable countries.

❑❑ **Do intentional or unintentional causes account for more firearm-related deaths?**

Intentional, which account for 94% (with subcategories of suicide = 48%, and homicide = 46%). Unintentional firearm injuries account for about 5%. Only 1% of firearm deaths occur as a result of legal intervention. The number of firearm-related fatalities has more than doubled over the last 30 years.

❑❑ **What are some risk factors for homicide?**

Most homicide victims are killed by someone they know, someone of the same race, and usually during an argument or fight. Drugs and alcohol are important co-factors, as is the presence of a handgun.

❑❑ **What are the relative risks for suicide and homicide if a gun is kept in the home?**

If there is a gun in the home, a suicide is 5 times more likely to occur (9 times more likely if a loaded handgun is available). A homicide is 3 times more likely to occur, and the victim is 43% more likely to be a member of the family than an intruder. In the case of domestic violence, a gun at home increases the risk of homicide 20 fold.

❑❑ **What is the clinical significance of the increased availability of semi-automatic weapons?**

Between 1982 and 1992, the percentage of gunshot victims with multiple gunshot wounds increased from 5% to 20%. The rate of spinal cord injuries from GSWs quadrupled. This trend has resulted in an increased number of major organ injuries, complications, and surgeries, as well as in a greater severity of injury and a higher probability of death.

☐☐   **In addition to the history, physical, laboratory tests, and collection of physical evidence, what else needs to be done in a case of sexual abuse of a child?**

File a report with child protective services and law enforcement agencies. Provide emotional support to the child and family. Give a return appointment for follow-up of STD cultures and testing for pregnancy, HIV, or syphilis, as indicated. Assure follow-up for psychological counseling by connecting the child/family to the appropriate services in your area.

☐☐   **What is the minimum recommended age for administration of measles, mumps and rubella (MMR) vaccine in the United States?**

12 months.

☐☐   **There are two types of polio vaccine licensed for administration in the United States: oral and intramuscular. Which one carries a risk of vaccine-induced poliomyelitis?**

Oral polio vaccine, which is a live attenuated vaccine. The intramuscular vaccine is inactivated.

☐☐   **What illnesses are more likely to occur among children exposed to second-hand tobacco smoke, compared to children not exposed?**

Asthma, pneumonia, bronchitis, otitis media, pharyngitis, and possibly meningitis.

☐☐   **How many months must elapse between the third and fourth DPT immunizations in the recommended childhood immunization schedule?**

6 months.

☐☐   **Children should ride in approved car seats until they are at least how many pounds?**

40 pounds.

☐☐   **Consider two vaccines, one inactivated and one live attenuated. Which vaccine is more likely to cause fever and rash within 10 days after administration?**

The live attenuated vaccine. Most side effects of inactivated vaccines tend to occur 1-3 days after administration.

☐☐   **To reduce the risk of neural tube defects in their offspring, prospective mothers should assure adequate periconceptional intake of what substance?**

Folic acid.

☐☐   **You are seeing a child with recurrent episodes of otitis media and cough. What environmental exposure history should you elicit?**

Exposure to cigarette smoke in the household.

☐☐   **What is the drug of choice for prophylaxis of most household contacts of a child with meningococcal meningitis?**

Rifampin.

☐☐   **An asymptomatic one year-old child presents for her first health care maintenance visit since she was 2 months old. She has been living in a deteriorated apartment building in a small city in New England. What screening blood test should you order?**

Blood lead level.

❏❏ An 8 year-old boy has recently acquired a pet iguana. This may place the household at increased risk of what disease?

Salmonellosis.

❏❏ A 15 month-old child who has not yet received MMR vaccine recently received immunoglobulin to prevent hepatitis A (postexposure prophylaxis). What is the suggested interval before measles vaccination?

3 months.

❏❏ You receive laboratory confirmation of hepatitis A infection in an 18 month old child who attends day care. What is recommended to prevent further spread of the infection?

Immune globulin .02 ml/kg to all susceptible day care contacts.

❏❏ What is the minimum interval required between oral polio virus doses?

4 weeks, but preferably 6 weeks.

❏❏ How many doses of varicella vaccine are recommended for adolescents 13 years and older?

2 doses at least 4 weeks apart.

❏❏ Name two modifiable risk factors for sudden infant death syndrome (SIDS).

Prone sleeping position, maternal smoking, lack of breastfeeding.

❏❏ Name two health consequences of iron deficiency anemia.

Reduced resistance to infection, fatigue, decreased intellectual performance.

❏❏ Name three health consequences of childhood obesity.

Hypertension, hyperinsulinemia, low self-esteem, increased adult mortality.

❏❏ Perinatal administration of zidovudine (ZDV) to HIV-infected mothers and their newborns has been shown to reduce risk of perinatal HIV transmission by how much?

About two-thirds (from 24% down to about 8%).

❏❏ Bicycle helmets appear to reduce the risk of bicycle-related head injury by about how much?

80%.

❏❏ From 1970 to 1990, have suicide rates among adolescents aged 15-19 in the United States increased, decreased, or stayed the same?

Increased. From 5.9 to 11.1 per 100,000.

❏❏ Give two characteristics of news stories about suicide that might increase suicide contagion.

Simplistic explanations of suicide, describing technical details of suicide, glorifying the person that committed suicide.

❏❏ What proportion of high-school aged adolescents in the United States smoke or use smokeless tobacco?

About 33%.

❏❏ What intervention at a national and state level has significantly reduced cigarette smoking?

The increase of cigarette price.

❑❑   **What are three clinical manifestations of kwashiorkor (severe protein malnutrition)?**

Fatigue, edema, dermatitis, sparse and reddened or greyish hair.

❑❑   **Should MMR vaccine be given intramuscularly, subcutaneously, or intradermally?**

Subcutaneously.

❑❑   **You are seeing a two-month old child whose 5 year-old brother is immunodeficient. Should you administer OPV (oral poliovirus vaccine) to the two-month old?**

No. Administer IPV.

❑❑   **Can MMR vaccine be safely administered to a child who has developed a non-anaphylactic mild red rash after eating eggs?**

Yes.

❑❑   **What approximate proportion of American 16 year-olds are sexually active?**

50%

❑❑   **In the United States, can a minor be treated for a sexually transmitted disease without parental consent?**

Yes.

❑❑   **You have just diagnosed syphilis in a 17 year-old girl. After assuring appropriate patient education and treatment, what should you do next?**

Notify public health department for contact tracing and treatment.

❑❑   **What is the leading cause of death among infants (less than one year of age) in the United States?**

Congenital anomalies.

❑❑   **Injuries accounted for 4% of infant deaths in the United States in 1995. What was the leading cause of injury deaths among these infants?**

Suffocation.

❑❑   **What is the leading cause of death among children aged 1 - 14 years in the United States?**

Motor vehicle traffic injuries.

❑❑   **What is the most important factor for reducing infectious disease transmission in day care centers?**

Hand-washing.

❑❑   **You have diagnosed an E coli O157:H7 infection in an 18 month old child who attends day care. When should you allow the child to return to day care?**

After diarrhea resolves and two stool cultures are negative.

❑❑   **A 4 year-old child who attends day care has impetigo. When should the child be allowed to return to day care?**

24 hours after treatment has been initiated.

❑❑   **A 4 year-old child who attends day care has streptococcal pharyngitis. When should this child be allowed to return to day care?**

24 hours after treatment has been initiated and after the child has been afebrile for 24 hours.

❑❑   **A three-year old girl has varicella. When should she be allowed to return to day care?**

6 days after the onset of the rash or sooner if all lesions have dried and crusted.

❑❑   **A 15 month-old boy has a mild case of hepatitis A. When should he be allowed to return to day care?**

1 week after onset of illness or jaundice.

❑❑   **Should an immunocompetent child with erythema infectiosum (Parvovirus B19 infection) be excluded from day care?**

No. Little or no virus is present in respiratory secretions by the time that the erythema infectiosum rash appears.

❑❑   **Can a PPD skin test for tuberculosis infection be planted the same day that you administer measles vaccine?**

Yes.

❑❑   **If a PPD skin test and measles vaccine are not adminesterd on the same day, how long after measles vaccination should you wait before administering the PPD skin test?**

4 to 6 weeks.

RANDOM PEARLS

"Errors, like straws, upon the surface flow; he who would search for pearls must dive below."
- John Dryden

☐☐   **What condition does boggy blue turbinates and eosinophils indicate?**

Allergic rhinitis.

☐☐   **What are the major distant sequelae of untreated streptococcal infections?**

Acute glomerulonephritis and rheumatic heart disease.

☐☐   **Which antibiotic most commonly produces the diarrhea associated with clostridium difficile?**

Ampicillin. Vancomycin and metronidazole are the antibiotic treatments of choice.

☐☐   **What is the first line of therapy for a migraine headache?**

Ergotamine derivatives. Second line therapies include Sumatriptan (Imitrex), phenothiazine, NSAIDs, and opiates.

☐☐   **What kinds of exercise will most likely trigger an asthma attack in patients with exercise-induced asthma?**

High intensity exercise for more than 5–6 minutes.

☐☐   **Which strain of influenza is most virulent?**

Influenza A.

☐☐   **Which organism is typically responsible for causing bacterial conjunctivitis?**

Staphylococcus. The second most common organism is Streptococcus.

☐☐   **What is the most common cause of portal hypertension in children?**

Extrahepatic portal vein occlusion.

☐☐   **Which virus causes herpangina?**

Coxsackievirus Group A. A sore throat, fever, malaise, and vesicular lesions on the posterior pharynx or the soft palate are often seen with this disease.

☐☐   **A complication of central sleep apnea in a child is:**

Sudden infant death syndrome (SIDS). Affected children develop morning cyanosis. However, children can be treated with theophylline.

☐☐   **What is the most probable age of presentation of malrotation in children? What is a common complication, and what signs and symptoms are usually present?**

1) Malrotation usually occurs in children under 12 months of age. 2) Volvulus is a common complication. The signs and symptoms typically include vomiting, blood streaked stools, and abdominal pain.

☐☐   **Describe the common features of a slipped femoral capital epiphysis.**

Injury usually occurs in adolescence. The rupture typically presents with an insidious development of knee or thigh pain and a painful limp. Frequently hip motion is limited, particularly that of internal rotation. Anteroposterior and frog-leg lateral films of both hips aid evaluation.

❑❑   **What are the two most common causes of fatal anaphylaxis?**

1) Drug reactions (95% of which are due to penicillin). Parenteral administration results in the deaths of approximately 300 people/year.
2) Hymenoptera stings cause fatal anaphylaxis in 100 people/year.

❑❑   **Which type of hypersensitivity reaction is responsible for anaphylaxis?**

Type I (IgE mediated).
Hypersensitivity Reaction Mediator Examples:
Type 1: Immediate IgE binds allergen, includes mast cells and basophils (e.g. food allergy, asthma),
Type 2: Cytotoxic IgG and IgM antibody reactions to antigen on cell surface activates complement and killers Blood transfusion rxn (e.g. ITP, hemolytic anemia),
Type 3: Immune complex (e.g. Arthrus Complexes activate complement Tetanus toxoid in sensitized persons, Post streptococcal glomerulonephritis),
Type 4: Cell mediated (e.g. delayed hypersensitivity, Activated T-lymphocytes, Skin tests).

❑❑   **What four pseudonyms are associated with regional enteritis?**

1) Crohn's disease.
2) Terminal ileitis.
3) Regional enteritis.
4) Granulomatous ileocolitis.

❑❑   **What symptoms are associated with presentation of regional enteritis?**

Fever, abdominal pain, weight loss, and diarrhea. Fistulas, fissures, and abscesses may also be noted. Ulcerative colitis, on the other hand, usually presents with bloody diarrhea.

❑❑   **What is the IM treatment for acute streptococcal pharyngitis?**

1.2 million units of benzathine penicillin G. Use 0.6 million units of benzathine penicillin-G for children weighing less than 27 kg.

❑❑   **Describe the rash that is present with exanthem subitum (roseola).**

The rash is usually found on the trunk and the neck and is maculopapular.

❑❑   **What is the most common cause of death among children between 1–12 month(s) old?**

Sudden infant death syndrome (SIDS).

❑❑   **What is the most common site of Crohn's disease?**

The ileum. Crohn's disease can actually involve any part of the GI tract from the social end to the antisocial end. It is segmental, often involving granuloma formation along with inflammatory reactions. Crohn's disease has two incidence peaks, one in the 15–22 year old age group and a second in the 55–60 year old age group.

❑❑   **What are the signs and symptoms of Crohn's disease?**

Fever, diarrhea, right lower quadrant pain with mass possible, fistulas, rectal prolapse, perianal fissures, and abscesses. Arthritis, uveitis, and liver disease are also associated with this condition.

❑❑   **What systemic diseases are associated with Crohn's disease?**

Pyoderma gangrenosum, uveitis, episclerosis, scleritis, arthritis, erythema nodosum, and nephrolithiasis.

❏❏   **What contrast x-ray findings are associated with Crohn's disease?**

The segmental involvement in the colon with an abnormal mucosal pattern and fistulas, often without involvement of the rectum. A narrowing of the small intestine may also be displayed.

❏❏   **What are the principal signs and symptoms of ulcerative colitis?**

Fever, weight loss, tachycardia, panniculitis, and six bloody bowel movements per day.

❏❏   **Does toxic megacolon commonly occur with ulcerative colitis or with Crohn's disease?**

Toxic megacolon is a very common, serious complication of ulcerative colitis.

❏❏   **Does cancer more often develop with ulcerative colitis or with Crohn's disease?**

Ulcerative colitis. Think of toxic megacolon and cancer. Avoid Antidiarrheal agents.

❏❏   **What are the two most common causes of acute diarrhea?**

Rotavirus and Norwalk agent.

❏❏   **What is the most common cause of diarrhea in a child less than one year old?**

Rotavirus.

❏❏   **Which cause of diarrhea is most commonly associated with seizures?**

Shigella.

❏❏   **What induces rose spots and watery diarrhea, as well as high fever and relative bradycardia?**

Salmonella. This condition is particularly common in IV drug abusers with new pet turtles!

❏❏   **What is the treatment for individuals infected with Salmonella?**

Supportive care without antibiotics. However, if a severe fever is exhibited, antibiotic therapy may be warranted.

❏❏   **What is the most common food–borne pathogen?**

Staphylococcus. This pathogen produces diarrhea and vomiting within 6–12 hours after ingestion.

❏❏   **Which type of infectious gastroenteritis is associated with the consumption of seafood?**

Vibrio parahaemolyticus.

❏❏   **Which type of diarrhea is profuse and bloody but does not involve vomiting?**

Entamoeba histolytica. Diarrhea that is not necessarily bloody and that is associated with contaminated meat may be due to Clostridium perfringens.

❏❏   **What is the most common parasitic cause of diarrhea in the U.S.?**

Giardia. Infected individuals presents with foul-smelling, floating stools; abdominal pain; and profuse diarrhea. The parasite may be identified with a positive string test or duodenal aspiration for trophozoites.

❏❏   **What types of defects cause left to right shunt murmurs?**

ASD, VSD, and PDA.

❏❏   **What type of defect produces diminished pulses in the lower extremities of a pediatric patient?**

Coarctation of the aorta.

❏❏   **Which fairly common conditions produce cardiac syncope in pediatrics?**

Aortic stenosis, which is not cyanotic, and tetralogy of Fallot, which is.

❏❏   **What are two unique clinical findings of tetralogy of Fallot (TOF)?**

A boot shaped heart on a chest x-ray and exercise intolerance which is relieved by squatting.

❏❏   **What are the signs and symptoms of aortic stenosis in a child?**

Exercise intolerance, chest pain, and a systolic ejection click with a crescendo, decrescendo murmur radiating to the neck with a suprasternal thrill. No cyanosis!

❏❏   **What are the signs of left-sided heart failure in an infant?**

Increased respiratory rate, shortness of breath, and sweating during feeding.

❏❏   **What is the single most common cause of CHF in the second week of life?**

Coarctation of the aorta.

❏❏   **What is the most common cause of impetigo?**

Group A ß-hemolytic streptococcus.

❏❏   **What is the most common cause of bullous impetigo?**

Staphylococcus aureus.

❏❏   **What is the most common cause of orbital infections?**

Staphylococcus aureus. Periorbital infections are usually caused by H. influenzae.

❏❏   **What is the most common cause of pediatric bacteremia?**

Streptococcus pneumonia.

❏❏   **What is the most common cause of viral pneumonia in the pediatric patient?**

RSV.

❏❏   **What is the most common type of asthma in children?**

Extrinsic asthma which is a type I. An immediate hypersensitivity reaction mediated by IgE is induced by this condition. Common causes include molds and pet dander.

❏❏   **How do steroids function in the treatment of asthma?**

Steroids increase cAMP, decrease inflammation, and aid in restoring the function of ß-adrenergic responsiveness to adrenergic drugs.

❏❏   **Which two viral illnesses are prodromes for Reye syndrome?**

Varicella (chicken pox) and influenzae B.

❏❏   **What are the signs and symptoms of Reye syndrome.**

Irritability, combativeness, and lethargy, right upper quadrant tenderness, history of influenzae B or recent chicken pox, papilledema, hypoglycemia, and seizures. Lab results reveal hypoglycemia, an ammonia level greater than 20 times normal, and a bilirubin level that is normal.

❏❏   **Describe the five stages of Reye syndrome.**

Stage I: Vomiting, lethargy, and liver dysfunction.
Stage II: Disorientation, combativeness, delirium, hyperventilation, increased deep tendon reflexes, liver dysfunction, hyperexcitable, tachypnea, fever, tachycardia, sweating, and pupillary dilatation.

Stage III: Coma, decorticate rigidity, increased respiratory rate, and a mortality rate of 50%.
Stage IV: Coma, decerebrate posturing, no ocular reflexes, loss of corneal reflexes, and liver damage.
Stage V: Loss of deep tendon reflexes, seizures, flaccidity, respiratory arrest, and 95% mortality.

❏❏   **In the pediatric esophagus, where is a foreign body most commonly lodged?**

The cricopharyngeal narrowing.

❏❏   **Do household pets transmit Yersinia?**

Yes, especially puppies.

❏❏   **What is the most common cause of an urinary tract infection in a female child?**

E. coli.

❏❏   **What is the most common cause of intrinsic renal failure?**

Acute tubular necrosis.

❏❏   **A baby boy is brought to the emergency department with vomiting and persistent crying for two hours. On exam, a testicle is tender and enlarged. What is the most common cause?**

A testicular torsion.

❏❏   **A child presents with bluish discoloration of the gingiva. What diagnosis should you suspect?**

Chronic lead poisoning. Expect the erythrocyte protoporphyrin level to be elevated with this condition.

❏❏   **What disorder is most likely to be confused with erythema nodosum?**

Cellulitis.

❏❏   **What is erythema nodosum?**

An inflammatory disease of the skin and subcutaneous tissue which is characterized by tender red nodules. The nodules are usually found in the pretibial area. This condition typically affects young adults; primary causes are streptococcal infections and sarcoidosis. The most common cause in children is UTI, especially with Streptococci. Other causes include leprosy, TB, psittacosis, ulcerative colitis, and drug reaction.

❏❏   **What is the most common dysrhythmia in a child?**

Paroxysmal atrial tachycardia.

❏❏   **What is the classic EKG for Wolff-Parkinson-White syndrome?**

A change in the upstroke of QRS, the delta wave.

❏❏   **Which agent is usually responsible for the onset of endemic encephalitis?**

Arbovirus.

❏❏   **How many days after a measles vaccine could a fever and a rash be expected to develop?**

7–10 days.

❏❏   **What is the most common complication of acute otitis media?**

Tympanic membrane perforation. Other complications include mastoiditis, cholesteatoma, and intracranial infections.

❏❏   **Describe the symptoms and signs of myasthenia gravis.**

Weakness and fatigability with ptosis, diplopia, and blurred vision are the initial symptoms in 40–70% of the patients. Bulbar muscle weakness is also prevalent with dysarthria and dysphagia.

❑❑   **Describe the signs and symptoms of Guillain-Barré disease.**

Guillain-Barré disease classically presents with symmetrical weakness in the legs, which ascends to include the arms or trunk. Distal weakness is usually greater than proximal. The onset of the disease rarely involves the cranial nerves.

❑❑   **What is that little bone seen behind the tympanic membrane?**

The malleus.

❑❑   **What disease should be suspected in a patient with a 2 week history of lower limb weakness?**

Guillain-Barré usually causes an ascending weakness which begins in the lower extremities. Conversely, the weakness is descending with botulism poisoning. Cranial nerves are typically affected first with myasthenia gravis.

❑❑   **Deep tendon reflexes are usually maintained in which of the following diseases: Myasthenia gravis, Guillain-Barré, or Eaton-Lambert syndrome?**

Myasthenia gravis. Reflexes are usually depressed in Eaton-Lambert syndrome and absent in Guillain-Barré.

❑❑   **Describe a typical patient with intussusception.**

Intussusception usually occurs in children between the ages of 3 months to 2 years. The majority are 5-10 months old and it is more common in boys. The area of the ileocecal valve is typically the source of the problem.

❑❑   **What is the current therapeutic regimen for treatment of meningitis in a neonate?**

Initially, ampicillin and aminoglycoside were favored for treating the neonate with meningitis. However, today recommendations include ampicillin and cefotaxime. A combination of these two antibiotics should be used infants up to 2 months of age to cover coliform, Group B Streptococci, Listeria, and Enterococcus. In children older than 2 months and up to 6 years, cefotaxime alone is indicated.

❑❑   **Which type of streptococci causes acute post streptococcal glomerulonephritis?**

Group A ß-hemolytic Streptococci.

❑❑   **What signs and symptoms are prevalent with post streptococcal glomerulonephritis?**

A physical exam may reveal facial edema and decreased urinary output, these are the most common findings. Urine may also be dark. Other laboratory results include normochromic anemia due to hemodilution, increased sedimentation rate, numerous RBC's and WBC's in the urine with casts, and hyperkalemia. Hospitalization is advised.

❑❑   **Name the 5 major modified Jones criteria.**

1) Erythema Marginatum.
2) Polyarthritis.
3) Subcutaneous Nodules.
4) Carditis.
5) Chorea.
Remember: Dr. Jones, the EM Physician, is SNoring, she Can't Come.
Other criteria include rheumatic fever or rheumatic heart disease, arthralgias, fever, prolonged PR interval on an EKG, C reactive protein, elevated sedimentation rate, or antistreptolysin O titer.

□□   **What disorder is present when the modified Jones criteria are met?**

Rheumatic fever.

□□   **Describe the symptoms and signs of varicella (chicken pox).**

The onset of varicella rash is 1–2 days after prodromal symptoms of slight malaise, anorexia, and fever. The rash begins on the trunk and scalp, appearing as faint macules and later becoming vesicles.

□□   **Describe the signs of roseola infantum.**

Roseola infantum usually affects children ages 6 months to 3 years. It is characterized by a high fever that begins abruptly and lasts 3–5 days, possibly precipitating febrile seizures. A rash appears as the temperature drops to normal.

□□   **How is the normal systolic blood pressure (SBP) for pediatric patients (toddlers and up) calculated?**

Average SBP (mm Hg) = (patient's Age x 2) + 90.
Low normal limit SBP (mm Hg) = (patient's Age x 2) + 70.
SBP for a term newborn is about 60 mm Hg.

□□   **How does a child present with erythema infectiosum (fifth disease or slapcheek syndrome)?**

Fifth disease typically does not infect infants or adults. There are no prodromal symptoms. The illness usually begins with the sudden appearance of erythema of the cheeks, followed by a maculopapular rash on the trunk and extremities that evolve into a lacy pattern.

□□   **What is the initial antibiotic treatment for a child with epiglottitis?**

The most likely cause of this condition is H. influenzae. Therefore, the child should be treated with a second or third generation cephalosporin. (Ed.Note.- Since the widespread use of the HiB vaccine, the epidemiology, causative organism, and treatment will change. As of the writing of this text, this is still the correct answer, but this will soon change)

□□   **What organism commonly causes a septic joint in a child?**

Staphylococcus aureus.

□□   **What organism commonly causes a septic joint in an adolescent?**

Neisseria gonorrhoeae.

□□   **What organism most commonly causes bacterial pneumonia, except for in the first week of life?**

Streptococcus pneumoniae.

□□   **What is the most common cause of abdominal pain in children?**

Constipation.

□□   **What is the most common cause of an intestinal obstruction in children under 2 years of age?**

Intussusception.

□□   **What is the effect on serum sodium as glucose increases by 100?**

Serum sodium decreases by 1.7 mEq/l.

□□   **Describe the key features of the Rocky Mountain Spotted Fever (RMSF) rash.**

RMSF is caused by Rickettsia rickettsii and is transmitted by Ixodidae ticks. Patients become sick with a high fever, headache, chills, and muscular pain. Around the fourth day of fever a rash begins on the wrists and ankles and spreads centripetally.

☐☐ **Describe the scarlet fever rash.**

The rash has a sandpaper type texture and begins on the face, neck, chest, and abdomen. It then spreads to extremities. Patients may also have strawberry tongue.

☐☐ **Syncope is a characteristic symptom of what valvular disease?**

Aortic stenosis.

☐☐ **Describe a patient with Chlamydial pneumonia.**

Chlamydial pneumonia is usually seen in children 2–6 weeks of age. The patient is afebrile and does not appear toxic.

☐☐ **A patient has had 3 days of diarrhea which was abrupt in onset. The patient reports slimy green, malodorous stools that contain blood. In addition, the patient is febrile. What is the most likely cause?**

Salmonella.

☐☐ **What is the drug treatment for Campylobacter?**

Erythromycin or tetracycline.

☐☐ **In a child, does coarctation of the aorta typically cause cyanosis?**

No.

☐☐ **What is the drug treatment for persistent E. coli?**

Trimethoprim with sulfamethoxazole (TMP/SMX).

☐☐ **What is the drug treatment for Giardia lamblia?**

Quinacrine or metronidazole or furazolidone.

☐☐ **What is the drug treatment for Salmonella?**

Ampicillin, TMP/SMX, Chloramphenicol.

☐☐ **What is the drug treatment for Yersinia?**

TMP/SMX, tetracycline, third generation cephalosporin.

☐☐ **What are the 8 common clinical presentations of pediatric heart disease?**

1) Cyanosis.
2) Pathologic murmur.
3) Abnormal pulses.
4) CHF.
5) HTN.
6) Cardiogenic shock.
7) Syncope.
8) Tachyarrhythmias.

☐☐ **What is Addison's disease?**

Deficiency or absence of mineralocorticoid (aldosterone). This results in increased sodium excretion. Potassium is retained. The urine cannot concentrate, which can lead to severe dehydration, hypotension, and circulatory collapse. Deficiency of cortisol (also produced in the adrenal cortex) leads to metabolic disturbances, weakness, hypoglycemia, and deceased resistance to infection.

❏❏   **What are some signs and symptoms of Thrombotic Thrombocytopenic Purpura (TTP)?**

Thrombocytopenia, purpura, and microangiopathic hemolytic anemia. Patient with TTP presents with fever, fluctuating neurologic signs, and renal complications. If the disease goes untreated, it is almost uniformly fatal. Therapy includes steroids, splenectomy, plasmapheresis and exchange, and antiplatelet agents, such as dipyridamole and aspirin.

❏❏   **How low does the platelet count drop before spontaneous bleeding occurs?**

Below 50,000/mm3 spontaneous bleeding may occur. CNS bleeds usually do not occur until counts drop below 10,000/mm3.

❏❏   **What are the 5 key lab findings in DIC?**

1) Increased PT.
2) Increased PTT.
3) Increased fibrin degradation products.
4) Decreased fibrinogen.
5) Decreased platelet levels.

❏❏   **What are the classic findings of shaken baby syndrome?**

1) Failure to thrive.
2) Lethargy.
3). Seizures.
4) Retinal hemorrhages.
5) CT may show subarachnoid hemorrhage or subdural hematoma from torn bridging veins.

❏❏   **T/F: High fever in neonates with bacterial pneumonia usually follows a period of general fussiness and decreased feeding.**

True.

❏❏   **Chlamydia pneumonia is more likely to occur in the neonate after how many weeks of age?**

Three weeks.

❏❏   **Conjunctivitis is an associated finding in about what percentage of neonates with chlamydia pneumonia?**

About 50%.

❏❏   **Neonates with chlamydia pneumonia are usually tachypneic with a bad cough; are they febrile?**

Usually not.

❏❏   **Newborns should stop losing weight how many days after birth?**

About 6 days.

❏❏   **T/F: A neonate's stool color can be an important sign.**

False. Unless blood is evident, stool color is insignificant.

❏❏   **What is the difference between vomiting and regurgitation?**

Very little once it's on you! Vomiting is caused by forceful diaphragmatic and abdominal muscle contraction. Regurgitation occurs without effort.

□□ **Is regurgitation dangerous in an otherwise thriving neonate?**

No. However, it can be dangerous for newborns with failure to thrive or respiratory problems, and it may be associated with chronic aspiration.

□□ **Projectile vomiting in the neonate is often associated with pyloric stenosis. When this is the case, such vomiting becomes a prominent sign at what age?**

2–3 weeks.

□□ **What is the name for diarrhea associated with sepsis, otitis media, UTI or any other systemic disease?**

Parenteral diarrhea.

□□ **T/F: Bacterial and parasitic etiologies of diarrhea in the neonate are rare.**

True.

□□ **What are some entities in the differential diagnosis of bloody diarrhea in the neonate?**

Necrotizing enterocolitis, bacterial enteritis, allergic reactions to milk, and iatrogenic causes secondary to antibiotics.

□□ **Neonates with necrotizing enterocolitis are sick. What are some of the signs of sepsis to look for?**

Poor feeding, lethargy, fever, jaundice, abdominal distention, and poor color.

□□ **What should be considered in the case of a neonate who has never passed stool?**

Meconium ileus or plug, Hirschsprung's disease, intestinal stenosis, or atresia.

□□ **Anal stenosis, hypothyroidism, and Hirschsprung's disease can all present with what clinical sign?**

Constipation that was not present at birth but which began before the infant was 1 month old.

□□ **Describe the signs and symptoms of a slipped capital femoral epiphysis. What x-ray tests are necessary for its diagnosis?**

Gradual onset of hip pain and stiffness with restriction of internal rotation. Patient may walk with a limp. X-ray analysis should include both the anterior-posterior and lateral views of both hips. The slip of the epiphyseal plate posteriorly is best seen on the lateral view.

□□ **Describe a patient with intussusception.**

Patients are most likely very young. 70% of patients have intussusception within the first year of life. In children, the cause is thought to be secondary to lymphoid tissue at the ileocecal valve; in adults, it is thought to be caused by local lesions, Meckel's diverticulum, or tumor. On exam, bowel sounds are usually normal. Intussusception typically involves the terminal ileum. Meckel's diverticulum is the single most common intrinsic bowel lesion involved.

□□ **Should salmonella be treated?**

Only if symptomatic infection persists. Treat with ampicillin, TMP/SMX, or Chloramphenicol.

□□ **What is the most common cause of acute food-borne disease?**

Staphylococcus aureus and the enterotoxins it produces.

□□ **What are the common features of Vibrio parahaemolyticus?**

This condition is caused by organisms associated with oysters, clams, and crabs. Symptoms include cramps, vomiting, dysentery, and explosive diarrhea. Severe infections are treated with tetracycline and Chloramphenicol.

❏❏ **A patient presents with a symmetric weakness that has progressed over several days and associated paresthesia. Diminished reflexes are noted. What is the diagnosis?**

Guillain-Barré syndrome. Other signs and symptoms are diminished reflexes, minimal loss of sensation, paresthesias, and leg weakness.

❏❏ **How is Guillain-Barré syndrome diagnosed in the office?**

Suspect the diagnosis based on signs and symptoms, but confirmation requires nerve conduction studies performed as an inpatient.

❏❏ **What is the most common cause of food-borne viral gastroenteritis?**

Norwalk virus commonly found in shell fish.

❏❏ **What are some common entities in the differential diagnosis of a limp or gait abnormality in a child?**

Legg-Calvé-Perthes disease (avascular necrosis of the femoral head), Osgood-Schlatter disease, avulsion of the tibial tubercle, infection, toxic transient tenosynovitis, patellofemoral subluxation, chondromalacia patella, slipped capital femoral epiphysis, septic arthritis, metatarsal fracture, proximal stress fracture, and toddler fracture (spiral tibia fracture).

❏❏ **What is the usual cause of facial cellulitis in children less than 3 years of age?**

H. influenzae.

❏❏ **What is the most common site of aseptic necrosis?**

The hip.

❏❏ **A child presents with a history of fever, conjunctival hyperemia, and erythema of the mucus membranes with desquamation. What is the diagnosis?**

Kawasaki's Disease. Remember, Kawasaki's disease may have lesions resembling erythema multiforme.

❏❏ **What findings mark the presentation of a patient with rapidly progressive glomerulonephritis?**

Hematuria (most common), edema (periorbital), HTN, ascites, pleural effusion, rales, and anuria.

❏❏ **When can one auscultate the fetal heart?**

Ultrasound: 6 weeks.
Doppler: 10–12 weeks.
Stethoscope: 18–20 weeks.

❏❏ **Describe a Brudzinski sign.**

Flexion of the neck produces flexion of the knees.

❏❏ **Describe Kernig's sign.**

Extension of the knees from the flexed thigh position results in strong passive resistance.

❏❏ **What hypersensitivity skin rashes are noted with phenytoin use?**

Lupus-like and Stevens-Johnson syndrome.

❏❏ **What are the potential, often rare, complications of Mycoplasma pneumonia?**

Non-pulmonary: Hemolytic anemia, aseptic meningitis, encephalitis, Guillain-Barré syndrome, pericarditis, and myocarditis.
Pulmonary: ARDS, atelectasis, mediastinal adenopathy, pneumothorax, pleural effusion, and abscess.

☐☐ **What is normal systolic blood pressure in a newborn?**

60 mmHg.

☐☐ **After the first month of life, what is the number # 1 cause of meningitis and the # 1 cause of pneumonia in children?**

Meningitis: H. influenzae.
Pneumonia: Streptococcus pneumoniae. H. influenzae is the second most common cause.

☐☐ **Discuss infantile spasms.**

Onset is by 3–9 months of age. It typically lasts seconds, and may occur in single episodes or bursts. The EEG is often abnormal. 85% of these patients will be mentally handicapped.

☐☐ **Erythema multiforme can be associated with which anticonvulsants?**

Phenobarbital, phenytoin, and carbamazepine.

☐☐ **Hepatic failure is commonly associated with what anticonvulsant?**

Valproic acid.

☐☐ **Name four enterotoxin-producing organisms that can cause food poisoning.**

Clostridium, staphylococcus aureus, vibrio cholerae, and E. coli.

☐☐ **Antibiotics should be avoided with what infectious diarrhea?**

Salmonella. Exceptions include severe cases of diarrhea in the very young, the immunocompromised, or those with enteric fever (where the infecting strain is S. typhi or is otherwise in the bloodstream).

☐☐ **Name 3 disorders associated with decreased DTRs.**

Guillain-Barré, tic paralysis due to Dermacentor andersoni (Wood Tick) bite, and diphtheria exotoxin.

☐☐ **What is the most likely cause of CHF in a premature infant?**
PDA.

☐☐ **What is the most likely cause of CHF in the first 3 days of life?**

Transposition of the great vessels which leads to cyanosis and failure.

☐☐ **What is the most likely cause of CHF in the first week of life?**

Hypoplastic left ventricle.

☐☐ **What is the most likely cause of CHF in the second week of life?**

Coarctation of the aorta.

☐☐ **Do you treat Shigella with antibiotics?**

In general, yes.

☐☐ **What kind of tick transmits Rocky Mountain Spotted Fever (RMSF)?**

The female andersoni tick. It transmits Rickettsia rickettsii.

☐☐ **What is the most common symptom in RMSF?**

Headache occurs in 90% of patients.

□□   **Describe the rash of RMSF.**

It is a macular rash, 2–6 mm in diameter, located on the wrists and palms and spreading to the soles and trunk.

□□   **What tick transmits Lyme disease?**

The Ixodes dammini tick.
Spirochete Borrelia burgdorferi is diagnosed by culture on Kelly's medium.

□□   **Describe the skin lesion seen in Lyme disease.**

A large distinct circular skin lesion called erythema chronicum migrans. It is an annular erythematous lesion with central clearing.

□□   **What is the causative organism of otitis externa?**

Pseudomonas.

□□   **What is the most common congenital valvular disease?**

Bicuspid aortic valve.

□□   **What makes the first heart sound?**

Closure of the mitral valve and left ventricular contraction.

□□   **The second heart sound?**

Closure of the pulmonary and aortic valves.

□□   **The third heart sound?**

This is caused by the deceleration of blood flowing into the ventricle when the ventricle reaches its final stages of filling.

□□   **The fourth heart sound?**

Vibrations of the left ventricular muscle, the mitral valve, and the left ventricular flow tract cause this.

□□   **What is a common pathological cause of an S3?**

Congestive heart failure.

□□   **What are the pathological causes of an S4?**

Decreased left ventricular compliance due to acute ischemia is the most common cause. Others include aortic stenosis, subaortic stenosis, HTN, coronary artery disease, myocardiopathy, anemia, and hyperthyroidism.

□□   **Time for a food question! There are 9 questions in this book that deal with either strawberry tongue, strawberry cervix, currant jelly sputum, or currant jelly stool. Describe the pathology associated with each of these.**

Strawberry tongue: Scarlet fever and Kawasaki's disease.
Strawberry cervix: Trichomonas.
Currant jelly sputum: Klebsiella and (less commonly) type 3 Pneumococcus.
Currant jelly stool: Intussusception.

APPENDIX A

Recommended Childhood Immunization Schedule United States, January - December 1999

Vaccines[1] are listed under routinely recommended age. | Bars | indicate range of recommended ages for immunization. Any dose not given at the recommended age should be given as a "catch-up" immunization at any subsequent visit when indicated and feasible. (Ovals) indicate vaccines to be given if previously recommended doses were missed or given earlier than the recommended minimum age.

Age ▶ Vaccine ▼	Birth	1 mo	2 mos	4 mos	6 mos	12 mos	15 mos	18 mos	4-6 yrs	11-12 yrs	14-16 yrs
Hepatitis B[2]	Hep B	Hep B									
			Hep B		Hep B					(Hep B)	
Diphtheria, Tetanus, Pertussis[3]			DTaP	DTaP	DTaP		DTaP[3]		DTaP	Td	
H. influenzae type b[4]			Hib	Hib	Hib	Hib					
Polio[5]			IPV	IPV	Polio[5]				Polio		
Rotavirus[6]			Rv[6]	Rv[6]	Rv[6]						
Measles, Mumps, Rubella[7]						MMR			MMR[7]	(MMR[7])	
Varicella[8]						Var				(Var[8])	

Approved by the Advisory Committee on Immunization Practices (ACIP), the American Academy of Pediatrics (AAP), and the American Academy of Family Physicians (AAFP)

1. This schedule indicates the recommended ages for routine administration of currently licensed childhood vaccines. Combination vaccines may be used whenever any components of the combination are indicated and its other components are not contraindicated. Providers should consult the manufacturers' package inserts for detailed recommendations.

2. ***Infants born to HBsAg-negative mothers*** should receive the 2nd dose of hepatitis B vaccine at least 1 month after the 1st dose. The 3rd dose should be administered at least 4 months after the 1st dose and at least 2 months after the 2nd dose, but not before 6 months of age for infants.

   Infants born to HBsAg-positive mothers should receive hepatitis B vaccine and 0.5 mL hepatitis B immune globulin (HBIG) within 12 hours of birth at separate sites. The 2nd dose is recommended at 1-2 months of age and the 3rd dose at 6 months of age.

   Infants born to mothers whose HBsAg status is unknown should receive hepatitis B vaccine within 12 hours of birth. Maternal blood should be drawn at the time of delivery to determine the mother's HBsAg status; if the HBsAg test is positive, the infant should receive HBIG as soon as possible (no later than 1 week of age).

   All children and adolescents (through 18 years of age) who have not been immunized against hepatitis B may begin the series during any visit. Special efforts should be made to immunize children who were born in or whose parents were born in areas of the world with moderate or high endemicity of HBV infection.

3. DTaP (diphtheria and tetanus toxoids and acellular pertussis vaccine) is the preferred vaccine for all doses in the immunization series, including completion of the series in children who have received 1 or more doses of whole-cell DTP vaccine. Whole-cell DTP is an acceptable alternative to DTaP. The 4th dose (DTP or DTaP) may be administered as early as 12 months of age, provided 6 months have elapsed since the 3rd dose and if the child is unlikely to return at age 15-18 months. Td (tetanus and diphtheria toxoids) is recommended at 11-12 years of age if at least 5 years have elapsed since the last dose of DTP, DTaP, or DT. Subsequent routine Td boosters are recommended every 10 years.

4. Three *H. influenzae* type b (Hib) conjugate vaccines are licensed for infant use. If PRP-OMP (PedvaxHIB and COMVAX [Merck]) is administered at 2 and 4 months of age, a dose at 6 months is not required. Because clinical studies in infants have demonstrated that using some combination products may induce a lower immune response to the Hib vaccine component, DTaP/Hib combination products should not be used for primary immunization in infants at 2, 4, or 6 months of age, unless FDA-approved for these ages.

5. Two poliovirus vaccines currently are licensed in the United States: inactivated poliovirus vaccine (IPV) and oral poliovirus vaccine (OPV).

   The ACIP, AAP, and AAFP now recommend that the first two doses of poliovirus vaccine should be IPV. The ACIP continues to recommend a sequential schedule of two doses of IPV administered at ages 2 and 4 months, followed by two doses of OPV at 12-18 months and 4-6 years. Use of IPV for all doses also is acceptable and is recommended for immunocompromised persons and their household contacts.

   OPV is no longer recommended for the first two doses of the schedule and is acceptable only for special circumstances such as: children of parents who do not accept the recommended number of injections, late initiation of immunization which would require an unacceptable number of injections, and imminent travel to polio-endemic areas. OPV remains the vaccine of choice for mass immunization campaigns to control outbreaks due to wild poliovirus.

6. Rotavirus (Rv) vaccine is shaded and italicized to indicate: 1) health care providers may require time and resources to incorporate this new vaccine into practice; and 2) the AAFP feels that the decision to use rotavirus vaccine should be made by the parent or guardian in consultation with their physician or other health care provider. The first dose of Rv vaccine should not be administered before 6 weeks of age, and the minimum interval between doses is 3 weeks. The Rv vaccine series should not be initiated at 7 months of age or older, and all doses should be completed by the first birthday.

7. The 2nd dose of measles, mumps, and rubella vaccine (MMR) is recommended routinely at 4-6 years of age but may be administered during any visit, provided at least 4 weeks have elapsed since receipt of the 1st dose and that both doses are administered beginning at or after 12 months of age. Those who have not previously received the second dose should complete the schedule by the 11- to 12-year-old visit.

8. Varicella vaccine is recommended at any visit on or after the first birthday for susceptible children, ie, those who lack a reliable history of chickenpox (as judged by a health care provider) and who have not been immunized. Susceptible persons 13 years of age or older should receive 2 doses, given at least 4 weeks apart.

BIBLIOGRAPHY

BOOKS/ARTICLES:

Aaron CK, Bania TC: Insecticides: Organophosphates and Carbamates. In Goldfranks, LR (ed): Goldfrank's Toxicologic Emergencies. East Norwalk, CT, Appleton and Lange, 1994, pp 1105-1116.

Adler, J.N. & Plantz, S.H. Emergency Medicine Pearls of Wisdom. (4th Ed.). Watertown: Mt. Auburn Press, 1997.

Advanced Cardiac Life Support. Dallas: American Heart Association, 1996.

Advanced Trauma Life Support. Chicago: American College of Surgeons, 1990.

Anderson, J.E. Grant's Atlas of Anatomy (8th Ed.). Baltimore: Williams & Wilkins, 1983.

Auerbach, P.S. Management of Wilderness and Environmental Emergencies (2nd Ed.). St. Louis: C.V. Mosby Company, 1989.

Bakerman, S. ABCs of Interpretive Laboratory Data (2nd Ed.). Greenville: Interpretive Laboratory Data, Inc., 1984.

Barkin, R.M. Emergency Pediatrics (3rd Ed.). St. Louis: C.V. Mosby Company, 1990.

Berkow, R. The Merck Manual (15th Ed.). Rahway: Merck Sharp & Dohme Research Laboratories, 1987.

Bork, K. Diagnosis and Treatment of Common Skin Diseases. Philadelphia: W.B. Saunders Company, 1988.

Bryson, P.D. Comprehensive Review in Toxicology (2nd Ed.) Aspen Publishers, Inc., 1989

Dambro, M.R. Griffith's 5 Minute Clinical Consult. Williams and Wilkins, 1996.

DeGowin, E.L. Bedside Diagnostic Examination (4th Ed.). New York: Macmillan Publishing Co. Inc., 1981.

Diagnostic and Treatment Guidelines on Domestic Violence, AMA Publication.

Diagnostic and Treatment Guidelines on Sexual Assault, AMA Publication.

Firearm Violence: Community Diagnosis and Treatment, Publication and slide show of Physicians for Social Responsibility

Fitzpatrick, T.B. Color Atlas and Synopsis of Clinical Dermatology. New York: McGraw-Hill Publishing Company, 1990.

Harris, J.H. The Radiology of Emergency Medicine (2nd Ed.). Baltimore: Williams and Wilkins, 1981.

Harrison, T.R. Principles of Internal Medicine (11th Ed.). New York: McGraw-Hill Book Company, 1987.

Harwood-Nuss, A. The Clinical Practice of Emergency Medicine. Philadelphia: J.B. Lippincott Company, 2nd. Ed, 1996.

Hoppenfeld, S. Physical Examination of the Spine and Extremities. Norwalk: Appleton-Century-Crofts, 1976.

Leaverton, P.E. A Review of Biostatistics (3rd Ed.). Boston: Little Brown and Company, 1986.

Marriott, H.J.L. Practical Electrocardiography (7th Ed.). Baltimore: Williams and Wilkins, 1983.

Moore, K.L. Clinically Oriented Anatomy. Baltimore: Williams & Wilkins, 1982.

Nelson, Waldo E. Textbook of Pediatrics. Philadelphia: W.B. Saunders Company, 1996.

Perkins, E.S. An Atlas of Diseases of the Eye (3rd Ed.). London: Churchill Livingstone, 1986.

Physicians' Desk Reference (50th Ed.). Oradell: Medical Economics Company Inc., 1996.

Plantz, SH. Emergency Medicine PreTest, Self-Assessment and Review, McGraw- Hill, 1990.

Rivers, C.S. Preparing for the Written Board Exam in Emergency Medicine. Milford: Emergency Medicine Educational Enterprises, Inc. 1997.

Robbins, S.L. Pathologic Basis of Disease (3rd Ed.). Philadelphia: W.B. Saunders Company, 1984.

Rosen, P. Emergency Medicine Concepts and Clinical Practice (3rd Ed.). St. Louis: Mosby Year Book, 1992.

Rowe, R.C. The Harriet Lane Handbook (11th Ed.). Chicago: Year Book Medical Publishers, Inc., 1987.

Simon, R.R. Emergency Orthopedics The Extremities (2nd Ed.). Norwalk: Appleton & Lange, 1987.

Simon, R.R. Emergency Procedures and Techniques (2nd Ed.). Baltimore: Williams and Wilkins, 1987.

Slaby, F. Radiographic Anatomy. New York: John Wiley & Sons, 1990.

Squire, L.F. Fundamentals of Radiology (3rd Ed.). Cambridge: Harvard University Press, 1982.

Stedman, T.L. Illustrated Stedman's Medical Dictionary (24th Ed.). Baltimore: Williams & Wilkins, 1982.

Stewart, C.E. Environmental Emergencies. Baltimore: Williams and Wilkins, 1990.

Textbook of Pediatric Advanced Life Support. Dallas: American Heart Association, 1988.

The Hand Examination and Diagnosis (2nd Ed.). London: Churchill Livingstone, 1983.

The Hand Primary Care of Common Problems (2nd Ed.). London: Churchill Livingstone, 1990.

The Physician's Guide to Domestic Violence, Salber and Taliaferro, Volcano Press, 1995

Tintinalli, J.E. Emergency Medicine A Comprehensive Study Guide (4th Ed.). New York: McGraw-Hill, Inc., 1996.

Tsang T, Demby AM. Penile fracture with urethral injury. The Journal of Urology, 1992;147:466-468.

Weinberg, S. Color Atlas of Pediatric Dermatology (2nd Ed.). New York: McGraw-Hill, 1990.

Weiner, H.L. Neurology for the House Officer (4th Ed.). Baltimore: Williams & Wilkins, 1989.

Wilkins, E. W. Emergency Medicine (3rd Ed.). Baltimore: Williams & Wilkins, 1989.

COURSES/CONFERENCES:

Eye Diseases and Emergencies, Chicago, IL 1991.

ENT Diseases and Emergencies, Chicago, IL 1991.

CRIT Course, Springfield, MA 1992.

Interactive Board Review, Boca Raton, FL 1992.

Selected Topics in Emergency Medicine. Sponsored by MGH and Brigham and Women's Hospitals and Harvard Medical School, Boston, MA 1995 and 1996.

Update on New Techniques and Review of Established Principles of Management of Cerebrovascular Emergencies. Sponsored by MGH Brain Aneurysm/AVM Center, Neurointensive Care Unit and ED, Boston, MA 1996.